principles of
CLINICAL ELECTROCARDIOGRAPHY

6
Edition

principles of

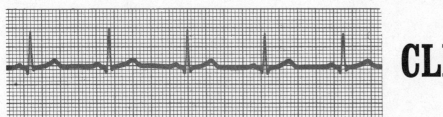

CLINICAL

ELECTROCARDIOGRAPHY

by

MERVIN J. GOLDMAN, MD
Associate Clinical Professor of Medicine
University of California School of Medicine, San Francisco

Lange Medical Publications
Los Altos, California

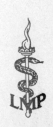

1967

A Concise Medical Library for Practitioner and Student

Physician's Handbook, 14th Edition, 1966 $5.00
    M. A. Krupp, N. J. Sweet, E. Jawetz, E. G. Biglieri

Handbook of Medical Treatment, 10th Edition, 1966 $5.50
    M. J. Chatton, S. Margen, H. Brainerd, Editors

Handbook of Pediatrics, 7th Edition, 1967 $5.50
    H. K. Silver, C. H. Kempe, H. B. Bruyn

Handbook of Poisoning: Diagnosis & Treatment, 5th Edition, 1966 $5.00
    R. H. Dreisbach

Current Medical References, 5th Edition, 1967   Approx. $8.00
    M. J. Chatton, P. J. Sanazaro, Editors

Handbook of Surgery, 3rd Edition, 1966 $5.50
    J. L. Wilson, J. J. McDonald, Editors

Handbook of Obstetrics & Gynecology, 2nd Edition, 1966 $5.50
    R. C. Benson

Correlative Neuroanatomy and Functional Neurology $6.50
    13th Edition, 1967
    J. G. Chusid, J. J. McDonald

Review of Physiological Chemistry, 11th Edition, 1967 $6.50
    H. A. Harper

Review of Medical Microbiology, 7th Edition, 1966 $6.50
    E. Jawetz, J. L. Melnick, E. A. Adelberg

Principles of Clinical Electrocardiography, 6th Edition, 1967 $6.00
    M. J. Goldman

General Urology, 5th Edition, 1966 $6.50
    D. R. Smith

General Ophthalmology, 4th Edition, 1965 $6.00
    D. Vaughan, R. Cook, T. Asbury

Current Diagnosis & Treatment, 1967 $9.50
    H. Brainerd, S. Margen, M. J. Chatton, Editors

Review of Medical Physiology, 3rd Edition, 1967 $7.00
    W. F. Ganong

Preface

It is the author's intention to present in this volume the basic concepts of electrocardiography and their clinical application. He realizes that material so presented must be simplified and that an exhaustive and detailed treatment of the subject matter to be covered will not be possible.

Emphasis has been placed on the unipolar leads. To one who first learned electrocardiography by memorizing patterns in the bipolar standard leads and later followed the development of unipolar electrocardiography, the latter offers a more logical approach to the subject material. Vector analysis of the electrocardiogram offers an intelligent means of understanding the electrical potentials generated from the heart. There should be no major disagreement between vector and unipolar electrocardiographic analysis. Both are descriptive of the same phenomena, the former offering an evaluation of the electrical potentials as oriented in space and the latter as reflected in the resulting electrocardiographic pattern.

The unitarian concept of the atrial arrhythmias and the theory of accelerated conduction are admittedly not universally accepted. However, the author feels that these are the most acceptable theories of the above phenomena available at the present time.

The author cannot too strongly emphasize the fact that the electrocardiogram is a laboratory test only. Like all laboratory findings, an abnormal electrocardiographic tracing is significant only when interpreted in the light of clinical findings. Ideally, the person best qualified to interpret the electrocardiogram is the physician caring for the patient.

The chapter on Spatial Vectorcardiography and corrected orthogonal lead systems is intended to give the reader an insight into this relatively new field and not as a comprehensive discussion of the subject.

For the Sixth Edition we have added sections on the internodal atrial pathways, electrical depolarization of the heart, and cell to cell conduction as explained by electron microscopic studies.

We are most gratified with the acceptance this Review has received among students and physicians both here and abroad. Spanish, Italian, Japanese, and Greek translations are now available.

Mervin J. Goldman

San Francisco, California
May, 1967

Table of Contents

Chapter   1   **Introduction to Electrocardiography** · 1
    Usefulness of the Electrocardiogram 1
    Electrocardiographic Apparatus 2
    Bipolar Standard Leads 2
    Bipolar Chest Leads 4
    Unipolar Leads 4
        Improvised Unipolar Leads Using an Indifferent Electrode 5
        Unipolar Extremity Leads 6
        Unipolar Precordial (Chest) Leads 9
        Unipolar Esophageal Leads 13
        Relation Between Unipolar Extremity Leads and Standard
            Bipolar Leads 14
    Technical Difficulties Affecting the Electrocardiogram 16

Chapter   2   **Electrophysiology of the Heart** · 17
    Intracellular Potentials 17
    Electrical Potentials Produced by Normal Muscle 20
    The Electrogram 21

Chapter   3   **Definitions of Electrocardiographic Configurations** · · · · · · · · · · · · 25
    Normal Electrocardiographic Complexes 25
    Normal Interval Values 27
    Normal Segments and Junctions 28
    Voltage Measurements 29

Chapter   4   **The Cardiac Vector** · 31
    Frontal Plane Vectors 31
    Horizontal Plane Vectors 37
    Sagittal Plane Vectors 38
    Value of Vector Analysis 38

Chapter   5   **Normal Electrocardiographic Complexes** · · · · · · · · · · · · · · · · · 39
    Electrical Conduction Through the Heart 41
    Atrial Complexes 43
    Ventricular Complexes 45
        Unipolar Electrocardiograms on the Exposed Ventricle 45
            Left Ventricular Epicardial Complex 45
            Right Ventricular Epicardial Complex 45
            Transitional Zone Ventricular Epicardial Complex 48
            Left Ventricular Cavity Complex 49
            Right Ventricular Cavity Complex 50
            "Back-of-the-Heart" Complexes 51
        Application of the Complexes Described Above to Clinical
            Electrocardiography 52
        The Bipolar Electrocardiogram 53
            Normal Complexes in Standard Bipolar Leads 53
            Ventricular Complexes 54
        Summary of the Electrophysiology of the Normal Heart and the
            Production of the Normal Electrocardiogram 54

Chapter   6   **Effect of Heart Position on the Electrocardiogram** · · · · · · · · · ·   63
    Rotation on the Anteroposterior Axis 65
     Variation in Patterns in Unipolar Extremity Leads Due to
      Rotation on the Anteroposterior Axis 75
    Rotation on the Long Axis 76
    Rotation on the Transverse Axis 78
    Effect of Deep Respiration on the Rotational Patterns 80

Chapter   7   **The Electrocardiogram in Infants and Children; Normal Variants**
    of the Adult Electrocardiogram · · · · · · · · · · · · ·   81
    Fetal Electrocardiography 81
    Normal Electrocardiographic Patterns in Infants and Children 81
    Dextrocardia 83
    Technical Dextrocardia 85
    Unusual Normal Variants 86
     ST Segment Elevation in Precordial Leads 86
     ST Segment Elevation and T Wave Inversion 87
    Anxiety Reaction 88
    Bipolar vs. Unipolar Chest Leads 89

Chapter   8   **Hypertrophy Patterns** · · · · · · · · · · · · · · · · · ·   90
    Atrial Hypertrophy 90
    Ventricular Hypertrophy 95
     Ventricular Strain 97
     Left Ventricular Hypertrophy 98
      Electrocardiographic Patterns of Left Ventricular
       Hypertrophy 98
      Left Ventricular Strain 106
      Summary of Electrocardiographic Criteria of Left
       Ventricular Hypertrophy 107
     Right Ventricular Hypertrophy 108
      Right Ventricular Strain 113
      Summary of Electrocardiographic Criteria of Right
       Ventricular Hypertrophy 117
     Combined Right and Left Ventricular Hypertrophy 118

Chapter   9   **Bundle Branch Block** · · · · · · · · · · · · · · · · · ·   120
    Right Bundle Branch Block 121
     Summary of Electrocardiographic Criteria of Right Bundle
      Branch Block 130
    Left Bundle Branch Block 131
     Summary of Electrocardiographic Criteria of Left Bundle
      Branch Block 138

Chapter 10   **Coronary Artery Disease: Myocardial Anoxia** · · · · · · · · ·   139
    Electrocardiographic Patterns Resulting From
     Myocardial Anoxia 143
    Exercise Tests 145
    Anemia 148
    Pseudodepression vs. Coronary ST Depression 149
    Summary of Electrocardiographic Criteria of Myocardial Anoxia 150

Chapter 11 **Coronary Artery Disease: Myocardial Infarction** · · · · · · · · · · · · · 151
      Mechanism of the Electrocardiographic Pattern 152
        The Abnormal Q Wave and the QS Complex 152
        QRS Patterns of Infarction 153
        The ST Segment Changes 156
        The T Wave Changes 157
      Localization of Myocardial Infarction by Electrocardiographic
        Patterns 158
        Anterior Wall Infarction 159
        Summary of Electrocardiographic Criteria of Anterior
          Myocardial Infarction 171
        Posterior Wall Infarction (and Inferior Wall Infarctions) 172
        Summary of Electrocardiographic Criteria of Posterior and
          Inferior Wall Infarction 181
      Subendocardial Infarction 182
      Multiple Infarcts 185
      Ventricular Aneurysm 189
      Differential Diagnosis of Myocardial Infarction 190
      Infarction Associated With Bundle Branch Block 192
      Effect of Further Coronary Insufficiency on the Infarct Pattern 196

Chapter 12 **Normal Cardiac Rhythm and the Atrial Arrhythmias** · · · · · · · · · 197
      Physiology of Cardiac Rhythm 197
      Effect of the Autonomic Nervous System on Cardiac Rhythm 198
      Effect of Digitalis, Quinidine, and Procainamide on Cardiac
        Rhythm 198
      Normal and Abnormal Cardiac Rhythms 199
      Sinus Rhythms 200
      Abnormal Atrial Rhythms 203
        Atrial Premature Beats 203
        Wandering Pacemaker 206
        Paroxysmal Atrial Tachycardia 207
        Atrial Flutter 211
        Atrial Fibrillation 215
        Summary of the Atrial Arrhythmias 219

Chapter 13 **Disturbances of Atrioventricular Conduction** · · · · · · · · · · 220
      Atrioventricular Block 220
      Atrioventricular Nodal Rhythms 228
      Atrioventricular Nodal Tachycardia 234

Chapter 14 **The Ventricular Arrhythmias** · · · · · · · · · · · · · · · 235
      Intraventricular Conduction Defect 235
      Ventricular Premature Beats 236
      Ventricular Tachycardia 245
      Ventricular Fibrillation 250

Chapter 15 **The Pararrhythmias** · · · · · · · · · · · · · · · · 253
      Parasystole 253
      A-V Dissociation With Interference 255

Chapter 16 **Accelerated Conduction** · · · · · · · · · · · · · · · 258

Chapter 17 **Miscellaneous Abnormal Electrocardiographic Patterns** · · · · · · · · · · 267
     Pericarditis 267
     Myocarditis 271
     Hyperthyroidism 272
     Myxedema 272
     Traumatic Heart Disease 273
     Neuromuscular Diseases 273
     Malignancy Involving the Heart 274
     Refrigeration 274
     Effects of Drugs on the Electrocardiogram 275
      Digitalis 275
      Quinidine 279
      Emetine 281
      Tartar Emetic 281
      Nicotine (Smoking) 282
      Procainamide 282
     Cerebral Disease 282
     Effects of Electrolyte Disturbances on the Electrocardiogram 283
      Hyperkalemia 283
      Hypokalemia 286
      Electrocardiogram as a Guide to Potassium Levels 288
      Hypercalcemia 289
      Hypocalcemia 289
     Electrical Alternans 290
     Left Ventricular Conduction Defects 291
      Left Intraventricular Block 291
      Peri-infarction Block 293
     Electrical Depolarization of the Heart 296

Chapter 18 **An Introduction to Spatial Vectorcardiography** · · · · · · · · · · · · 301
     Orientation of the Vectorcardiographic Illustrations 304
     The Normal Adult Spatial Vectorcardiogram 305
     Specific Conditions Illustrated:
      Correlation of the Normal Adult Spatial Vectorcardiogram
       and Resulting Electrocardiogram 306
      Normal Adult Vectorcardiogram 311
      Left Ventricular Hypertrophy 312
      Left Bundle Branch Block 314
      Right Ventricular Hypertrophy 316
      Right Bundle Branch Block 318
      Right Bundle Branch Block vs. Right Ventricular Hypertrophy 320
      Accelerated Conduction 321
      Anterior Myocardial Infarction 322
      Inferior Myocardial Infarction 324
      Inferior and Posterior Myocardial Infarction 325
      Inferior Wall Infarction vs. Normal Record 326
     Ventricular Gradient 327

Chapter 19 **Interpretation of the Electrocardiogram** · · · · · · · · · · · · · · 328

Appendix: Interpretation of Abnormalities of the Adult Twelve-Lead
 Electrocardiogram · 367

References · 383

Index · 387

Direction of Electrical Axis · · · · · · · · · · · · · · · · · · · 396

Table and Scale for Determining Heart Rate · · · · · · · · · · · Inside back cover

Chapter 1

INTRODUCTION TO ELECTROCARDIOGRAPHY

The electrocardiogram (Ecg. or EKG) is a graphic recording of the electrical potentials produced in association with the heart beat. The heart muscle is unique among the muscles of the body in that it possesses the quality of automatic rhythmic contraction. The impulses which precede contraction arise in the conduction system of the heart. These impulses result in excitation of the muscle fibers throughout the myocardium. Impulse formation and conduction produce weak electric currents which spread through the entire body. By applying electrodes to various positions on the body and connecting these electrodes to an electrocardiographic apparatus, the electrocardiogram is recorded. The connections of the apparatus are such that an upright deflection indicates positive potential and a downward deflection indicates negative potential.

USEFULNESS OF THE ELECTROCARDIOGRAM

Since the advent of unipolar electrocardiography, the accuracy of electrocardiographic diagnosis has been greatly increased. The electrocardiogram is of particular value in the following clinical conditions:

A. Atrial and ventricular hypertrophy.

B. Myocardial Infarction: Unipolar extremity leads, multiple chest leads, and esophageal leads have greatly increased the incidence of correct diagnoses.

C. Arrhythmias: Not only can more exact diagnoses be made, but unipolar electrocardiography has also contributed substantially to our basic understanding of the origin and conduction of abnormal rhythms.

D. Pericarditis.

E. Systemic diseases which affect the heart.

F. Effect of cardiac drugs, especially digitalis and quinidine.

G. Disturbances in electrolyte metabolism, especially potassium abnormalities.

Caution to the Beginner:
It must always be borne in mind that the electrocardiogram is a laboratory test only and is not a sine qua non of heart disease diagnosis. A patient with an organic heart disorder may have a normal electrocardiogram, and a perfectly normal individual may show nonspecific electrocardiographic abnormalities. All too often a patient is relegated to the status of a cardiac invalid solely on the basis of some electrocardiographic abnormality. On the other hand, a patient may be given unwarranted assurance of the absence of heart disease solely on the basis of a normal electrocardiogram. The electrocardiogram must always be interpreted in conjunction with the clinical findings. In general, the person best qualified to interpret the electrocardiogram is the physician caring for the patient.

ELECTROCARDIOGRAPHIC APPARATUS

In modern electrocardiography two types of apparatus are used, the string galvanometer and the radio amplifier. The former records its pattern on photographic paper which must then be developed. It requires more experience to operate, and caution must be taken to prevent damage to the valuable string. The radio amplifier has been combined with a direct writer; it is a compact, light, and mobile unit which is very simple to operate, and there is much less chance of damaging the machine by technical errors of operation. It has the additional advantage of producing an instantaneous recording, thus making the record immediately available for interpretation.

In recent years another apparatus, the cardioscope, has been used in clinical medicine. This produces a constant electrocardiographic pattern on a fluorescent screen but does not give a permanent record unless connected to one of the above-mentioned machines. It is of particular value in the constant electrocardiographic monitoring of patients with myocardial infarction or serious arrhythmias (as in medical intensive care or coronary care units) and during surgery.

BIPOLAR STANDARD LEADS

The bipolar standard leads (I, II and III) are the original leads selected by Einthoven to record the electrical potentials in the frontal plane. Electrodes are applied to the left arm, right arm, and left leg. Proper skin contact must be made by rubbing electrode paste on the skin. The L. A. (left arm), R. A. (right arm), and L. L. (left leg) leads are then attached to their respective electrodes. By turning the selector dial to 1, 2, and 3, the three standard leads (I, II, and III) are taken.

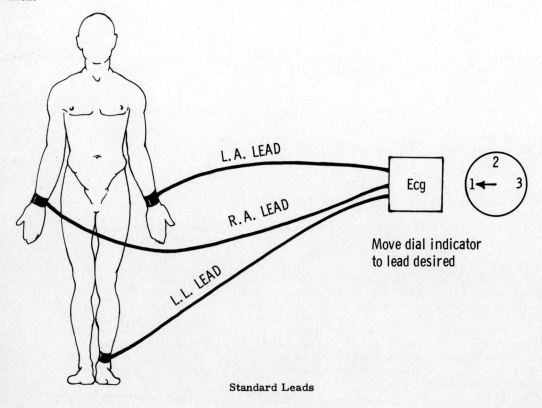

Standard Leads

Most modern electrocardiographs also have a right leg electrode and lead. This acts as a ground wire and plays no role in the production of the electrocardiogram. If the machine does not have this feature it may be necessary to run a ground wire from the bed or the machine to an appropriate ground (water pipe or steam pipe) to eliminate electrical interference.

Electrical Potential:

The bipolar leads represent a difference of electrical potential between two selected sites.

Lead I = Difference of potential between the left arm and the right arm (L. A. – R. A.).
Lead II = Difference of potential between the left leg and the right arm (L. L. – R. A.).
Lead III = Difference of potential between the left leg and the left arm (L. L. – L. A.).

The relation between the three leads is expressed algebraically by Einthoven's equation: lead II = lead I + lead III. This is based on Kirchoff's law, which states that the algebraic sum of all the potential differences in a closed circuit equals zero. If Einthoven had reversed the polarity of lead II (i. e., R. A. – L. L.), the three bipolar lead axes would result in a closed circuit (see p. 15), and leads I + II + III would equal zero. However, since Einthoven did make this alteration in the polarity of the lead II axis, the equation becomes: I – II + III = 0. Hence II = I + III.

The electrical potential as recorded from any one extremity will be the same no matter where the electrode is placed on the extremity. The electrodes are usually applied just above the wrists and ankles. If an extremity has been amputated, the electrode can be applied to the stump. In a patient with an uncontrollable tremor, a more satisfactory record may be obtained by applying the electrodes to the upper portions of the limbs.

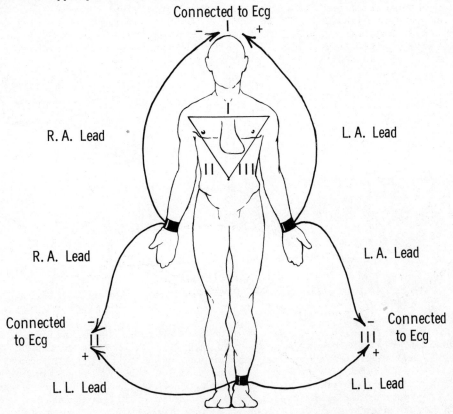

Connections for Bipolar Standard Leads I, II, and III

Following the use of bipolar standard leads, which recorded electrical potentials in the frontal plane of the body, bipolar chest leads were introduced to record the potentials in the horizontal plane.

BIPOLAR CHEST LEADS

Bipolar chest leads demonstrate differences of potential between any given position on the chest (C) and one extremity. Before unipolar electrocardiography was introduced, the left leg (F) was used as the "indifferent" electrode and the leads were called CF leads. Less commonly, the right arm (CR leads) or the left arm (CL leads) was used. It was assumed that the left leg (or right or left arm) was so remote from the heart that it would act as an "indifferent" electrode and not interfere with the chest potential. However, it is now realized that the potentials in the extremities can appreciably alter the pattern of the chest lead. For this reason CF, CR, and CL leads are not frequently used today.

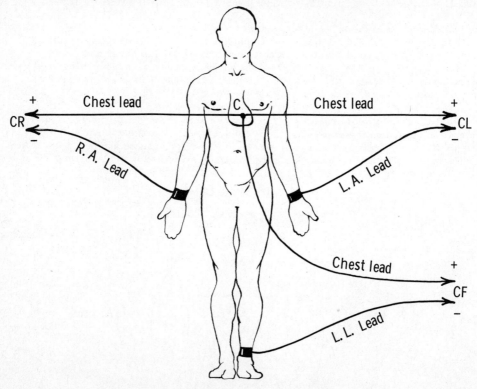

Connections for Bipolar Chest Leads CR, CL, and CF

UNIPOLAR LEADS
[EXTREMITY LEADS, PRECORDIAL (CHEST) LEADS, ESOPHAGEAL LEADS]

Unipolar leads (VR, VL, VF, multiple chest leads "V," and esophageal leads "E") were introduced into clinical electrocardiography by Wilson in 1932. The frontal plane unipolar leads (VR, VL, VF) bear a definite mathematical relationship to the standard (I, II, III) bipolar leads (see p. 14). The precordial (V) leads record potentials in the horizontal plane without being influenced by actual potentials from an "indifferent" electrode used in recording bipolar chest leads. One concept must be clearly understood: A unipolar precordial (or esophageal) lead does not record only the electrical potential from a small area of the underlying myocardium; it records all of the electrical events of the entire cardiac cycle as viewed from the selected lead site.

All modern electrocardiograph machines are constructed so that augmented extremity leads can be taken with the same hookup as used for standard leads by turning the selector dial to aVR, aVL, and aVF. Unipolar chest leads are taken by applying the chest lead and its electrode to any desired position on the chest and turning the selector dial to the V position. Multiple chest leads are taken by changing the position of the chest electrode (see diagram on p. 10). Unipolar esophageal leads are taken by attaching the esophageal lead to the chest lead and turning the selector dial to the V position. (See diagram on p. 13.)

A universal lead selector is available for a three-lead electrocardiograph apparatus. With this unit attached, the standard, unipolar extremity, and chest leads can be taken by simply rotating the selector dial as is done with the newer electrocardiograph machines.

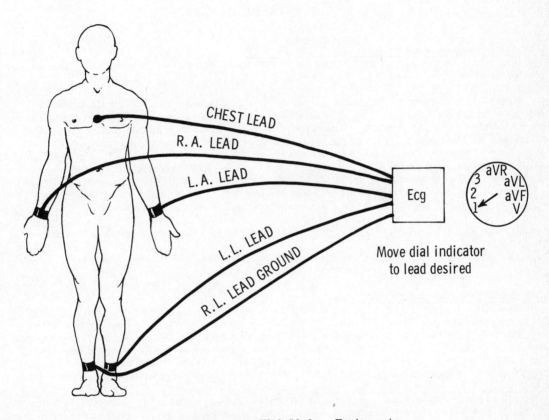

Unipolar Leads With Modern Equipment

IMPROVISED UNIPOLAR LEADS USING AN INDIFFERENT ELECTRODE

If a modern electrocardiograph machine or universal lead selector is not available, an electrocardiograph that can record standard leads I, II, and III can be used to obtain perfectly satisfactory unipolar leads. To do so one first constructs an indifferent electrode. This is easily made by fastening three separate lengths of insulated copper wire (each about four feet in length) together at one end with a battery clip. This end becomes the central terminal (T). The three free ends are connected to the L.A., R.A., and L.L. electrodes. The central terminal is con-

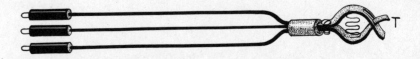

Indifferent Electrode

nected to the R. A. lead of the electrocardiograph. The L. A. lead becomes the exploring electrode for any desired unipolar lead. All such leads are taken with the selector dial on lead I.

In principle, the unipolar leads attempt to represent actual local potentials and not differences in potential. Since it is generally accepted that the sum of the potentials of the three extremity leads is zero (R. A. + L. A. + L. L. = 0), the connection of these three extremity leads (the central terminal) will for all clinical purposes result in a zero potential.

UNIPOLAR EXTREMITY LEADS

Unipolar Nonaugmented Extremity Leads VR, VL, VF:
These have been replaced by the augmented extremity leads aVR, aVL, and aVF and are not commonly taken.

Using the indifferent electrode (R. A. + L. A. + L. L.) as one terminal and placing another electrode on the right arm, a bipolar lead can be taken. This represents the difference between the potential of the right arm and the zero potential of the central terminal (R. A. − 0 = R. A.). Therefore the "actual" potential of the right arm is recorded. Although it is technically a bipolar lead, it represents a unipolar lead since one of the potentials is zero. This is designated as VR (vector of right arm). The left arm (VL) and left leg (VF) potentials are obtained in the same way. The selector dial is set at lead I (see diagram on p. 7).

  A. To take VR, the L. A. lead of the machine is attached to an electrode placed on the right arm at a different site from the R. A. electrode connected to the central terminal.

  B. To take VL, the L. A. lead of the machine is attached to an electrode on the left arm.

  C. To take VF, the L. A. lead of the machine is attached to an electrode on the left leg.

Augmented Extremity Leads aVR, aVL, aVF:
By a slight change in technic from above (this is automatically accomplished by all modern electrocardiograph machines), the amplitude of the deflections of VR, VL, and VF can be increased by about 50%. * These leads are called augmented unipolar extremity leads and are designated as aVR, aVL, and aVF. It must be emphasized that the only difference between leads VR, VL, and VF and leads aVR, aVL, and aVF is this difference in amplitude. In routine electrocardiographic practice the augmented leads have replaced the nonaugmented unipolar extremity

---

*Using lead aVR as an example, this can be shown as follows. Since aVR represents a difference of potential between the right arm (R. A. or VR) and the average of the potential of the left leg and left arm, the following equation (1) can be established:

$$(1)\ aVR = R.A. - \left[\frac{L.L. + L.A.}{2} \right]$$

By changing signs in (1):

$$(2)\ aVR = R.A. + \left[- \frac{L.L. + L.A.}{2} \right]$$

From Einthoven's equation it is known that:

$$(3)\ R.A. + L.A. + L.L. = 0.$$

By subtracting L. A. + L. L. from both sides of (3):

$$(4)\ R.A. = - (L.A. + L.L.)$$

By substituting equation (4) in (2):

$$(5)\ aVR = R.A. + \left[\frac{R.A.}{2} \right] = \tfrac{3}{2}\,R.A.\ (or\ \tfrac{3}{2}\,VR)$$

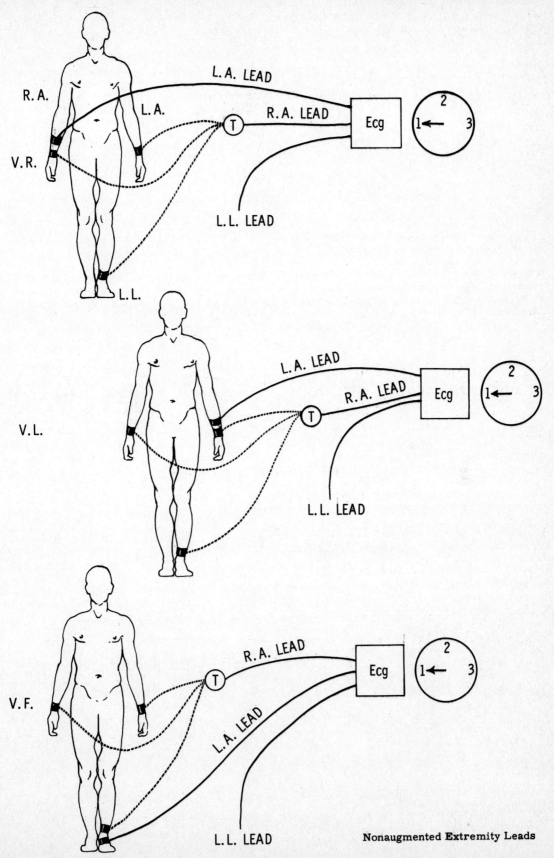

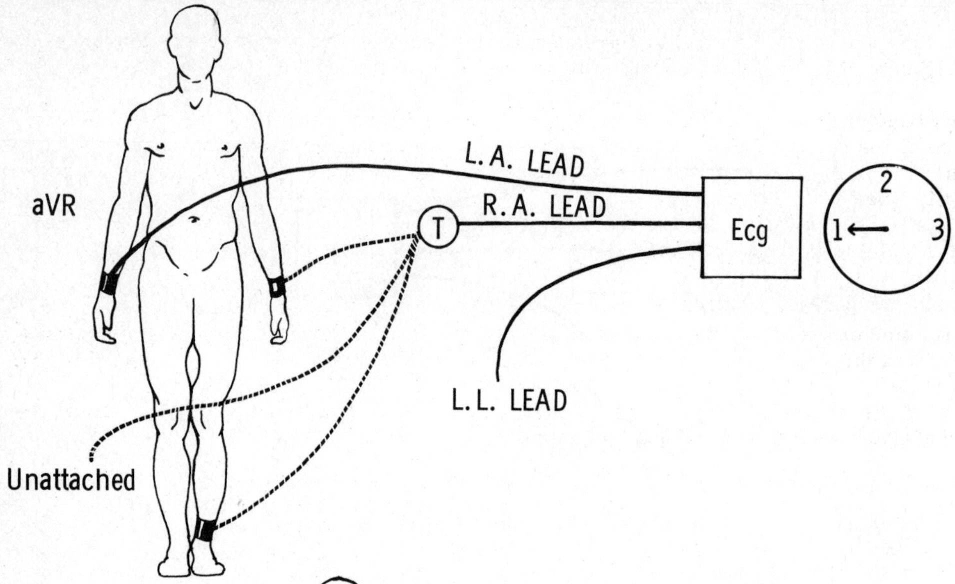

aVR

L.A. LEAD

R.A. LEAD

T

Ecg

2
1 ← 3

L.L. LEAD

Unattached

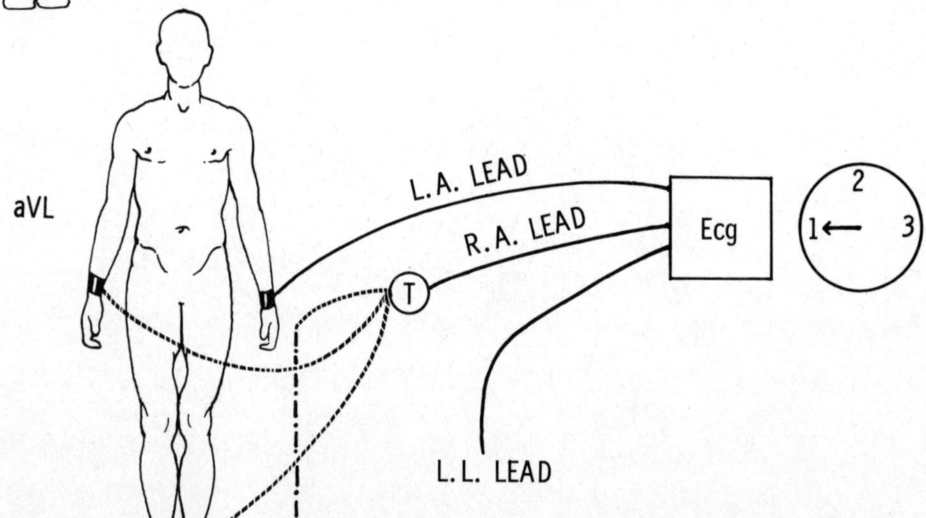

aVL

L.A. LEAD

R.A. LEAD

T

Ecg

2
1 ← 3

L.L. LEAD

Unattached

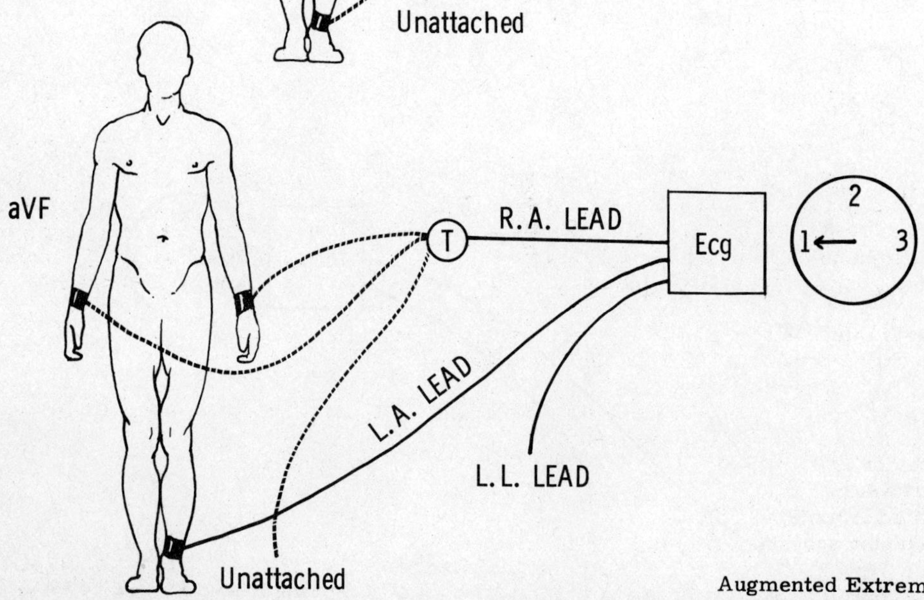

aVF

T

R.A. LEAD

Ecg

2
1 ← 3

L.A. LEAD

L.L. LEAD

Unattached

leads because they are easier to read. (Hereafter in this text, the term "extremity leads" will refer to the augmented leads.)

As in the nonaugmented leads, the three wires of the indifferent electrode are connected to the three extremities (L.A., R.A., and L.L.); the central terminal is connected to the R.A. lead of the machine; the L.A. lead of the machine becomes the exploring electrode; the selector dial is set on lead I. (See p. 8.)

A. To take aVR, the indifferent lead to the right arm is removed and left unattached, and the L.A. lead of the machine is attached to the R.A. electrode.

B. To take aVL, the indifferent lead to the left arm is removed and left unattached, and the L.A. lead of the machine is attached to the L.A. electrode. (Of course, the indifferent electrode removed from the right arm in taking aVR has been replaced.)

C. To take aVF the indifferent lead to the left leg is removed and left unattached, and the L.A. lead of the machine is attached to the left leg electrode.

Nonaugmented | Augmented

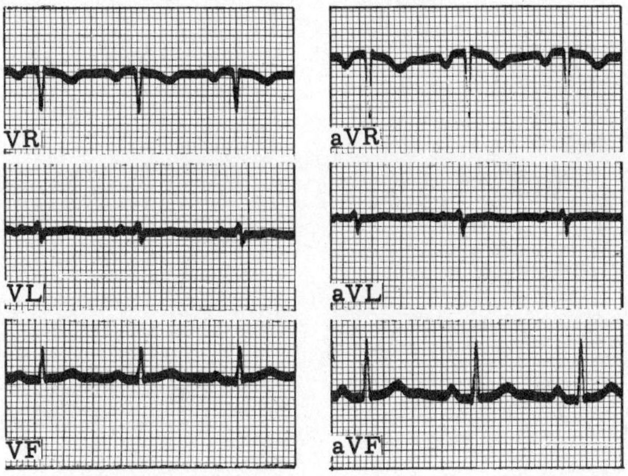

Comparison of Nonaugmented and Augmented Extremity Leads. All the above leads are taken on the same individual. Note that the pattern in comparable leads is the same; the only difference is that the augmented extremity leads are of greater voltage (approximately $3/2$).

UNIPOLAR PRECORDIAL (CHEST) LEADS

These are obtained by turning the selector to V on the dial or, in the older machines, by using the directions which follow.

The indifferent electrode leads remain connected to the three extremities. The central terminal is attached to the R.A. lead of the machine. The selector dial is set on lead I. The L.A. lead of the machine is attached to an electrode which can be applied to the desired chest positions, producing multiple unipolar chest leads. (See p. 12, top.) This results in a V lead. The common precordial positions used (as recommended by the American Heart Association) are as follows:

V_1: Fourth intercostal space at the right sternal border.
V_2: Fourth intercostal space at the left sternal border.
V_3: Equidistant between V2 and V_4.
V_4: Fifth intercostal space in the left midclavicular line. All subsequent leads (V_5 to V_9) are taken in the same horizontal plane as V_4.
V_5: Anterior axillary line.
V_6: Midaxillary line.
V_7: Posterior axillary line.
V_8: Posterior scapular line.

[Cont'd. on p. 13.]

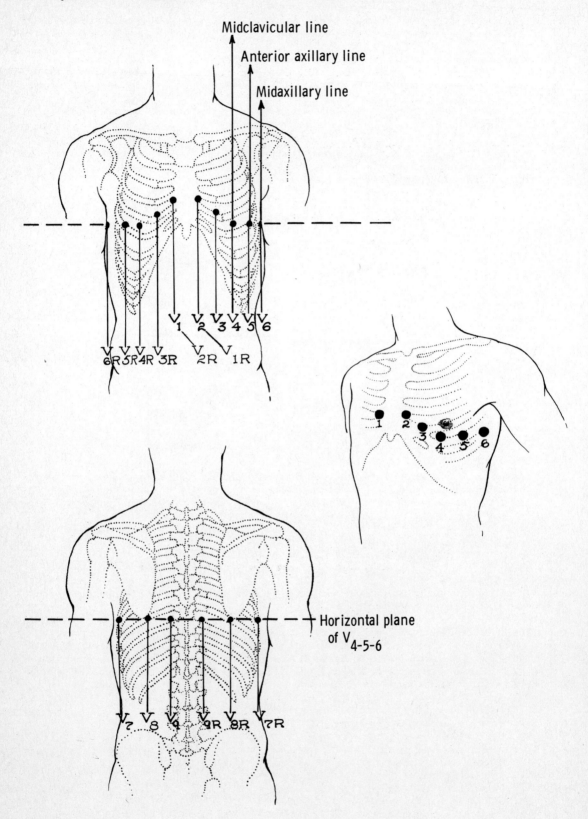

Locations of Unipolar Precordial Leads

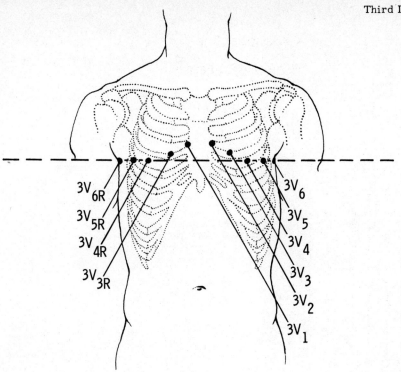

$3V_{6R}$
$3V_{5R}$
$3V_{4R}$
$3V_{3R}$

$3V_6$
$3V_5$
$3V_4$
$3V_3$
$3V_2$
$3V_1$

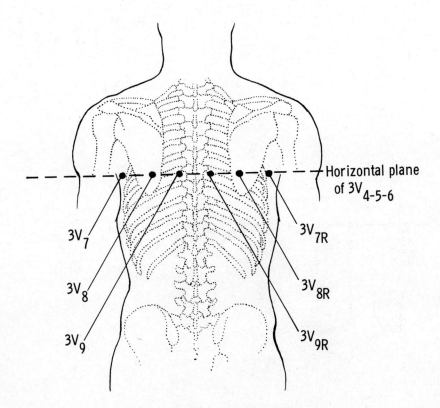

Horizontal plane
of $3V_{4-5-6}$

$3V_7$
$3V_8$
$3V_9$

$3V_{7R}$
$3V_{8R}$
$3V_{9R}$

Third Interspace Leads

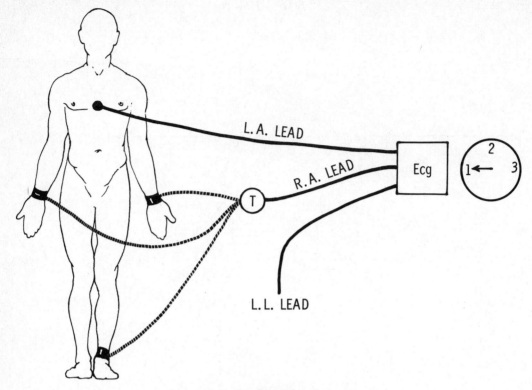

Unipolar Chest Leads

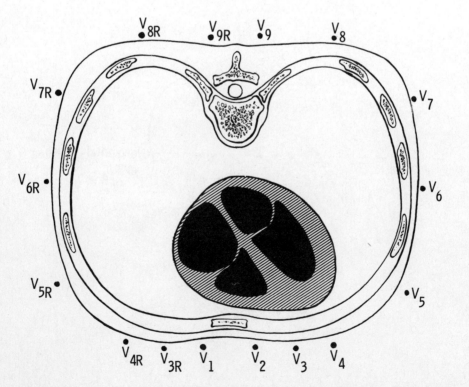

Transverse Section of Thorax Illustrating Position of the Unipolar Chest Leads

V_9 : Left border of the spine.

V_{3R-9R}: Taken on the right side of the chest in the same location as the left-sided leads V_{3-9} . V_{2R} is therefore the same as V_1 .

$3V_{1-9}$: Taken one interspace higher than V_{1-9} ; these are the third interspace leads.   The same terminology can be applied to leads taken in other interspaces, e.g., $2V_{1-9}$, $6V_{1-9}$, etc.

$3V_{3R-9R}$: Right precordial leads taken one interspace higher than V_{3R-9R}.

VE: Taken over the ensiform cartilage.

The usual routine electrocardiogram consists of 12 leads: I, II, III; aVR, aVL, aVF; and V_1 through V_6 .

UNIPOLAR ESOPHAGEAL LEADS

Esophageal leads can be taken by attaching an esophageal lead to the V (chest) lead of the newer machine or the left arm lead of the improvised machine, using the indifferent electrode.

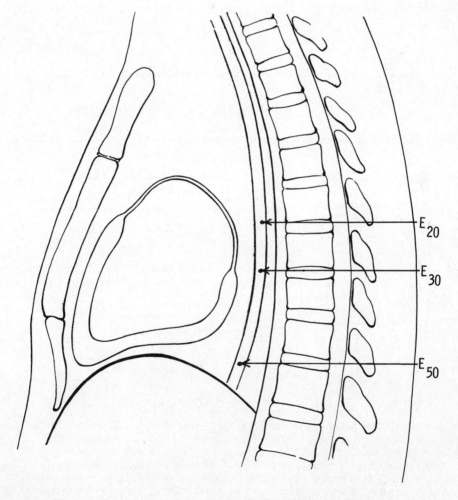

Sagittal View of Thorax Illustrating Position of the Unipolar Esophageal Leads

Esophageal leads are taken from within the esophagus. A nasal catheter through which is threaded a wire with an electrode attached to its tip can be passed through the nares into the esophagus. Using this as one terminal and the zero potential as the other terminal, a unipolar esophageal lead can be obtained. This is designated as an E lead. The nomenclature of the lead is derived from the distance in centimeters from the tip of the nares to the electrode. Thus E_{50} represents a unipolar esophageal lead at a distance of 50 cm. from the nares. Leads E_{40}-E_{50} usually reflect the posterior surface of the left ventricle; leads E_{15}-E_{25} the atrial area; and leads E_{25}-E_{35} the region of the atrioventricular groove. Since these positions vary tremendously with individual differences in body size and shape and heart position, no interpretation should be made from a single esophageal lead; an entire series of low to high esophageal levels must be studied for proper evaluation. For more accurate localization of the position of the esophageal electrode, fluoroscopy may be used.

Esophageal leads are especially useful in recording the atrial complexes, which are greatly magnified at this location, and exploring the posterior surface of the left ventricle.

RELATION BETWEEN UNIPOLAR EXTREMITY LEADS AND STANDARD BIPOLAR LEADS

Leads I, II, III, aVR, aVL, and aVF all represent frontal plane vectors (see p. 31). As stated on p. 3:

$$I = VL - VR\ (L.A. - R.A.) \quad II = VF - VR\ (L.L. - R.A.) \quad III = VF - VL\ (L.L. - L.A.)$$

Since the augmented extremity leads are $3/2$ the nonaugmented extremity leads, the equations are changed to:

$$I = 2/3\ (aVL - aVR) \qquad II = 2/3\ (aVF - aVR) \qquad III = 2/3\ (aVF - aVL)$$

The relationship of the extremity leads to the standard leads is derived from Einthoven's formula:

1. $VR + VL + VF = 0.$
2. $VR = - VL - VF.$
3. Adding 2VR to equation (2),
   $3VR = - VL - VF + 2VR.$
4. $VR = \dfrac{- VL - VF + 2VR}{3}$

5. $VR = \dfrac{-VL + VR - VF + VR}{3}$
6. $VR = - \dfrac{(VL - VR) + (VF - VR)}{3}$
7. $VR = - \dfrac{I + II}{3}$

In the same manner the relationships of the extremity leads to the standard leads can be derived. The nonaugmented leads are multiplied by $3/2$ to give the other augmented leads.

$$VR = - \frac{I + II}{3} \qquad aVR = - \frac{I + II}{3} \times \frac{3}{2} = - \frac{I + II}{2}$$

$$VL = \frac{I - III}{3} \qquad aVL = \frac{I - III}{3} \times \frac{3}{2} = \frac{I - III}{2}$$

$$VF = \frac{II + III}{3} \qquad aVF = \frac{II + III}{3} \times \frac{3}{2} = \frac{II + III}{2}$$

Bipolar and unipolar leads are not of equal lead strength. A nonaugmented unipolar lead is 58% of the lead strength of a bipolar lead. An augmented unipolar lead is 87% (i.e., $3/2 \times 58\%$) of the lead strength of a bipolar lead. Therefore, the above equations must be corrected by these factors. When the strength (voltage) of an augmented unipolar lead is determined from bipolar lead values, the latter is corrected by multiplying the result by 0.87. When the strength of a bipolar lead is determined from augmented unipolar lead values, the latter is corrected by multiplying by 1.15 (100/87).

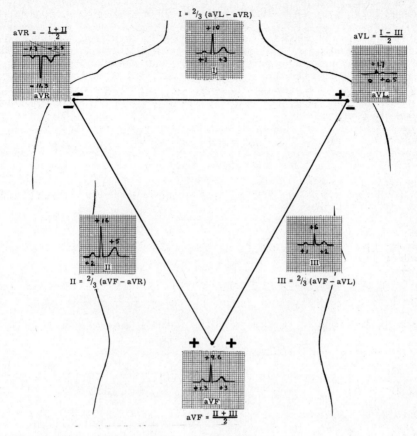

$$I = {}^2/_3 \, (aVL - aVR)$$

$$aVR = -\frac{I + II}{2}$$

$$aVL = \frac{I - III}{2}$$

$$II = {}^2/_3 \, (aVF - aVR)$$

$$III = {}^2/_3 \, (aVF - aVL)$$

$$aVF = \frac{II + III}{2}$$

Illustration of Relationship of Unipolar Limb and Standard Leads.   In order for the determinations to be accurate the leads should be taken simultaneously.

EXAMPLE - see electrocardiogram above.

The measured voltages of the individual R waves in the six leads are as follows (method of measurement is given on p. 29):

I: R = +10   II: R = +16   III: R = +6   aVR: R = −11.3   aVL: R = +1.7   aVF: R = +9.6

To determine the voltage in augmented extremity leads from the actual measurements of the standard leads (only R will be calculated, but the same method is to be used for P and T):

$$aVR \;=\; -\frac{I + II}{2}(0.87) \;=\; -\left[\frac{10 + 16}{2}\right](0.87) \;=\; -11.3$$

$$aVL \;=\; \frac{I - III}{2}(0.87) \;=\; \left[\frac{10 - 6}{2}\right](0.87) \;=\; +1.7$$

$$aVF \;=\; \frac{II + III}{2}(0.87) \;=\; \left[\frac{16 + 6}{2}\right](0.87) \;=\; +9.6$$

To determine the voltage in standard leads from the actual measurement of the augmented extremity leads (again calculating only the R wave):

$$I \;=\; {}^2/_3 \, (aVL - aVR)\,(1.15) \;=\; {}^2/_3 \, (1.7 + 11.3)\,(1.15) \;=\; +10$$

$$II \;=\; {}^2/_3 \, (aVF - aVR)\,(1.15) \;=\; {}^2/_3 \, (9.6 + 11.3)\,(1.15) \;=\; +16$$

$$III \;=\; {}^2/_3 \, (aVF - aVL)\,(1.15) \;=\; {}^2/_3 \, (9.6 - 1.7)\,(1.15) \;=\; +6$$

TECHNICAL DIFFICULTIES AFFECTING THE ELECTROCARDIOGRAM

Attention to the following details will ensure against artifacts and poor technical records:

1. The patient must lie on a comfortable bed or examining table large enough to support his entire body. He must be completely relaxed in order to ensure a satisfactory tracing. It is best to explain the procedure to an apprehensive patient in order to relieve the fears and anxiety he may be experiencing. Any muscular motions or twitchings by the patient can alter the record.

2. Be certain there is good contact between the skin and the electrode. A poor contact can result in a poor record.

3. The machine must be properly standardized so that one millivolt will produce a deflection of one centimeter. Incorrect standardization will produce inaccurate voltage of the complexes and can lead to faulty interpretation.

4. The patient and the machine must be properly grounded to avoid alternating current interference.

A Technically Good Tracing

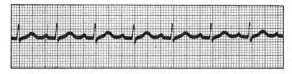

Effect of Muscle Twitchings

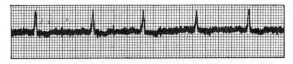

Effect of Poor Contact

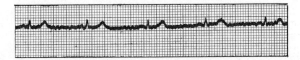

Effect of Standardization: (A) Proper standardization: 1 cm. deflection. **(B)** Overstandardization: 1.4 cm. deflection. This increases the voltage of the complexes. **(C)** Understandardization: 0.5 cm. deflection. This decreases the voltage of the complexes.

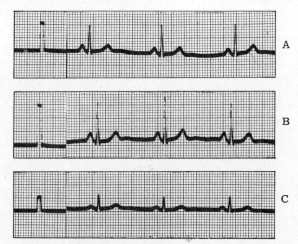

Effect of Alternating Current Interference

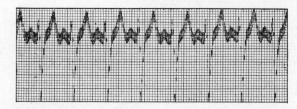

Chapter 2

ELECTROPHYSIOLOGY
OF THE HEART

INTRACELLULAR POTENTIALS

If one electrode is placed on the surface of a resting muscle cell and a second indifferent electrode is placed in a remote location, no electrical potential (i.e., zero potential) will be recorded because of the high impedance of the cell membrane. However, if the cell membrane is penetrated by a capillary electrode, a negative potential of about 90 millivolts (mv.) will be recorded. This is known as the membrane resting potential (MRP). The major factor which determines the MRP is the gradient of the potassium (K^+) ions across the cell membrane. The intracellular concentration of K^+ is approximately 150 mEq./L., and the extracellular concentration is approximately 5 mEq./L. This K^+ gradient of 30:1 is sufficient to explain the recorded MRP (-90 mv.). On the other hand an opposite gradient exists for the sodium (Na^+) ions. There is a relatively high extracellular Na^+ concentration in relation to intracellular Na^+ concentration. This Na^+ gradient, opposite in polarity to that of the K^+ gradient, does not appreciably alter the MRP because the cell membrane is considerably less permeable to the Na^+ ion than to the K^+ ion. It is estimated that the cell membrane in the resting state is 30 times more permeable to K^+ than to Na^+.

One must next try to explain the source of energy within the cell which allows for the high intracellular K^+ concentration and the negative MRP. Although, as stated above, the cell membrane, in the resting state, is 30 times less permeable to Na^+ than to K^+, the former does pass across the cell membrane. Most electrophysiologists believe that the energy for maintenance of the MRP is derived from the sodium ion. Theoretical considerations and some experimental evidence would seem to warrant the assumption that sodium enters the cell in an ionic form but leaves the cell in a nonionic form. This is referred to as the "active transport of sodium" or the "sodium pump." Thus it is thought that sodium ions enter the cell and produce the source of energy. The sodium ions then combine with some unknown intracellular substance, and this nonionic combination leaves the cell.

At the onset of depolarization of a muscle cell (e.g., a ventricular muscle cell) there is an abrupt change in the permeability of the cell membrane to sodium and potassium ions. Sodium ions enter the cell and result in a sharp rise of intracellular potential to positivity (approximately 20 mv.). This is associated with a migration of potassium ions outside the cell membrane. Following this rapid phase of depolarization (also known as phase 0) there is a relatively slow and gradual return of intracellular potential to the MRP. This is the phase of repolarization and is usually divided into three phases:

Phase 1: An initial rapid period of repolarization.

Phase 2: A plateau period of repolarization.

Phase 3: The last period of repolarization; a slow, gradual return of the intracellular potential to the MRP (MRP is known as Phase 4).

During repolarization, the sodium pump mechanism which has been "overwhelmed" by the rapid entry of sodium ions during depolarization again goes into operation, resulting in a rapid extrusion of sodium into the extracellular compartment. There is a more gradual return of potassium ions with restoration of the MRP at the end of repolarization.

The entire curve of intracellular potential, as illustrated below, is the monophasic action potential. The duration of this curve from the onset of depolarization to the termination of repolarization is the duration of action potential.

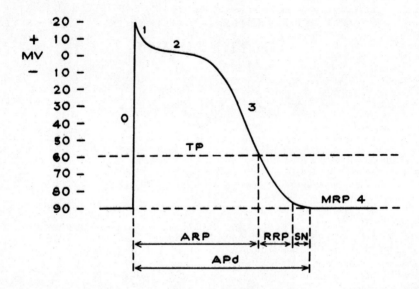

Diagram of the Action Potential of a Ventricular Muscle Cell. MRP = membrane resting potential; 0 = depolarization; 1, 2, 3 = phases of repolarization; 4 = diastolic phase = MRP; APd = duration of action potential; TP = threshold potential; ARP = absolute refractory period; RRP = relative refractory period; SN = supernormal period.

The monophasic action potential curve of an atrial muscle cell is different from that of a ventricular muscle cell. Phase 4 (MRP) and Phase 0 (depolarization) are similar, but the duration of repolarization, and hence the duration of action potential, is shorter in an atrial muscle cell. This is largely due to a shortening and steepening of the slope in Phase 2.

The monophasic action potential curve of a cell in the sinoatrial (S-A) node is markedly different from the above:

(1) There is a lower MRP (-60 to -70 mv.) at the onset of diastole.

(2) A prepotential is present in diastole (Phase 4). Instead of the MRP remaining at a constant level during diastole, as is typical of ventricular and atrial muscle cells, there is a gradual rise of the MRP during diastole. It is this prepotential which explains the automatic function of the sinus pacemaker.

(3) Depolarization is slower and does not reach sufficient positive potential to be recorded on a surface electrogram.

(4) The peak of the action potential is rounded, and repolarization is a single slow curve in which Phases 1, 2, and 3 cannot be defined.

The upper portion of the atrioventricular (A-V) node has an action potential curve similar to that of the S-A node. The configuration of the action potential of cells in the bundle of His and the Purkinje fibers is similar to that of a ventricular muscle cell except that some degree of prepotential is present which allows these centers to assume pacemaker activity under appropriate conditions. The duration of action potential is longer in a Purkinje fiber than in any other site. This is the result of prolongation of Phase 2 of repolarization.

Conduction Velocity:

The speed at which the electrical potential spreads through the heart varies considerably depending upon the inherent properties of different portions of the specialized conduction system and the myocardium. Velocity is most rapid in Purkinje fibers and slowest in the upper portion of the A-V node. The following figures are averages of many experiments done on various animal species: S-A node, 0.05 meters per second (M./sec.); atrial muscle, 0.8-1 M./sec.; bundle of His, 0.8-1 M./sec.; Purkinje fiber, 4 M./sec.; and ventricular muscle, 0.9-1 M./sec.

Excitation and Threshold Potential:

Excitation of cardiac muscle occurs when the stimulus reduces the transmembrane potential to a certain critical level, the threshold potential. This is approximately -60 mv. in atrial and ventricular muscle cells. Thus, excitation will result from a relatively weak stimulus if the MRP is lowered and therefore closer to the level of threshold potential (providing other factors such as membrane resistance are constant). Conversely, excitation will require a stronger stimulus if the MRP is increased and therefore farther removed from the level of threshold potential.

Refractoriness of Heart Muscle:

That period of time in the action potential curve during which no stimulus will propagate another action potential is known as the absolute refractory period. This period includes Phases 0, 1, 2 and a part of Phase 3. Following this there is a period during which a strong stimulus can evoke a response. This is the relative refractory period. It begins when the transmembrane potential in Phase 3 reaches the threshold potential level (about -60 mv.) and ends just before the termination of Phase 3. This is followed by a period of supernormal excitability (terminal part of Phase 3 and beginning of Phase 4), during which time a relatively weak stimulus can evoke a response.

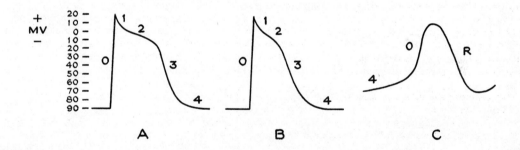

Diagrams of Action Potential Curves. A: Ventricular Muscle Cell. B: Atrial Muscle Cell. C: S-A Node. R = repolarization phase of S-A node, not divisible into Phases 1, 2, and 3.

Cell to Cell Conduction:

It had been assumed that cell to cell conduction and impulse transmission occurred through "intracellular bridges" between muscle cells. However, with electron microscopy it was shown that cells are bounded on all sides by membranes and no "bridges" are present. The membrane of the cell has a high resistance which should make electrical conduction impossible; for this reason chemical transmission was postulated. But it is now known that, although the cells have a true membrane along their longitudinal axes, the intercalated disks which cross the short axes of the cells are low resistance membranes. These disks have a resistance of $1/1000$ of cell membrane and thereby readily permit electrical transmission from cell to cell.

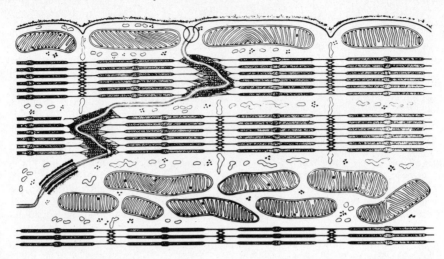

Diagrammatic Reconstruction of Mammalian Cardiac Muscle, Based on Electron Microscopic Findings. The ovoid structures are mitochondria; the parallel bars are muscle filaments. An intercalated disk is shown coursing downward and to the left from the top of the picture. It has a low resistance membrane which facilitates electrical cell to cell transmission. (Reproduced, with permission, from Sjöstrand et al.: J. Ultrastructure Research 1:271-87, 1958.)

ELECTRICAL POTENTIALS PRODUCED BY NORMAL MUSCLE

One can arrive at a basic understanding of the principles involved in electrocardiographic interpretation by an examination of the physiologic and electrical events which occur in isolated muscle strip experiments.

As stated above, if an electrode (E) is placed on the surface of a resting muscle strip and connected to a galvanometer, no deflection occurs since the entire surface of the muscle strip has zero potential owing to the high impedance of cell membranes.

When an isolated muscle strip is stimulated (S), the surface of the stimulated portion becomes electrically negative. As the impulse traverses the muscle strip there is a progressively advancing negative charge, whereas the portion of the muscle which has not as yet received the stimulus is electrically positive.

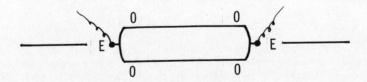

Resting Muscle; No Deflection

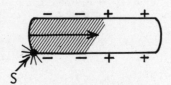

Stimulated Muscle

THE ELECTROGRAM

A tracing (electrogram) of the electrical potentials of a stimulated muscle strip is analogous to a unipolar electrocardiogram. There are two parts to the electrogram: (1) that produced during the passage of the stimulus (depolarization) and (2) that produced when the muscle returns to a resting state (repolarization).

Depolarization:
The initial spread of the stimulus through the muscle is known as depolarization. The direction in which a stimulus spreads through the muscle and the position of the electrode in relation to the spread of the stimulus determine the deflection of the tracing.
A. In a Single Muscle Strip:
    1. Upward deflection - The deflection will be upward if the stimulus spreads toward the electrode which is at the positively charged end of the muscle strip.

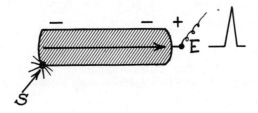

Upward Deflection

    2. Downward deflection - The deflection will be downward if the stimulus spreads away from the electrode which is at the negatively charged end of the muscle strip.

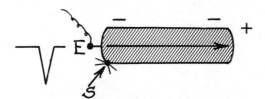

Downward Deflection

    3. Diphasic deflection - The deflection will be diphasic if the electrode overlies the midportion of the muscle strip. The initial deflection will be upward due to the advancing positive charge; the second deflection will be downward from the effect of the passing negative charge.

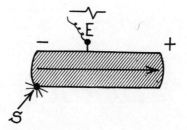

Diphasic Deflection

B. In a Double Muscle Strip:
   1. Muscles of equal size - If two muscle strips of approximately equal size are stimulated at a central point, a positive deflection (of depolarization) of equal magnitude will occur at either end.

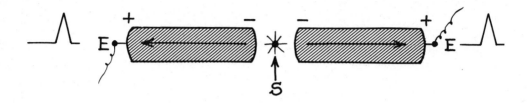

Two Muscle Strips of Equal Sizes

   2. Muscles of unequal size - If two muscle masses of markedly different sizes (analogous to the right and left ventricles) are stimulated at a central point, a large positive deflection will result over the larger muscle mass, and a small positive deflection followed by a deep negative deflection (or an entirely negative deflection) will result over the smaller muscle mass.

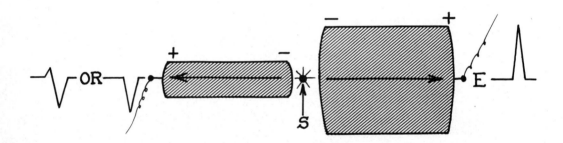

Two Muscle Strips of Markedly Different Sizes

Intrinsic Deflection (Ventricular Activation Time, V.A.T.):
   The time required for the spread of the impulse from the stimulated end to the opposite end of the muscle strip can be correlated with the electrogram by measuring the interval from the onset to the peak of the depolarization wave. In clinical electrocardiography this has been termed the intrinsic deflection or the ventricular activation time (V.A.T.).

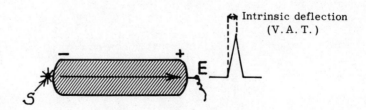

Intrinsic deflection
(V.A.T.)

Repolarization:
 The return of the stimulated muscle to the resting state is known as repolarization.

A. If repolarization occurs in a direction opposite that of depolarization, the deflection will be in the same direction as that produced by depolarization. Repolarization from right to left is illustrated in the following three diagrams:

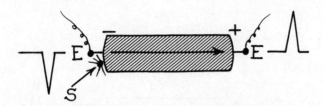

Depolarization From Left to Right

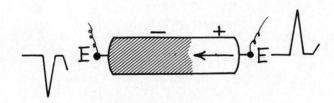

Repolarization Beginning From Right to Left

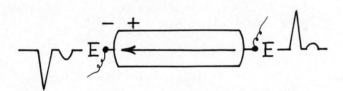

Repolarization Completed

Repolarization From Right to Left

B. If repolarization occurs in the same direction as that of depolarization, the deflection will be opposite that of depolarization. Repolarization from left to right is illustrated in the following three diagrams:

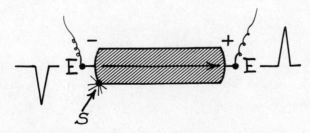

Depolarization from Left to Right

[Cont'd. on next page.]

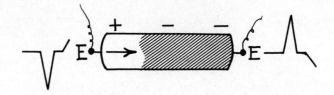

Repolarization Beginning from Left to Right

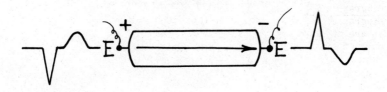

Repolarization Completed

Repolarization From Left to Right

Chapter 3

DEFINITIONS OF ELECTROCARDIOGRAPHIC CONFIGURATIONS

The Electrocardiographic Grid:

Electrocardiographic paper is a graph in which horizontal and vertical lines are present at 1 mm. intervals. A heavier line is present every 5 mm. Time is measured along the horizontal lines: 1 mm. = 0.04 sec.; 5 mm. = 0.2 sec. Voltage is measured along the vertical lines and is expressed as mm. In routine electrocardiographic practice the recording speed is 25 mm. per sec.

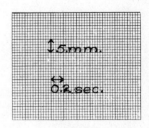

The above and all subsequent electrocardiographic illustrations are 70% of actual size.

NORMAL ELECTROCARDIOGRAPHIC COMPLEXES

Capital letters (Q, R, S) refer to relatively large waves (over 5 mm.); small letters (q, r, s) refer to relatively small waves (under 5 mm.).

P wave: The deflection produced by atrial depolarization.

T_a(or P_t) wave: The deflection produced by atrial repolarization. This deflection is usually not seen in the average 12-lead electrocardiogram.

Q (q) wave: The initial negative deflection resulting from ventricular depolarization. It precedes the first positive deflection (R).

R (r) wave: The first positive deflection during ventricular depolarization.

S (s) wave: The first negative deflection of ventricular depolarization which follows the first positive deflection (R).

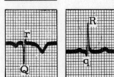
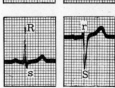

UPPER LIMITS OF THE NORMAL P-R INTERVALS*†

Rate	Below 70	71-90	91-110	111-130	Above 130
Large Adults	0.21	0.20	0.19	0.18	0.17
Small Adults	0.20	0.19	0.18	0.17	0.16
Children, ages 14 to 17	0.19	0.18	0.17	0.16	0.15
Children, ages 7 to 13	0.18	0.17	0.16	0.15	0.14
Children, ages 1½ to 6	0.17	0.165	0.155	0.145	0.135
Children, ages 0 to 1½	0.16	0.15	0.145	0.135	0.125

TABLE FOR DETERMINING HEART RATE‡

To find heart rate, select the figure in the column L which represents the cycle length in seconds measured on the electrocardiogram. The corresponding number in column R gives the rate per minute. Thus if the distance between P waves (or R waves) of two consecutive beats is .60, the heart rate is 100. Accurate values are obtained only if rhythm is regular.

L§	R**	L	R	L	R	L	R	L	R	L	R
.10	600	.33	182	.57	105	.80	75	1.07	56	1.82	33
.11	550	.34	177	.58	103	.81	74	1.09	55	1.86	32
.12	510	.35	173	.59	101	.82	73	1.11	54	1.92	31
.13	470	.36	168	.60	100	.83	72	1.13	53	2.00	30
.14	430	.37	164	.61	98	.84	71	1.15	52	2.06	29
.15	400	.38	158	.62	96	.85		1.17	51	2.15	28
.16	375	.39	155	.63	95	.86	70	1.20	50	2.22	27
.17	350	.40	150	.64	93	.87	69	1.23	49	2.30	26
.18	335	.41	145	.65	92	.88	68	1.25	48	2.40	25
.19	315	.42	142	.66	91	.89	67	1.27	47	2.50	24
.20	300	.43	138	.67	90	.90		1.29	46	2.60	23
.21	284	.44	136	.68	89	.91	66	1.33	45	2.70	22
.22	270	.45	133	.69	87	.92	65	1.36	44	2.84	21
.23	260	.46	129	.70	85	.93	64	1.38	43	3.00	20
.24	250	.47	127	.71	84	.94	63	1.42	42	3.15	19
.25	240	.48	125	.72	83	.95		1.45	41	3.35	18
.26	230	.49	123	.73	82	.96	62	1.50	40	3.50	17
.27	222	.50	120	.74	81	.97	61	1.55	39	3.75	16
.28	215	.51	117	.75	80	.98		1.58	38	4.00	15
.29	206	.52	115	.76	79	.99	60	1.64	37	4.30	14
.30	200	.53	113	.77	78	1.00		1.68	36	4.70	13
.31	192	.54	111	.78	77	1.01	59	1.73	35	5.10	12
.32	186	.55	109	.79	76	1.03	58	1.77	34	5.50	11
		.56	107			1.05	57			6.00	10

*From Ashman and Hull, Essentials of Electrocardiography. Copyright, 1937, by the Macmillan Company and used with their permission.
†Intervals measured in fractions of a second.
‡Modified after Ashman and Hull, ibid.
§L = Heart cycle length in seconds.
**R = Heart rate per minute.

R′ (r′) wave: The second positive deflection, i.e., the first positive deflection during ventricular depolarization which follows the S wave. The negative deflection following the r′ is termed the s′.

T wave: The deflection produced by ventricular repolarization.

U wave: A deflection (usually positive) seen following the T wave and preceding the next P wave. The exact cause of this wave is unknown. It is currently thought to be the result of the slow repolarization of the intraventricular conduction system (see p. 18).

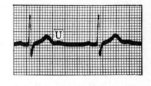

NORMAL INTERVAL VALUES

R-R interval: The R-R interval is the distance between two successive R waves. If the ventricular rhythm is regular, the interval in seconds (or fractions of a second) between the peaks of two successive R waves divided into 60 (seconds) will give the heart rate per minute. This is more easily determined by consulting the table on p. 26. If the ventricular rhythm is irregular, the number of R waves in a given period of time (e.g., 10 seconds) should be counted and the results converted into the number per minute. For example, if 20 R waves are counted in a ten-second interval, the ventricular rate is counted as 120 per minute.

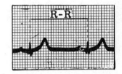

P-P interval: In regular sinus rhythm (see p. 200), the P-P interval will be the same as the R-R interval. However, when the ventricular rhythm is irregular or when atrial and ventricular rates are different but regular, the P-P interval should be measured from the same point on two successive P waves and the atrial rate per minute computed in the same manner as the ventricular rate.

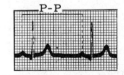

P-R interval: This measures the atrioventricular conduction time. It includes the time required for atrial depolarization and part of atrial repolarization (the late phase of atrial repolarization occurring during ventricular depolarization), plus the normal delay of excitation (approximately 0.07 sec.) in the atrioventricular node. It is measured from the onset of the P wave to the beginning of the QRS complex. Although the term P-R is in common use, P-Q would be more accurate. The normal value is in the range of 0.12 to 0.20 sec. (possibly up to 0.22 sec.). This must be correlated with the heart rate; normally, the slower the heart rate, the longer the P-R interval. A P-R interval of 0.2 sec. may be of no clinical significance with a heart rate of 60 but may well be significant with a heart rate of 100. The values vary also with age and body build (see p. 26).

QRS interval: This is the measurement of total ventricular depolarization time. It is measured from the onset of the Q wave (or R if no Q is visible) to the termination of the S wave. The upper limit of normal is 0.1 sec. Occasionally in precordial leads V_2 or V_3 this interval may be 0.11 sec.

QRS

Ventricular activation time (V. A. T.): The time it takes an impulse to traverse the myocardium from the endocardial to the epicardial surface is assumed to be reflected in a measurement from the beginning of the Q wave to the peak of the R wave. Such a measurement is only accurate when recorded directly from the surface of the heart (intrinsic deflection), preferably with closely placed bipolar electrodes. The accuracy and significance of this measurement diminishes with body surface unipolar recordings (intrinsicoid deflection).

V. A. T.

Q-T interval: This is measured from the onset of the Q wave to the end of the T wave. It measures the duration of electrical systole. The Q-T interval varies with the heart rate and must be corrected ($Q-T_c$). This is easily done by use of the nomogram on p. 29, which gives the $Q-T_c$ for a heart rate of 60. The normal $Q-T_c$ should not exceed 0.42 sec. in men and 0.43 sec. in women.

Q-T

Q-U interval: This measures the interval from the beginning of the Q wave to the end of the U wave. It has no known clinical significance. It must not be confused with the Q-T interval.

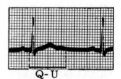

Q-U

S-T interval: The duration of the RS-T segment (see below).

NORMAL SEGMENTS AND JUNCTIONS

PR segment: That portion of the electrocardiographic tracing from the end of the P wave to the onset of the QRS complex. It is normally iso-electric.

PR segment

RS-T junction (J): The point at which the QRS complex ends and the RS-T segment begins.

RS-T segment (usually called the ST segment): That portion of the tracing from the J to the onset of the T wave. This segment is usually iso-electric but may vary from −0.5 to +2.0 mm. in precordial leads (see p. 86). It is elevated or depressed in comparison with that portion of the base line between the termination of the T wave and the beginning of the P wave (T-P segment).

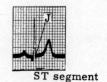

ST segment

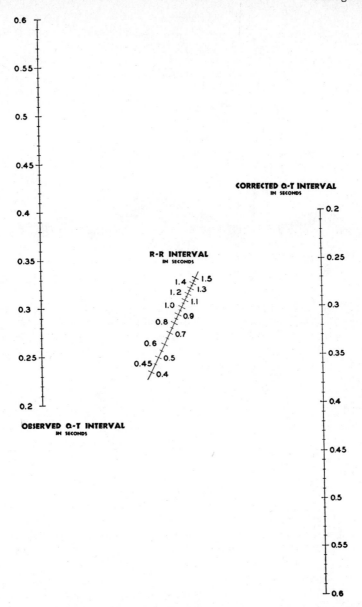

Nomogram for Rate Correction of Q-T Interval. Measure the observed Q-T interval and the R-R interval. Mark these values in the respective columns of the chart (left and middle). Place a ruler across these two points. The point at which the extension of this line crosses the third column is read as the corrected Q-T interval (Q-T$_c$). (Reproduced, with permission, from Kissin, et al.: Am. Heart J. **35**:990-2, 1948.)

VOLTAGE MEASUREMENTS

The voltage of upright deflections (upright P, R, upright T) is measured from the upper portion of the base line to the peak of the wave.

The voltage of negative deflections (inverted P, Q, S, inverted T) is measured from the lower portion of the base line to the nadir of the wave.

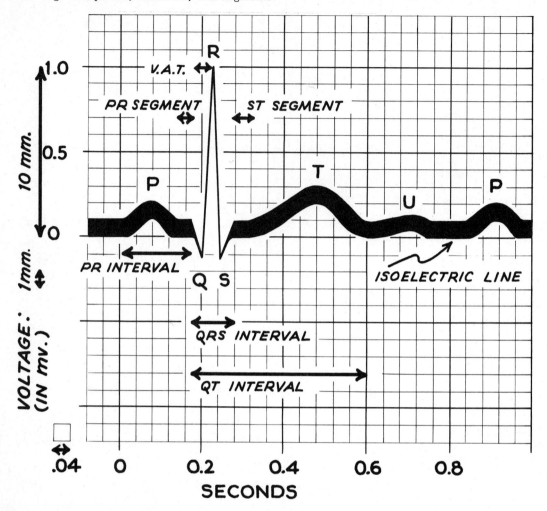

Diagram of Electrocardiographic Complexes, Intervals, and Segments

Chapter 4

THE CARDIAC VECTOR

"**Cardiac vector**" is a term used to designate all of the electrical events of the heart cycle. It has known magnitude and direction. The **instantaneous vector** represents the net electrical forces being propagated through the heart at a given instant. A **mean vector** of any given portion of the heart cycle (e.g., the QRS interval) represents the mean direction and magnitude for that period (e.g., the mean QRS vector).

The mathematical symbol of a vector is an arrow pointing in the direction of the net potential (positive or negative); the length of the arrow indicates the magnitude of the electrical force.

A vector can be drawn for atrial depolarization (P), ventricular depolarization (QRS), and ventricular repolarization (T). Each vector is constantly changing: starting at a central point, spreading through the heart, and then returning to the starting point. It therefore forms a three-dimensional loop, i.e., the spatial vectorcardiogram (see p. 301). Cathode ray oscilloscopes are now available which can record the vectorcardiogram in three planes: frontal, horizontal, and sagittal. However, the cost of the apparatus and our relative inexperience in interpretation renders the spatial vectorcardiogram impractical for routine clinical use.

FRONTAL PLANE VECTORS

The result of the electrical potentials of the entire cardiac cycle as reflected in the frontal plane of the body is the frontal plane vector. The Einthoven triangle diagrammatically illustrates the bipolar standard leads:

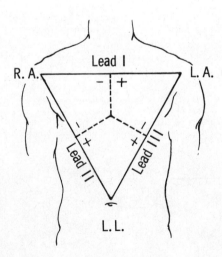

If a perpendicular is dropped from the center of each lead axis the intersection of these will theoretically represent the center of electrical activity.

Einthoven devised this equilateral triangle on the following assumptions:

(1) The "dipolar hypothesis." It is believed that each instantaneous vector is the result of an electrical potential which acts as a dipole, as illustrated in the following diagram:

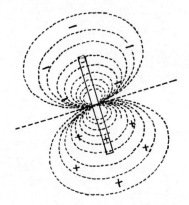

One half of the dipole is positive and the opposite half is negative. One half of the electrical field is positive, the other half negative. The greatest electrical potential, either positive or negative, will be along a line parallel with the dipole. Electrical potential along a line perpendicular to the dipole at its electrical center will be practically nil.

(2) The center of electrical activity of the heart is located in the anatomic center of the chest.
(3) Leads I, II, and III are all equidistant from the center of electrical activity.
(4) The human torso can be assumed to be spherical in shape.
(5) All body tissues and fluids can be assumed to be equally good conductors of electrical potential.

However, it is now recognized that assumptions (2), (3), (4), and (5) above are unwarranted, and even the dipolar hypothesis is still the subject of considerable controversy. Although for mathematical accuracy it is necessary to correct for these errors, the purposes of clarification will be best served by a simplified presentation of the concept of vector analysis; the more complicated but more correct analysis will be discussed later (see Chapter 18, p. 302) in relation to corrected orthogonal leads.

If the Einthoven triangle is modified so that the leads intersect at a central point, the lead potentials are seen to be placed as shown in the following diagram: (This does not alter the mathematical relationship of the leads.)

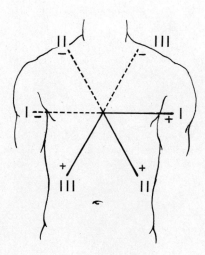

The frontal plane unipolar leads can be diagrammed as follows:

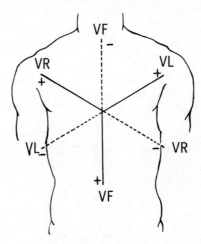

If the above two diagrams are superimposed, a hexaxial reference system can be drawn which illustrates all the six leads of the frontal plane.

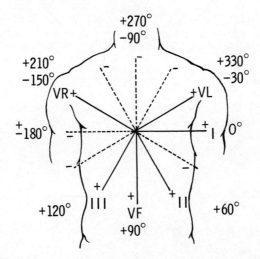

By convention the positive pole of lead I is designated as 0°, the negative pole of lead I as ± 180°, the positive pole of VF as +90°, the negative pole of VF as +270° or −90°, the positive pole of lead II as +60°, the positive pole of lead III as +120°, the positive pole of VR as +210° or −150°, and the positive pole of VL as +330° or −30°.

Polarity of Individual Frontal Plane Lead Axes:

If a perpendicular is drawn through the center of a given lead axis, any electrical force (i.e., vector) oriented in the positive half of the electrical field will record an upright deflection in that lead; any force oriented in the negative half of the electrical field will record a downward deflection.

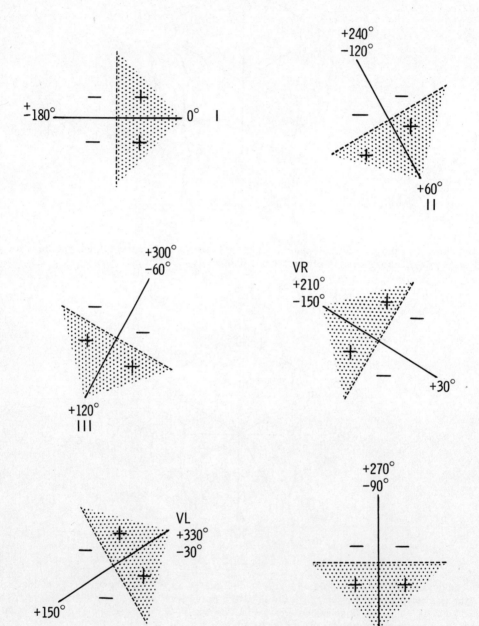

Direction of Mean Frontal Plane Axis:

    The mean QRS vector in the frontal plane can be approximated from standard leads by use of the above-described reference system (see p. 32). This is only an approximation, however, since it is determined by measurement of magnitude (i.e., voltage) alone whereas the true mean QRS vector must be determined from two factors: magnitude and time. The net amplitude and direction of the QRS complex in any two of the three standard leads are plotted along the axes of the two standard leads. Perpendicular lines are drawn at these locations. A line drawn from the center of the reference system to the intersection of the perpendiculars represents the approximate mean QRS vector. Its angle is the frontal plane axis.

Example:

I: R = +6 mm., S = −2 mm.

III: R = +2 mm., S = −5 mm.

The algebraic sum of R + S in I and III is determined

$$I = +6 - 2 = +4$$

$$III = +2 - 5 = -3$$

    The values +4 and −3 are plotted on the respective lead axes. Perpendiculars are drawn from each lead axis at these points. The resultant vector is oriented at an angle of −15°; its magnitude is approximately 4.1.

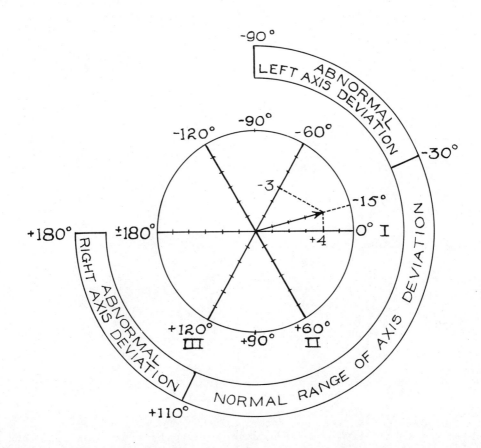

Thus, if one knows the direction and magnitude of a cardiac vector, one can derive its direction and magnitude in any of the frontal plane leads.

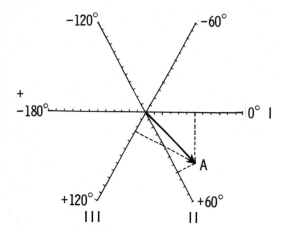

At left is illustrated a cardiac vector (A) whose angle in the frontal plane is +45°. The magnitude is indicated by the length of the arrow. On the scale used in this diagram the vector has an arbitrary magnitude of 8.6 units. If one draws a perpendicular from the tip of the arrow to each of the standard lead axes, the polarity (positive or negative) and magnitude for each lead can be determined. Thus, I = +6 units, II = +8 units, and III = +2.7 units.

Axis Deviation:

The angle of the mean frontal QRS vector determines the electrical axis. In the earlier days of electrocardiography the normal axis was considered to be 0 to +90°, right axis deviation +90 to +180°, and left axis deviation 0 to −90°. However, in order to facilitate the differentiation of normal and abnormal electrocardiograms the following criterion is now accepted: The normal axis lies between −30 and +110°; therefore left axis* deviation between −30 and −90°, and right axis deviation between +110 and ±180°, are abnormal. Within the range of normal (−30 to +110°), left axis deviation (+30 to −30°) represents a normal horizontal heart position in unipolar morphology; and right axis deviation (+75 to +110°) represents a normal vertical heart position (see pp. 65 and 67). See also diagram on p. 35.)

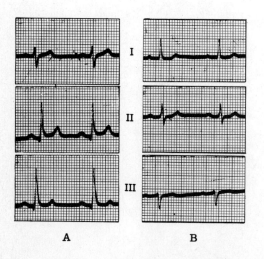

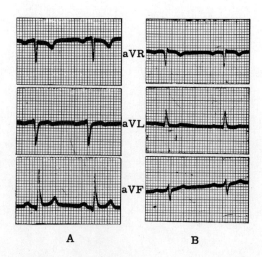

A: **Frontal Plane Axis = +96°; Vertical Heart Position**
B: **Frontal Plane Axis = −13°; Horizontal Heart Position**

---

*Although the term left axis is traditional, a more accurate term would be superior axis. Any force of unchanging magnitude which is oriented between −30° and −90° will be more superior than leftward. The greatest leftward magnitude will be represented on the 0° axis (lead I).

HORIZONTAL PLANE VECTOR

The unipolar precordial leads reflect the electrical potentials (i.e., the vector forces) in the horizontal plane. This can be diagrammed as follows:

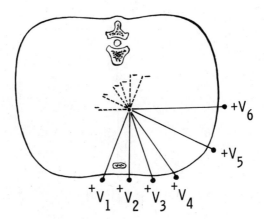

As has been illustrated for the frontal plane, a perpendicular can be drawn through the zero point of any unipolar precordial lead axis. Any electrical force oriented in the positive half of the electrical field will record a positive (upright) deflection in that lead; any force oriented in the negative half of the electrical field will record a negative (downward) deflection in that lead.

Examples:

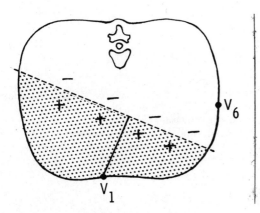

Polarity of V_1 Axis

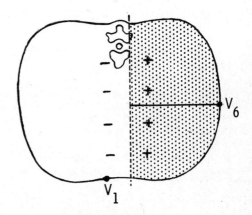

Polarity of V_6 Axis

SAGITTAL PLANE VECTOR

The unipolar esophageal leads reflect the electrical potentials in the sagittal plane. Following the principles as outlined above, a diagram can be drawn for the sagittal plane.

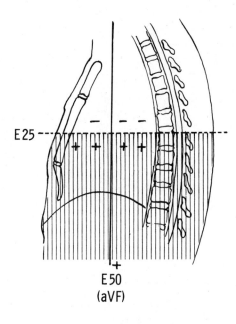

Polarity of the Long Axis

VALUE OF VECTOR ANALYSIS

Vector analysis of the electrocardiogram (vector electrocardiography) serves its most useful purpose in the teaching and understanding of the propagation of the electrical events of the cardiac cycle. It is the author's opinion that the details and interpretation of these phenomena can best be learned from the study of spatial vectorcardiography. For this reason, in Chapters 5 through 17, only brief mention will be made of vector analysis of the normal and abnormal electrocardiographic patterns. A more detailed and accurate concept of vector analysis will be deferred to the chapter on spatial vectorcardiography (Chapter 18).

Chapter 5

NORMAL ELECTROCARDIOGRAPHIC COMPLEXES

Anatomy and Physiology of the Conduction System:

The heart possesses the property of automatic and rhythmic contraction. It has the inherent ability to initiate and conduct impulses which stimulate muscular contraction. This ability is located in the specialized neuromuscular tissue known as the conduction system. The conduction system consists of (1) the sinoatrial (S-A) node, (2) the internodal atrial pathways, (3) the atrioventricular (A-V) node, (4) the bundle of His, (5) the right and left bundle branches, and (6) the Purkinje system.

Sinoatrial Node:

The heart beat is normally controlled by rhythmic impulses which arise in the sinoatrial node, and the latter is therefore the cardiac pacemaker. It consists of a bundle of specialized neuromuscular tissue measuring approximately 5 X 20 mm. which lies on the endocardial surface of the right atrium at the junction of the superior vena cava and the right atrial appendage. The impulse then spreads through both atria, producing the P wave.

Internodal Atrial Pathways:

Conduction through the atria occurs through three bundles of myocardium which contain Purkinje type fibers: (1) The anterior internodal tract (Bachmann) leaves the S-A node in a forward direction and curves about the superior vena cava and anterior wall of the right atrium.

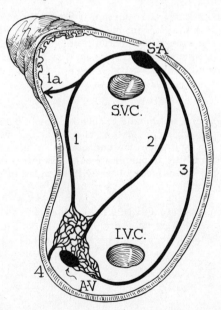

Schematic Diagram of Internodal Atrial Pathways, as Seen From Posterior Aspect of Right Atrium.
S. V. C. = superior vena cava; I. V. C. = inferior vena cava; S-A = sinoatrial node; A-V = atrioventricular node; 1 = anterior internodal tract; 1a = branch of anterior internodal tract to left atrium; 2 = middle internodal tract; 3 = posterior internodal tract; 4 = interconnecting fibers from all three tracts which bypass the A-V node.

39

There it divides into two bundles of fibers, one entering the left atrium and the other coursing over the anterior portion of the interatrial septum and descending obliquely behind the root of the aorta to enter the anterior-superior margin of the A-V node. (2) The middle internodal tract (Wenckebach) leaves the posterior margin of the S-A node, curves behind the superior vena cava, and courses along the posterior portion of the interatrial septum to enter the superior margin of the A-V node. (3) The posterior internodal tract (Thorel) leaves the posterior margin of the S-A node and follows the course of the crista terminalis and eustachian ridge to enter the posterior margin of the A-V node. Lateral extensions from this tract arborize over the dorsum of the right atrium. Between all three tracts there are interconnecting fibers that merge just above the A-V node. Some of these fibers do not enter the A-V node but bypass it; they can reenter the conducting system at a place distal to the A-V node.

Atrioventricular Node:

This bundle of specialized neuromuscular tissue measures 2 X 5 mm. It is located on the endocardial surface of the right side of the interatrial septum just inferior to the opening of the coronary sinus. The impulse which has spread through both atria enters the A-V node and is normally delayed for 0.07 sec.

Bundle of His:

The bundle of His is in direct continuity with the lower portion of the A-V node. It is approximately 20 mm. long and is located on the endocardial surface of the right side of the interatrial septum, immediately superior to the interventricular septum.

Bundle Branches:

The right and left bundle branches arise from the bifurcation of the lower portion of the bundle of His in the membranous portion of the interventricular septum. The right bundle is much longer than the left. The left, very shortly after its origin, divides into a superior and an inferior branch. The passage of the impulse through the bundle branches is not reflected in the electrocardiogram.

The midportion of the interventricular septum is normally activated from left to right. Purkinje fibers arise more proximally from the divisions of the left bundle than from the right bundle branch and enter the left side of the septum, which they activate initially. This wave of excitation from left to right produces the initial negativity of the left ventricular cavity and the initial positivity of the right ventricular cavity. (See pp. 42 and 58.)

Purkinje System:

After traversing the right and left bundle branches, the impulse passes into the multiple ramifications of the Purkinje system which cover the subendocardial surfaces of both ventricles. The impulse then travels perpendicularly from the endocardial to the epicardial surface of the myocardium. It is the propagation of the impulses through the Purkinje system into the ventricular myocardium which produces the remainder of the QRS complex (after activation of the interventricular septum from left to right). (See pp. 59 to 61.)

The anteroseptal region of the right ventricle is the earliest site of ventricular activation. The posterobasal region of the left ventricle, the pulmonary conus, and the uppermost portion of the I-V septum are activated last.

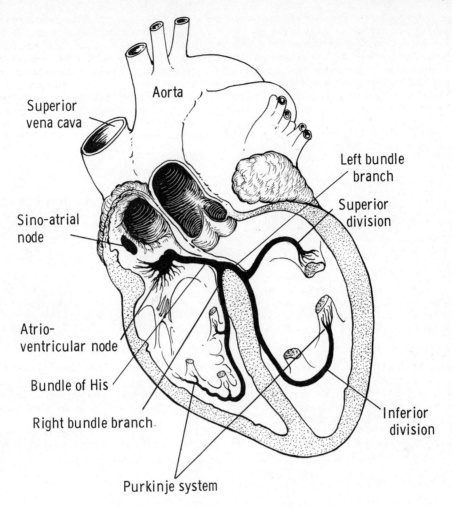

Illustration of Conduction System

ELECTRICAL CONDUCTION THROUGH THE HEART

The initial impulse in the cardiac cycle begins in the sinoatrial (S-A) node.

Atrial Activation:
    The impulse traverses the atrial musculature, producing the P wave, and then reaches the atrioventricular (A-V) node. Normally the impulse is "delayed" in the A-V node for 0.07 sec. before passing on to the bundle of His, the right and left bundles, the ramifications of the Purkinje system, and then into the ventricles. Conduction through this electrical pathway is much more rapid than through ordinary heart muscle.

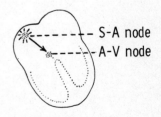

Atrial Activation

Ventricular Activation:

    Initial intraventricular activation occurs in the mid-portion of the I-V septum in a left to right direction. The anteroseptal region of the ventricular myocardium is the next site of activation. The major portion of ventricular activation then occurs through the myocardium of the left and right ventricles. The last parts to be activated are the posterobasal region of the left ventricle, the pulmonary conus, and the uppermost portion of the I-V septum. The spread of excitation through the myocardium is from the endocardial to the epicardial surface. Thus evolves the QRS complex.

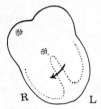
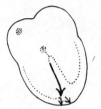
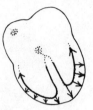
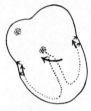

| Septal activation from left to right. | Activation of anteroseptal region of the ventricular myocardium. | Activation of major portion of ventricular myocardium from endocardial to epicardial surfaces. | Late activation of posterobasal portion of the left ventricle, the pulmonary conus, and the uppermost portion of the I-V septum. |

Ventricular Activation

Relation Between Electrical Conduction and Contraction:

    The passage of the electrical impulse through any given portion of the heart precedes the resulting contraction of that portion of the myocardium. The following diagram illustrates these time relationships.

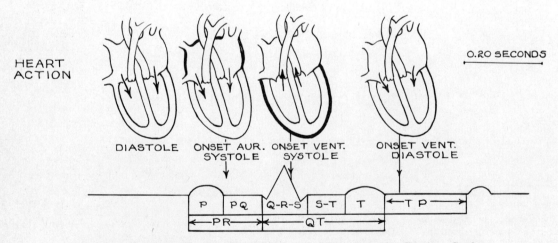

Relation Between Electrical and Mechanical Events in the Cardiac Cycle

ATRIAL COMPLEXES

The normal P wave in standard, extremity, and precordial leads is not over 0.11 sec. in duration or over 2.5 mm. in height. Since the spread of excitation from the S-A node to the A-V node is in a head-to-foot direction, the P is normally upright in leads I, II, aVF, and V_{3-9}. The P is normally inverted in aVR and frequently in V_1 (and at times in V_2). The P may be upright, diphasic, flat, or inverted in leads III and aVL. Thus the normal P vector is oriented inferiorly, to the left, and slightly anteriorly.

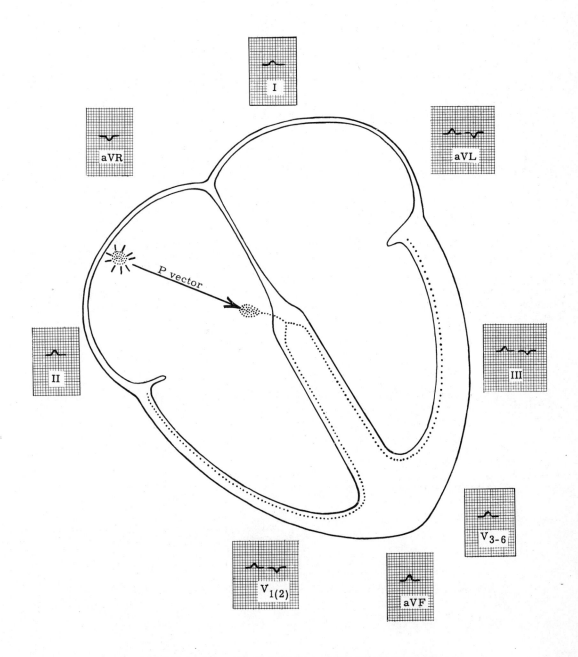

Direction of the Normal P Wave in the Various Leads

Esophageal leads will show P waves which are of greater amplitude than in any lead of the conventional 12-lead electrocardiogram. For the reason given above the P will be inverted in high esophageal levels (E_{10}-E_{25}), i.e., above the atrioventricular groove, and will be upright in low esophageal leads (E_{35}-E_{50}). In the region of the atrioventricular groove (E_{25}-E_{35}), the P wave will be a large, sharply peaked diphasic complex, simulating an RS complex of a ventricular lead.

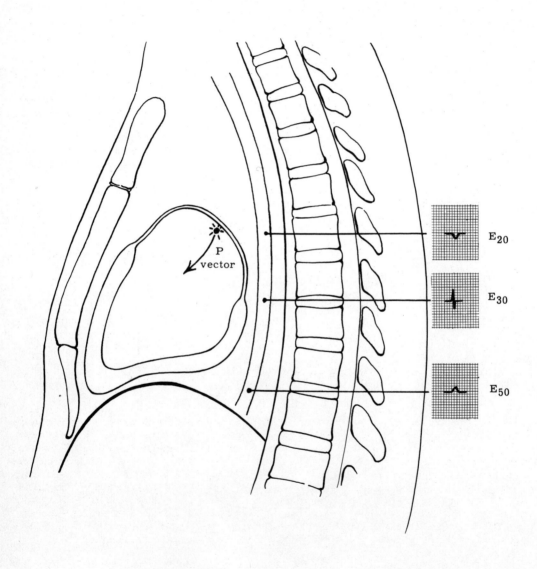

Direction of the Normal P Wave in Esophageal Leads

VENTRICULAR COMPLEXES

UNIPOLAR ELECTROCARDIOGRAMS ON THE EXPOSED VENTRICLE

Our knowledge of unipolar electrocardiography on the exposed heart is derived from animal work and direct electrocardiography performed during operations in which the human heart is exposed. It again must be emphasized that any such unipolar lead records all of the electrical events of the cardiac cycle (i.e., all the vector forces) and not merely those reflecting a small area of the underlying myocardium.

LEFT VENTRICULAR EPICARDIAL COMPLEX

Such a complex is recorded by placing an electrode directly over the left ventricle of the exposed heart. It records all of the electrical events of the cardiac cycle as viewed from this electrode site. The P wave is upright. The initial spread of excitation across the septum from left to right in a direction away from the exploring electrode (producing initial negativity of the left side of the septum which is transmitted through the left ventricular cavity and left myocardium) results in an initial downward deflection, the q wave. The spread of excitation through the large muscle mass of the left ventricle in the direction of the electrode produces a tall upright deflection, the R wave. If the electrode is so situated that the spread of excitation passes it to activate the remaining (posterobasal) portion of the left ventricle, a second small negative deflection will result, the s wave. Thus the typical pattern of a left ventricular epicardial lead is a qRs complex. The V.A.T. is not over 0.04-0.05 sec.

Following depolarization the complex usually returns to the iso-electric line, producing an iso-electric ST segment.

Repolarization results in an upright T wave which is asymmetrical, the upstroke being of longer duration than the downstroke. The T wave should be at least one-tenth as high as the R in the same complex.

RIGHT VENTRICULAR EPICARDIAL COMPLEX

This complex is recorded by placing an electrode directly over the right ventricle of an exposed heart. It records all of the electrical events of the cardiac cycle as viewed from this electrode site. The P wave may be upright, diphasic, or inverted. The spread of excitation through the interventricular septum from left to right in the direction of the exploring electrode (producing an initial positivity of the right side of the septum which is transmitted through the right ventricular cavity and right myocardium) produces an initial positive deflection, the r wave. Contributing to this initial upright deflection is the early activation of the right ventricular myocardium. The V.A.T. is not over 0.02-0.03 sec. Following this the major wave of excitation is spreading away from the exploring electrode into the large muscle mass of the left ventricle, which far exceeds the spread through the smaller mass of the right ventricle, resulting in a large downward deflection. Thus an rS complex is one typical form of right ventricular epicardial complex.

At times the initial r wave is not recorded, resulting in a completely negative deflection, or QS complex.

Occasionally (5%) the late activation of the posterobasal surface of the left ventricle and the region of the pulmonary conus, occurring in the direction of the exploring electrode, produces a second small upright deflection, an r' wave. Thus an rSr' complex or a Qr complex can occur.

The ST segment may be iso-electric or normally may be elevated 1-2 mm.

The T wave may be upright, flat, or inverted in the above complexes.

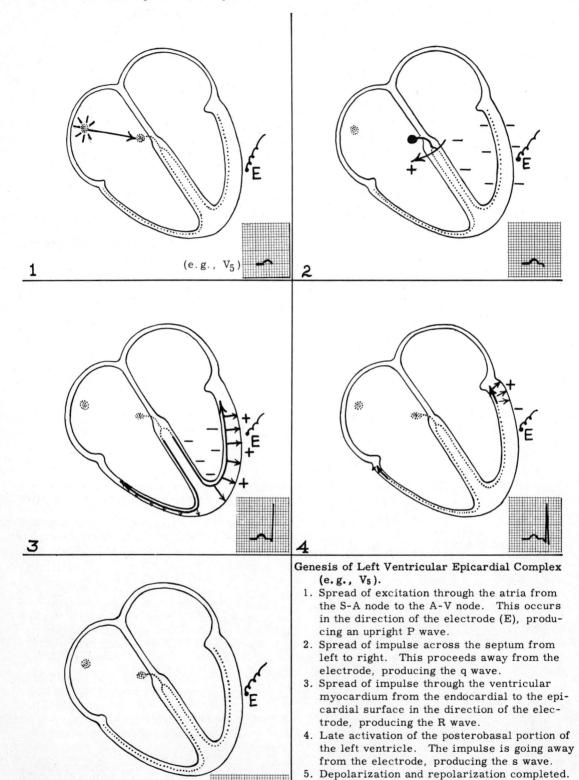

(e.g., V_5)

1

2

3

4

5

Genesis of Left Ventricular Epicardial Complex (e.g., V_5).

1. Spread of excitation through the atria from the S-A node to the A-V node. This occurs in the direction of the electrode (E), producing an upright P wave.
2. Spread of impulse across the septum from left to right. This proceeds away from the electrode, producing the q wave.
3. Spread of impulse through the ventricular myocardium from the endocardial to the epicardial surface in the direction of the electrode, producing the R wave.
4. Late activation of the posterobasal portion of the left ventricle. The impulse is going away from the electrode, producing the s wave.
5. Depolarization and repolarization completed. There is no satisfactory method of diagrammatically illustrating repolarization in the heart.

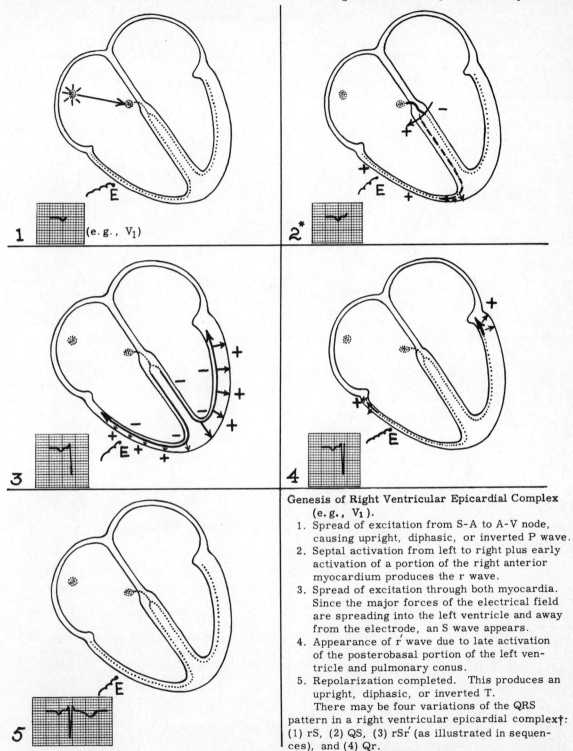

1 (e.g., V$_1$)

2*

3

4

5

Genesis of Right Ventricular Epicardial Complex (e.g., V$_1$).

1. Spread of excitation from S-A to A-V node, causing upright, diphasic, or inverted P wave.
2. Septal activation from left to right plus early activation of a portion of the right anterior myocardium produces the r wave.
3. Spread of excitation through both myocardia. Since the major forces of the electrical field are spreading into the left ventricle and away from the electrode, an S wave appears.
4. Appearance of r' wave due to late activation of the posterobasal portion of the left ventricle and pulmonary conus.
5. Repolarization completed. This produces an upright, diphasic, or inverted T.

There may be four variations of the QRS pattern in a right ventricular epicardial complex†: (1) rS, (2) QS, (3) rSr' (as illustrated in sequences), and (4) Qr.

In any of the above, either the P wave or the T wave may be upright, diphasic, or inverted.

*The early activation of the right anterior myocardium is illustrated only in this sequence diagram. It will be omitted in all other sequence illustrations since it contributes only to the production of a part of the r wave in a right ventricular epicardial complex.

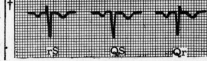

rS   QS   Qr

TRANSITIONAL ZONE VENTRICULAR EPICARDIAL COMPLEX

This complex is recorded by placing an electrode on the epicardial surface of the exposed heart overlying the interventricular septum. It records all the electrical events of the cardiac cycle as viewed from this electrical site. Since in many instances the direction of this vector force is perpendicular to the mean QRS vector, its magnitude (voltage) will be small and diphasic, resulting in an rs complex. The ST segment is iso-electric and the T wave upright.

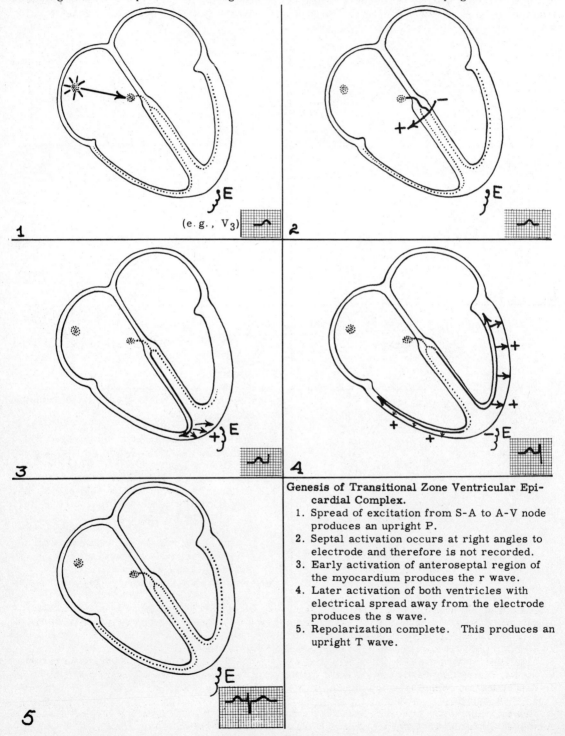

Genesis of Transitional Zone Ventricular Epicardial Complex.

1. Spread of excitation from S-A to A-V node produces an upright P.
2. Septal activation occurs at right angles to electrode and therefore is not recorded.
3. Early activation of anteroseptal region of the myocardium produces the r wave.
4. Later activation of both ventricles with electrical spread away from the electrode produces the s wave.
5. Repolarization complete. This produces an upright T wave.

LEFT VENTRICULAR CAVITY COMPLEX

This complex is recorded by actually inserting an electrode within the left ventricular cavity. The P wave is inverted if the electrode is above the A-V groove and upright if below. The initial septal activation as well as all subsequent myocardial activation is travelling away from the exploring electrode. Therefore, the entire ventricular depolarization complex will be a downward deflection, a QS complex. The ST segment is iso-electric, and the T is normally inverted. *

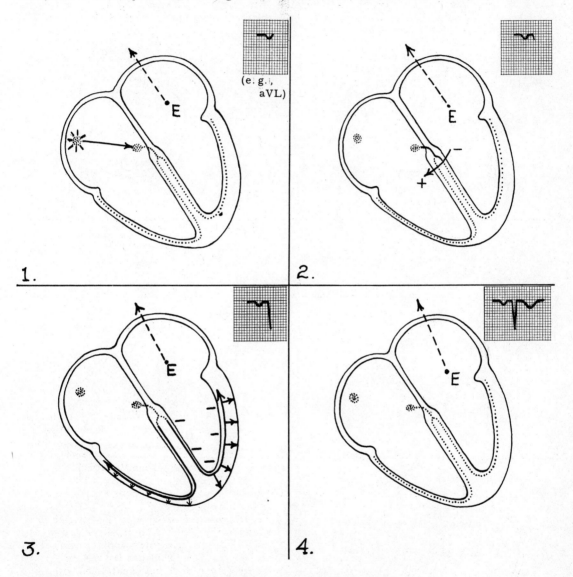

Genesis of Left Ventricular Cavity Complex (e. g., aVL in a Vertical Heart).
1. Spread of excitation from S-A to A-V node. Since the electrode in this diagram is above the A-V groove, the P wave is inverted.
2. Septal activation from left to right produces the first portion of the QS complex.
3. Activation of the left ventricular myocardium from endocardial to epicardial surfaces renders the left ventricular cavity negative and produces the remainder of the QS complex.
4. Repolarization complete. This produces an inverted T wave. *

*Studies by Prinzmetal, et al. (1955), indicate that the T wave may be normally upright in a left ventricular cavity lead. This is contrary to all previous information.

RIGHT VENTRICULAR CAVITY COMPLEX

This complex is recorded by actually placing an electrode within the right ventricular cavity. The P wave is inverted, diphasic, or upright. As a result of septal activation from left to right, an initial small r wave may be registered. Actually this occurs only if the electrode is in close proximity to the septum. As the excitation wave passes through the right myocardium from endo-cardial to epicardial surfaces and passes into the left ventricle, all impulses will be spreading away from the electrode, producing a deep negative deflection, the S wave. For the reason given above (see p. 45), a late r' may be recorded. Thus the complexes may be (1) rS (as shown in sequence), (2) QS, (3) rSr', or (4) Qr.*

The ST segment is iso-electric and the T wave inverted.

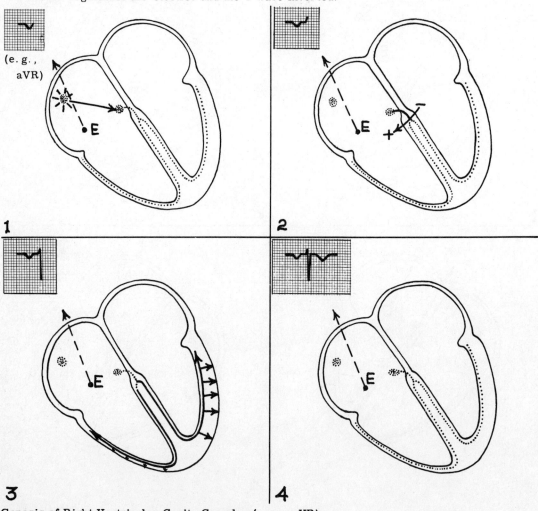

Genesis of Right Ventricular Cavity Complex (e.g., aVR).

1. Spread of excitation from S-A to A-V node. The electrode is above the level of the A-V groove, resulting in an inverted P wave.
2. Septal activation from left to right produces initial positivity of the right ventricular cavity and hence the r wave.
3. Spread of excitation from the endocardial to the epicardial surface of the right myocardium produces negativity of the cavity and therefore the S wave.
4. Repolarization complete. This produces an inverted T wave.

*The complexes not shown in the sequence are shown at right. (Left, QS; center, rSr'; right, Qr.)

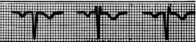

"BACK-OF-THE-HEART" COMPLEXES

These are recorded by placing an exploring electrode directly on the exposed epicardial surface of the posterior aspect of the heart at varying locations.

An electrode overlying the atrial level will reflect cavity potential, thus recording an inverted P, a QS complex, and an inverted T.

An electrode placed over or just inferior to the atrioventricular groove will record a summation of cavity and left ventricular epicardial potentials: a large diphasic P, a QR complex and an inverted T. This is the typical "back of the heart" complex.

An electrode overlying the posterior aspect of the left ventricle will show a typical left ventricular epicardial complex.

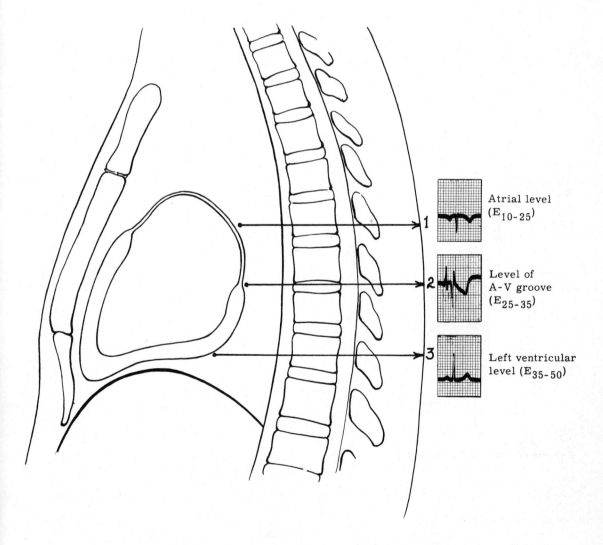

1   Atrial level (E_{10-25})

2   Level of A-V groove (E_{25-35})

3   Left ventricular level (E_{35-50})

Diagram of Back-of-Heart Patterns. (1) Atrial level. **(2)** Level of A-V groove. **(3)** Left ventricular level.

APPLICATION OF THE COMPLEXES DESCRIBED ABOVE
TO CLINICAL ELECTROCARDIOGRAPHY

The complexes described above have been obtained by actually applying the electrode to the surfaces or within the cavities of the heart. However, in clinical electrocardiography it must be remembered that all the electrodes, being on the surface of the body, are at varying distances from the heart. In unipolar electrocardiographic analysis the electrocardiographic patterns derived from body surface leads are correlated with the patterns developed from direct heart surface and cavity leads. Unipolar precordial and esophageal leads are much closer to the heart than unipolar extremity leads. The proximity of the former leads results in the major disagreement between the vector analysts and the unipolar lead analysts. The former believe that proximity leads offer no more information than can be obtained by a corrected lead system using remote leads. The unipolar lead analysts believe there may be local potentials recorded in proximity leads which are not evident in remote leads and that these may yield valuable clinical information.

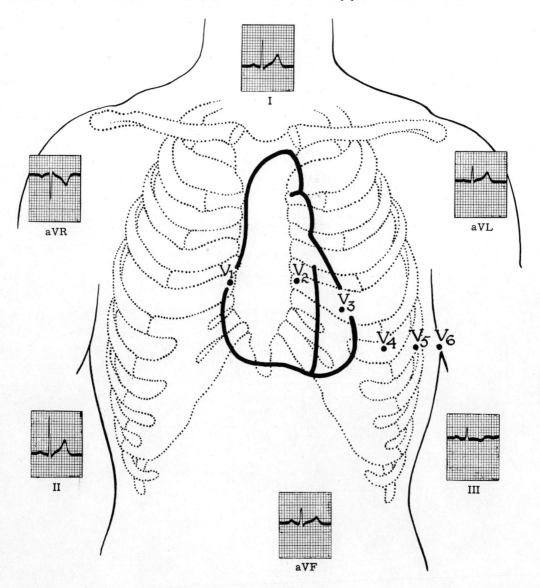

Frontal Plane Electrocardiographic Patterns. Standard leads I, II, and III; augmented unipolar extremity leads, aVR, aVL, and aVF. (Intermediate Heart Position.)

Standard leads I, II, and III and unipolar extremity leads aVR, aVL, and aVF record the electrocardiographic pattern in the frontal plane. The pattern will vary depending upon the heart position.

Unipolar precordial leads V_{1-6}, etc., record the electrocardiographic pattern (i. e., the cardiac vector) in the horizontal plane. An individual chest lead does not represent the electrical potentials of a localized area of underlying heart muscle but records all of the electrical events of the heart cycle as viewed from that particular lead site. However, owing to the proximity of the precordial lead to the surface of the heart, those electrical potentials which are being generated in the underlying heart muscle will be magnified whereas those potentials arising from more distant locations will be of lesser magnitude (amplitude).

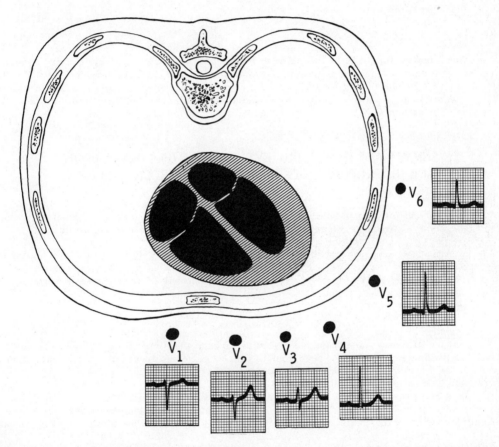

Horizontal Plane Electrocardiographic Patterns. As the electrode is advanced from V_1 to V_6, right ventricular epicardial complexes ($V_{1,2}$) change into left ventricular epicardial complexes ($V_{4,5,6}$). A transition zone pattern is seen in V_3.

THE BIPOLAR ELECTROCARDIOGRAM

NORMAL COMPLEXES IN STANDARD BIPOLAR LEADS

This discussion is purposely being placed after the discussion of unipolar complexes since the pattern in leads I, II, and III will merely be additional patterns of the frontal plane vector. In fact, some electrocardiographers no longer take these leads. However, since our knowledge of electrocardiography began with these standard leads it is well to be aware of their patterns, realizing that their value in electrocardiographic interpretation is complementary to that offered by the unipolar leads.

ATRIAL COMPLEXES (P WAVES): See p. 43.

VENTRICULAR COMPLEXES

QRS:
  The normal QRS interval has a duration of 0.05 to 0.1 sec. The direction of these complexes will depend upon the heart position, i.e., axis deviation (see p. 98).

ST Segment: (See p. 28.)

T Wave:
  This is normally upright in lead I. It may be upright, flat, diphasic, or inverted in lead III. The pattern in lead II will represent a summation of leads I and III. The presence of a T in lead I of lower amplitude than that in lead III can be a normal or abnormal finding. It will occur when the T is inverted in aVL. The decision as to whether this is normal or abnormal will depend on whether the T inversion in aVL is a part of a normal aVL or an abnormal aVL.

SUMMARY OF THE ELECTROPHYSIOLOGY OF THE NORMAL HEART AND THE PRODUCTION OF THE NORMAL ELECTROCARDIOGRAM

As the electrical impulse passes through the conduction system there is a constant changing of electrical potential which is reflected in the production of the electrocardiogram.

The pattern in any one lead of the normal electrocardiogram will depend on the relationship of the electrode to the cardiac vector. The patterns will therefore vary with heart position (see pp. 63 to 80). To illustrate the sequence of events in a conventional 12-lead electrocardiogram, a vertical heart position will be used.

Atrial Complex:
  The passage of the impulse from the S-A node through the atria to the A-V node produces the P wave. This impulse travels in a head-to-foot direction. The direction of the P wave in any given lead will therefore depend on its relation to the direction of this impulse.
  A. Unipolar Extremity Leads:
    1. aVR - The pattern of right arm potential is the same as the potential at the right shoulder, the arm merely acting as a conductor from the latter site. The impulse is therefore travelling away from this electrode and will result in a negative deflection, i.e., an inverted P wave.
    2. aVL - This lead reflecting left shoulder potential is so situated that the impulse is travelling away from it and therefore the P wave is inverted.
    3. aVF - The impulse is travelling toward the left foot electrode, and the P is therefore upright.

  B. Standard Leads: The pattern in these leads is a further reflection of the frontal plane vector. In a normal vertical heart, the P wave is upright in all three leads.

  C. Precordial Leads: The P wave in V_1 may be upright, diphasic, or inverted. The P wave may be inverted in V_2, but this is rare. The P wave is upright in leads V_{3-6}. (See p. 56.)

After the impulse reaches the A-V node it is normally delayed for 0.07 sec. before the impulse passes on to the bundle of His. This produces an iso-electric P-R segment in all leads. (See p. 57.)

Ventricular Complex (Early):

The initial impulse transmission in the ventricle is across the mid-portion of the interventricular septum from left to right. This produces initial positivity of the right ventricular cavity which is transmitted through the right ventricular myocardium; and initial negativity of the left ventricular cavity which is transmitted through the left ventricular myocardium.

A. Unipolar Extremity Leads:
1. aVR - This lead reflects right cavity potential and may record an initial small positive deflection, an r wave.
2. aVL - This lead reflects left cavity potential and will record a small negative deflection, a q wave.
3. aVF - This lead reflects left ventricular epicardial potential and will record an initial small negative deflection, a q wave.

B. Standard Leads: These reflect the pattern in extremity leads. A small q wave may be seen in leads I, II, and III.

C. Precordial Leads: Those leads reflecting right ventricular epicardial potential (V_{1-2}) will show an initial small positive deflection, the r wave. Those leads reflecting left ventricular epicardial potential (V_{4-6}) will show an initial small negative deflection, the q wave. (See p. 58.)

D. Vector Analysis: The initial QRS vector is oriented to the right, anteriorly, and usually superiorly. Therefore, in the frontal plane this vector (directed to the right and superiorly) results in a small negative deflection (q) in leads I, II, III, aVL, and aVF, and an upright deflection (r) in aVR. In the horizontal plane this vector (directed to the right and anteriorly) results in a small positive deflection (r) in V_{1-2} and a small negative deflection (q) in V_{4-6}.

Ventricular Complex (Late):

After activation of the mid-portion of the interventricular septum, the impulse passes down the right and left bundle branches into the Purkinje system, thereby activating the right and left ventricles. The impulses traverse the ventricular myocardium from the endocardial to the epicardial surface.

A. The first portion of the ventricular myocardium to be activated is the anteroseptal region of the right ventricle. This contributes to the r wave in right precordial leads (V_{1-2}). It has no appreciable influence on the pattern in other leads. (See p. 59.)

B. The major muscle mass of both the right and left ventricles is then activated. Since the impulse is spreading from the endocardium to the epicardium, both ventricular cavities will have a negative potential at this time. This will produce a negative wave in aVR which is an S wave since it is preceded by a positive deflection, the r wave, and hence an rS complex. It will similarly produce a negative wave in aVL. Since the initial deflection of septal activation was also negative, this completely negative wave is termed a QS complex.

Since the left ventricular muscle mass is much greater than the right there will be greater electrical potential spreading through the left ventricle than the right. This is analogous to the muscle strip illustration on p. 22. Left ventricular epicardial leads (aVF, V_{4-5-6}) will therefore record a tall upright deflection, the R wave, and right ventricular epicardial leads (V_{1-2}) will record deep S waves (see p. 60).

C. Vector Analysis: The major QRS vector is directed to the left, inferiorly, and slightly posteriorly. In the frontal plane the leftward and inferiorly directed vector produces an upright deflection (R) in leads I, II, III, and aVF, and a downward deflection (s) in aVR and (QS) in aVL. In the horizontal plane the leftward and posteriorly directed vector produces a downward deflection (S) in V_{1-2} and an upright deflection (R) in V_{4-6}.

D. The last portions of the ventricular muscle mass to be activated are the posterobasal portion of the left ventricle, the region of the pulmonary conus, and the uppermost portion of the I-V septum. This vector force is oriented to the right and superiorly. This produces a second small negative deflection in a left ventricular epicardial lead (aVF, V_{4-6}), an s wave, and, if oriented anteriorly, may produce a small second positive deflection, an r' wave, in leads aVR and V_1 (see p. 61).

Repolarization:

The sequences discussed above reflect ventricular depolarization. Following this, ventricular repolarization occurs. The sequence of events involved in ventricular repolarization are so complex that they cannot be illustrated. It is known that both the right and left ventricular cavities are negative during ventricular repolarization. The epicardial surface of the left ventricle is positive and that of the right ventricle may be positive or negative.

The ST segment will be iso-electric in all leads with the minor exceptions discussed on pp. 28 and 86.

The T wave will be inverted in aVR and aVL (right and left cavity potential), upright in aVF and left precordial leads V_{3-6}, may be upright or inverted in V_1, and is rarely inverted in V_2. (See p. 62.) The mean T vector is oriented to the left, inferiorly, and anteriorly.

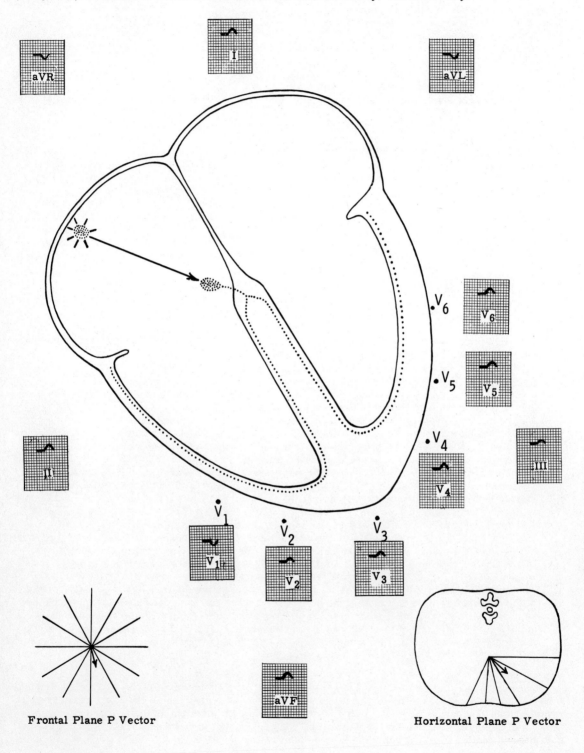

Frontal Plane P Vector

Horizontal Plane P Vector

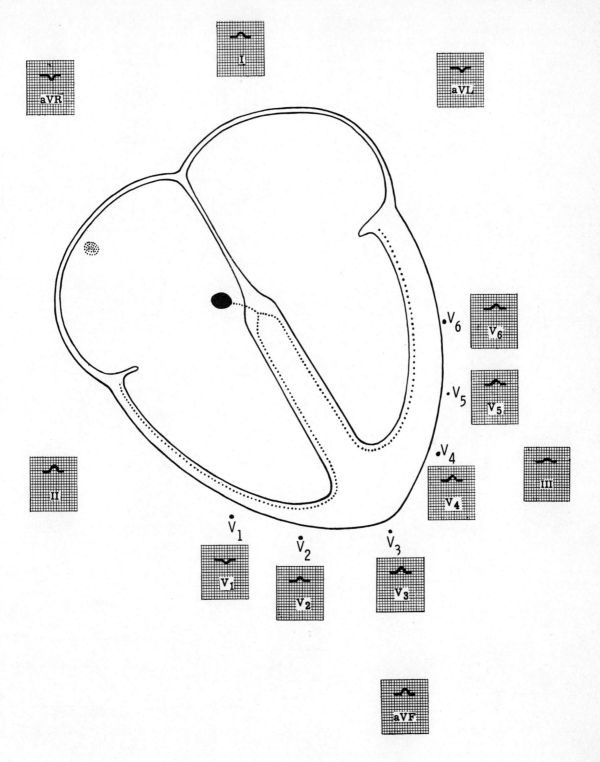

Completion of Atrial Complex and Delay of Impulse at A-V Node

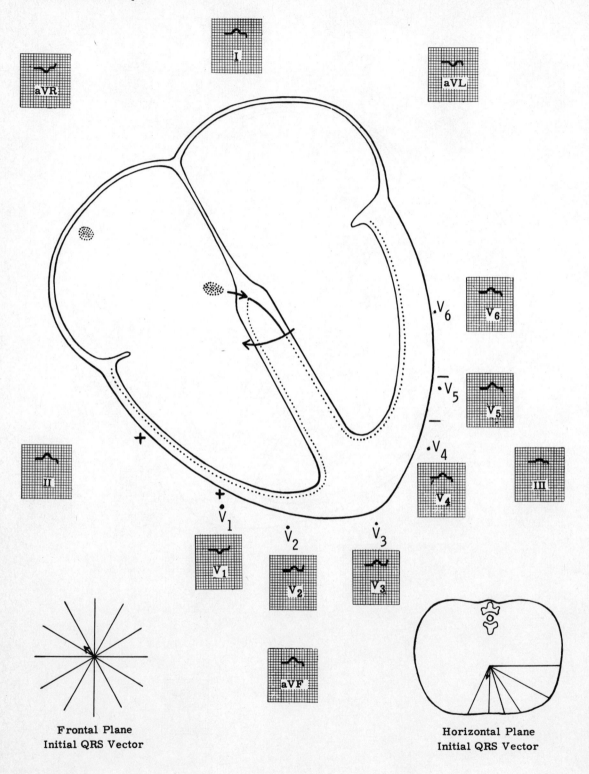

Frontal Plane
Initial QRS Vector

Horizontal Plane
Initial QRS Vector

Beginning of Ventricular Complex: Septal activation.

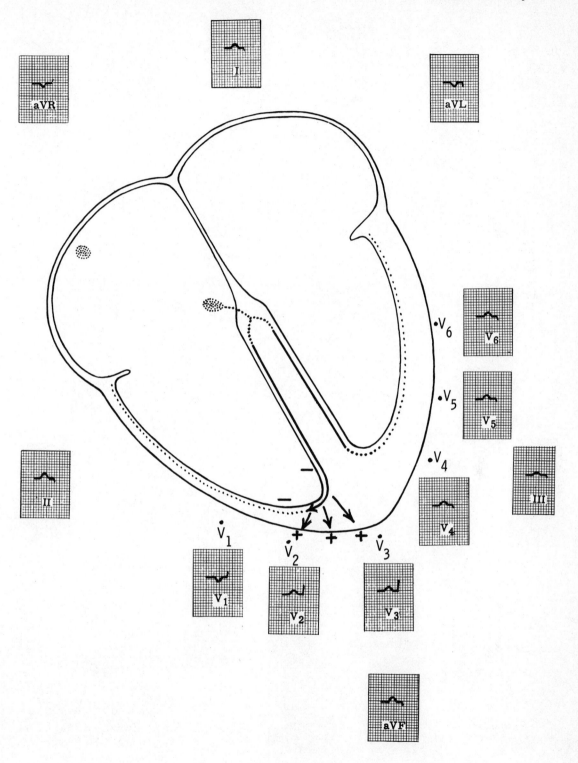

Early Activation of Anteroseptal Region of Myocardium

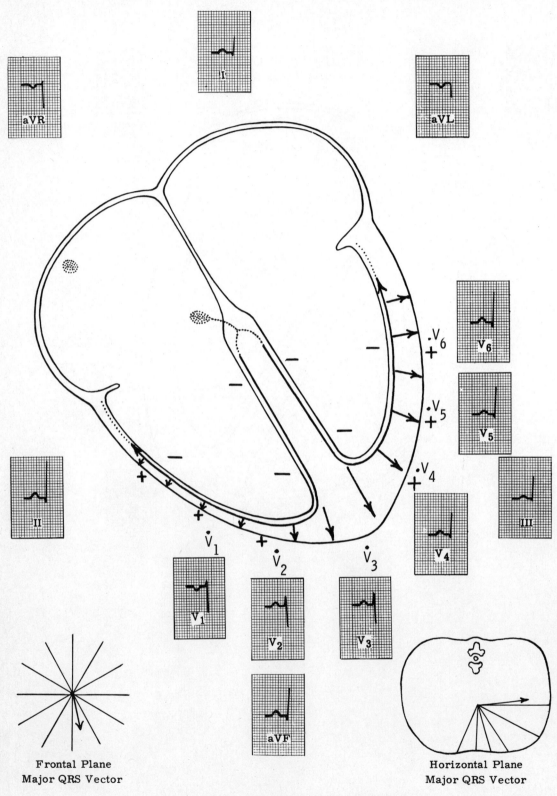

Frontal Plane
Major QRS Vector

Horizontal Plane
Major QRS Vector

Major Activation of Left and Right Ventricles

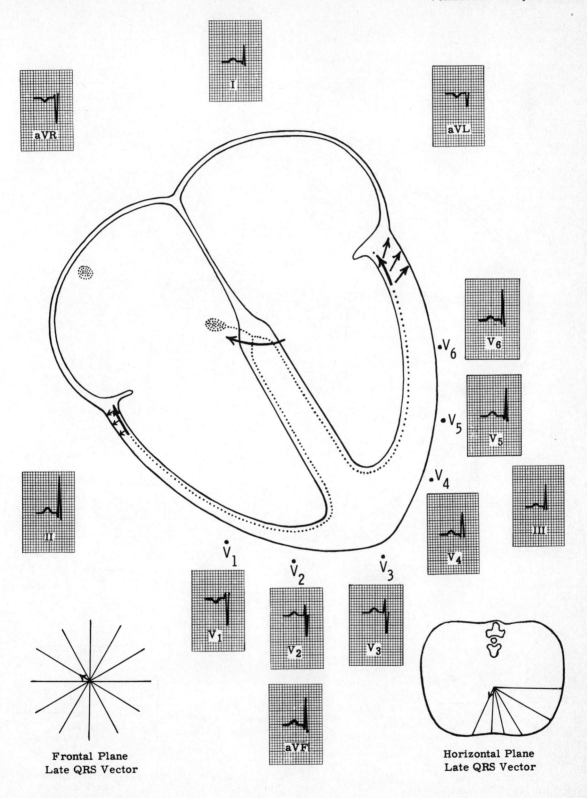

**Frontal Plane
Late QRS Vector**

**Horizontal Plane
Late QRS Vector**

Activation of Posterobasal Portion of Left Ventricle, Pulmonary Conus, and Uppermost Portion of I-V Septum.

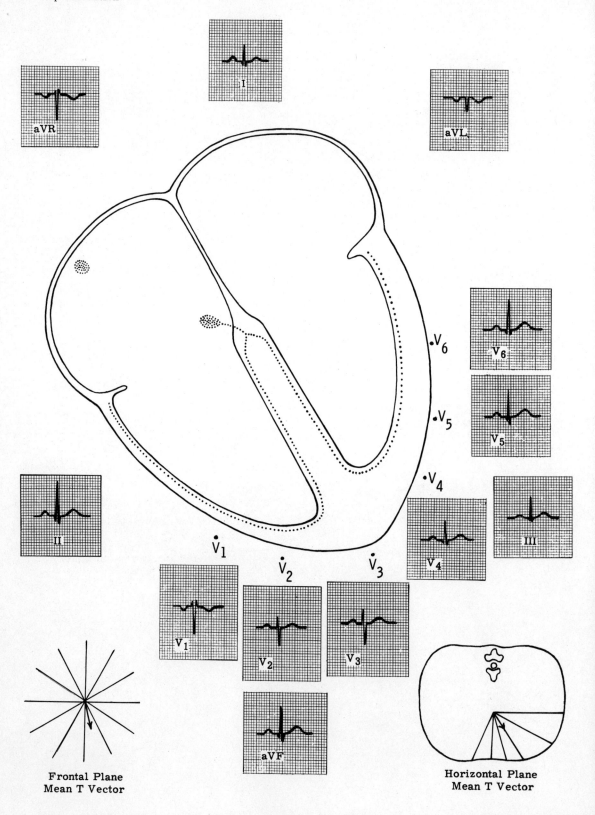

Frontal Plane
Mean T Vector

Horizontal Plane
Mean T Vector

Repolarization

Chapter 6

EFFECT OF HEART POSITION ON
THE ELECTROCARDIOGRAM

It must be understood that when one speaks of heart position as interpreted electrocardiographically, one refers to a pattern resulting from electrical spread of excitation. Although "electrical" heart position is not synonymous with anatomic position, "electrical" heart positions must be understood for proper interpretation of the normal and abnormal electrocardiogram.

Rotation of the heart may occur upon any one (or any combination) of the following three axes:

Rotation on the Anteroposterior Axis (Frontal Plane):
  A. Vertical.
  B. Horizontal.   D. Semi-vertical.
  C. Intermediate.   E. Semi-horizontal.

Rotation on the Long Axis (Horizontal Plane):
  A. Clockwise.
  B. Counterclockwise.

Rotation on the Transverse Axis (Sagittal Plane):
  A. Forward.
  B. Backward.

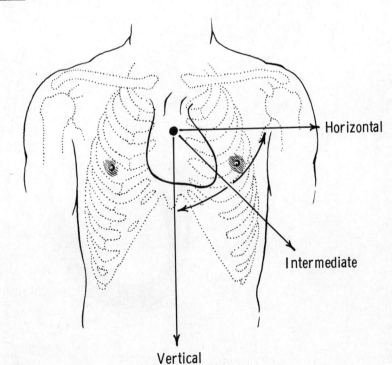

Rotation on the
Anteroposterior
Axis

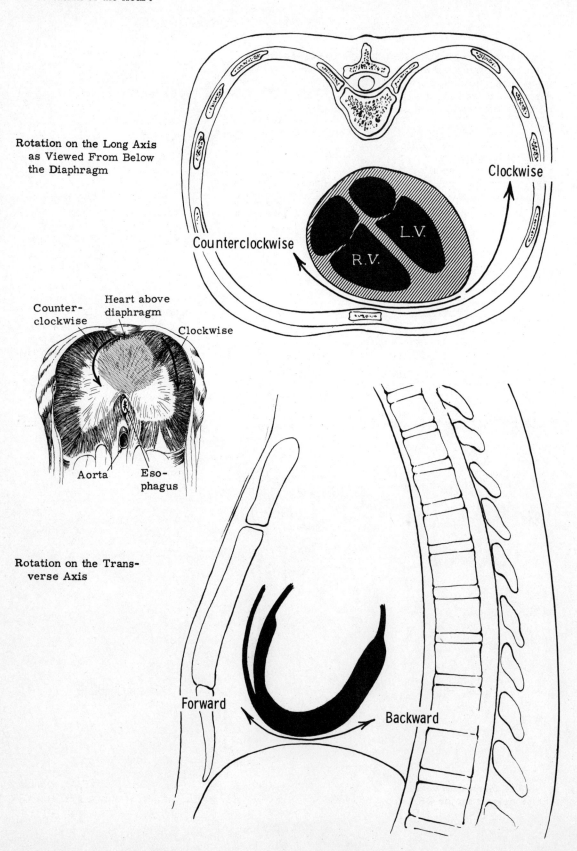

Rotation on the Long Axis
as Viewed From Below
the Diaphragm

Clockwise

Counterclockwise

L.V.

R.V.

Counter-
clockwise

Heart above
diaphragm

Clockwise

Aorta

Eso-
phagus

Rotation on the Trans-
verse Axis

Forward

Backward

ROTATION ON THE ANTEROPOSTERIOR AXIS

Electrocardiographically, this is the most significant of the three rotational patterns. The positions on this axis will be diagnosed by the patterns in the unipolar extremity leads and their resemblance to the patterns in V_1 and V_6. There are five subdivisions of this rotational pattern: vertical, horizontal, intermediate, semi-vertical, and semi-horizontal. For the sake of simplicity, "electrical" position will in part be explained in terms of the anatomical heart position.

This expresses in unipolar terminology the frontal plane axis.

Vertical Rotation:

The heart is so situated that a left ventricular epicardial complex will be recorded in aVF, a right ventricular cavity complex in aVR, and a left or right ventricular cavity complex or right ventricular epicardial complex in aVL. Thus aVF will resemble V_6 and aVL will resemble V_1.

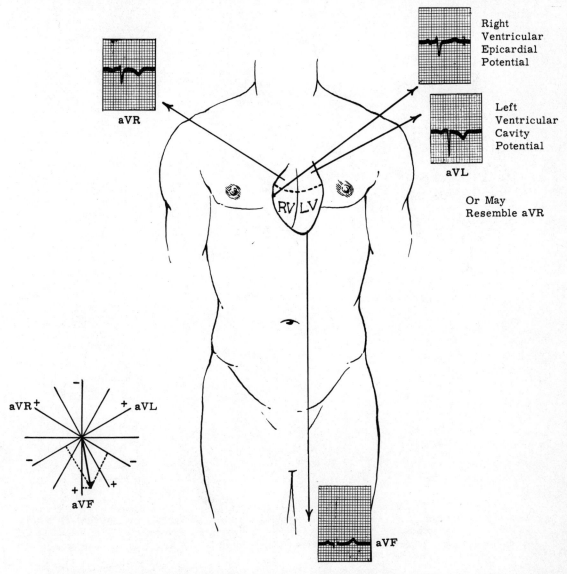

The mean QRS vector is oriented to the left and inferiorly, between +75° and +110°, resulting in an upright major QRS deflection in aVF and a downward major QRS deflection in aVL and aVR.

Vertical Heart

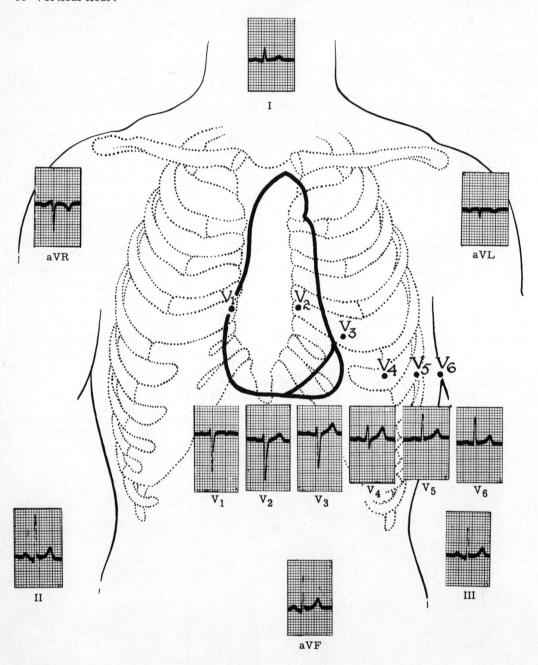

Vertical Heart Position. Left ventricular epicardial complex (upright P, qR, upright T) is seen in aVF, which resembles V₆; right cavity complex (inverted P, rS, inverted T) is seen in aVR; left cavity complex (inverted P, QS, inverted T) is seen in aVL. The frontal plane axis is +75°.

<u>Horizontal Rotation:</u>
A left ventricular epicardial complex is recorded in aVL (resembling V_6), either a right or left ventricular cavity complex in aVR, and a right ventricular epicardial complex in aVF (resembling V_1). This pattern is more commonly seen in heavy-set, broad-chested individuals.

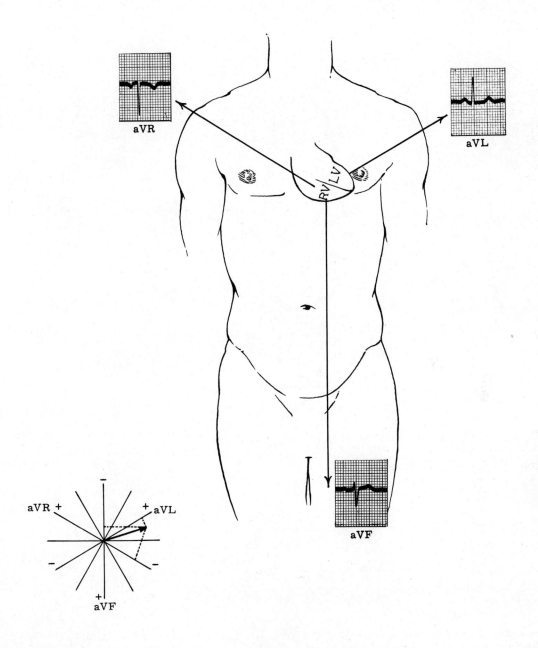

Horizontal Heart

The mean QRS vector is oriented to the left and superiorly, between 0° and -30°, resulting in an upright major QRS deflection in aVL and a downward major QRS deflection in aVR and aVF.

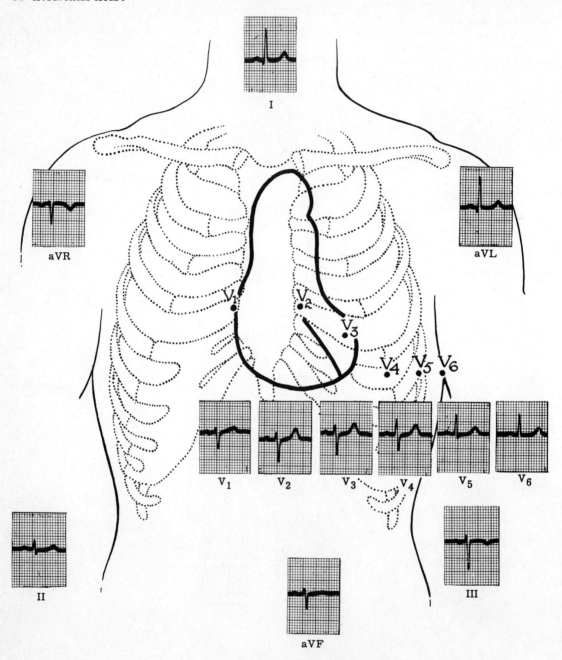

Horizontal Heart Position. Left ventricular epicardial complex (upright P, qR, upright T) is seen
in aVL, which resembles V_6; right ventricular epicardial complex (upright P, rS, upright T) is
seen in aVF, which resembles V_1; right cavity complex (inverted P, rS, inverted T) is seen in
aVR. The frontal plane axis is -20°.

Intermediate Rotation:

This is a midway position between vertical and horizontal. A left ventricular epicardial complex is recorded in both aVL and aVF (both resembling V_6). Either a right or left ventricular cavity complex is recorded in aVR.

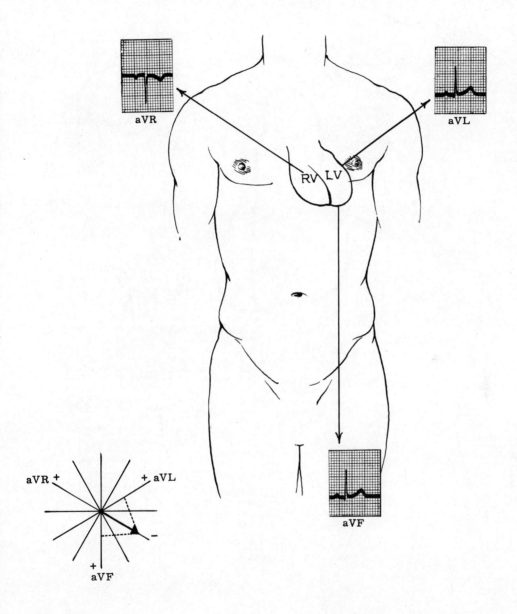

Intermediate Heart

Mean QRS vector is oriented to the left and inferiorly, halfway between the positive axes of aVF (+90°) and aVL (-30°). This results in an average frontal plane axis of +30° with a range of +15° to +45°. At +30° a positive QRS deflection of equal magnitude will be seen in aVL and aVF. Since the +30° axis is along the negative axis of aVR, the QRS deflection will be downward in aVR.

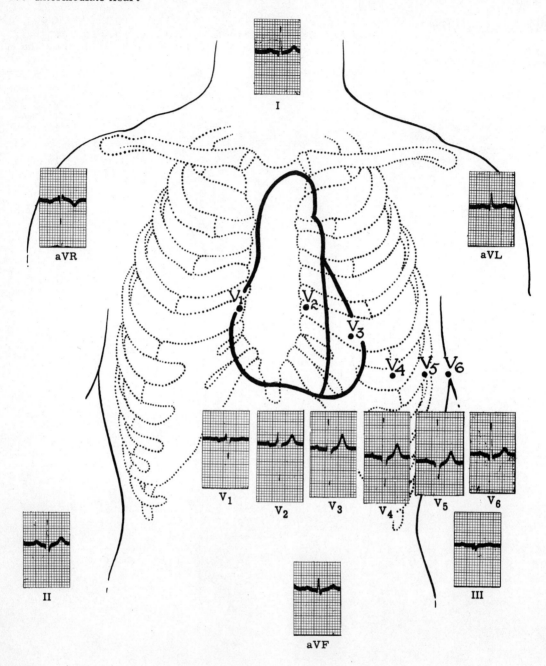

Intermediate Heart Position. Leads aVL and aVF both record left ventricular epicardial complex (upright P, qR in aVL, qRs in aVF; upright T) and resemble V₆; aVR records a right cavity complex (inverted P, rSr′, inverted T). The frontal plane axis is +27°.

Semi-vertical Rotation:

    A position midway between vertical and intermediate. Leads aVR and aVF are the same as in a vertical heart, but aVL consists of a small complex.

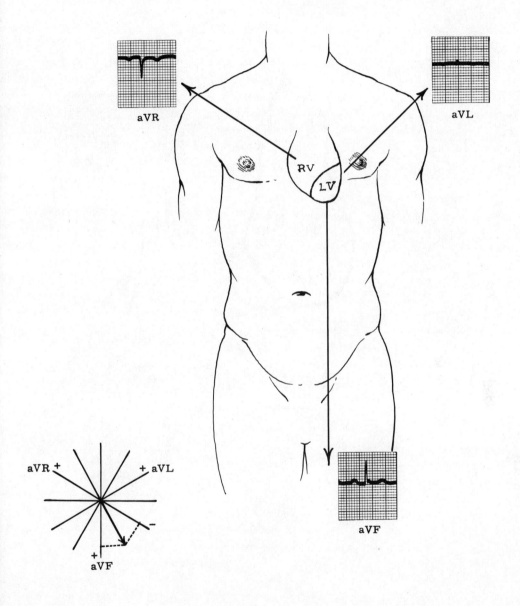

Semi-vertical Heart

    The mean QRS vector is oriented to the left and inferiorly. Since the QRS complex in aVL is very small, the major QRS vector is pointed 90° from the aVL axis (-30°), or +60°. This results in an upright QRS deflection in aVF and a downward deflection in aVR.

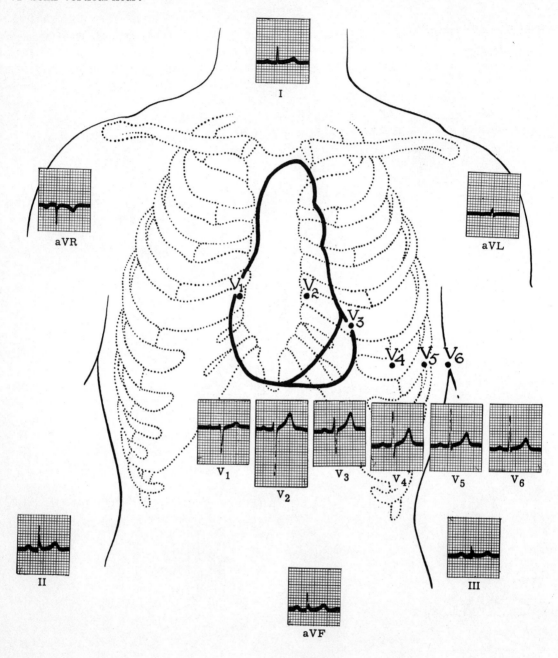

Semi-vertical Heart Position. Leads aVR and aVF are the same as in a vertical heart; however, lead aVL reveals a small complex. The frontal plane axis is +54°.

<u>Semi-horizontal Rotation:</u>
    A position midway between horizontal and intermediate. Leads aVR and aVL are the same as in a horizontal heart, but aVF consists of a small complex.

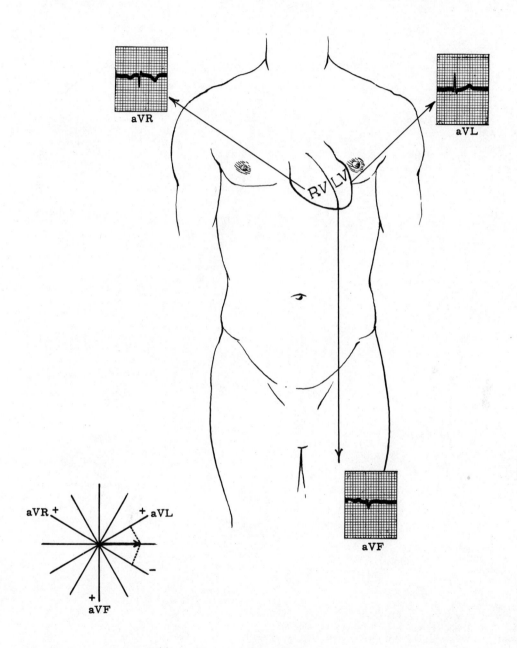

Semi-horizontal Heart

    The mean QRS vector is oriented to the left. Since aVF has a very small complex, the QRS vector is oriented 90° from the axis of aVF (+90°), or 0°. This results in an upright QRS in aVL and a downward QRS in aVR.

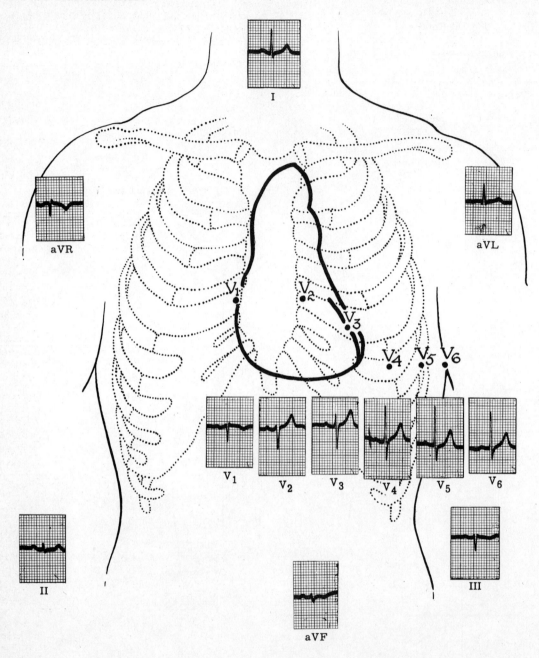

Semi-horizontal Heart Position. Leads aVL and aVR are the same as in a horizontal heart; however, aVF reveals a small complex. The frontal plane axis is -10°.

VARIATION IN PATTERNS IN UNIPOLAR EXTREMITY LEADS DUE TO ROTATION ON THE ANTEROPOSTERIOR AXIS

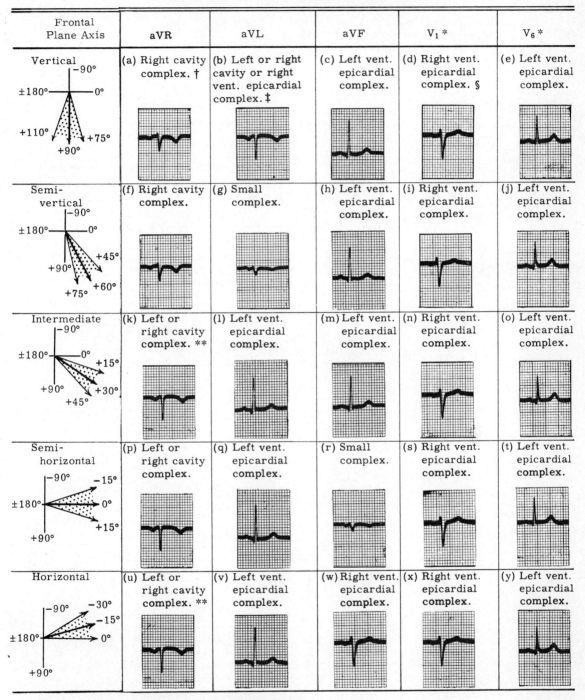

Frontal Plane Axis	aVR	aVL	aVF	V₁ *	V₆ *
Vertical	(a) Right cavity complex. †	(b) Left or right cavity or right vent. epicardial complex. ‡	(c) Left vent. epicardial complex.	(d) Right vent. epicardial complex. §	(e) Left vent. epicardial complex.
Semi-vertical	(f) Right cavity complex.	(g) Small complex.	(h) Left vent. epicardial complex.	(i) Right vent. epicardial complex.	(j) Left vent. epicardial complex.
Intermediate	(k) Left or right cavity complex. **	(l) Left vent. epicardial complex.	(m) Left vent. epicardial complex.	(n) Right vent. epicardial complex.	(o) Left vent. epicardial complex.
Semi-horizontal	(p) Left or right cavity complex.	(q) Left vent. epicardial complex.	(r) Small complex.	(s) Right vent. epicardial complex.	(t) Left vent. epicardial complex.
Horizontal	(u) Left or right cavity complex. **	(v) Left vent. epicardial complex.	(w) Right vent. epicardial complex.	(x) Right vent. epicardial complex.	(y) Left vent. epicardial complex.

*Assuming no unusual rotation on the long axis.
†See electrocardiogram on p. 47 for variations.
‡Or (a) or (d).
§See electrocardiogram on p. 44 for variations.
**Or (a).

ROTATION ON THE LONG AXIS

Rotation on this axis may be clockwise or counterclockwise. The direction of rotation is defined by its appearance as viewed from the inferior surface of the heart looking upward from below the diaphragm. This rotational pattern is diagnosed by the appearance of the precordial leads. In an average case the transitional zone is in the neighborhood of V_4.

Clockwise Rotation:

With clockwise rotation the transitional zone is displaced to the left, so the typical left ventricular epicardial pattern does not appear until V_{7-9}. With marked degrees of clockwise rotation a tall R may be seen in aVR, producing a QR pattern.

The mean QRS vector is oriented more posteriorly and superiorly.

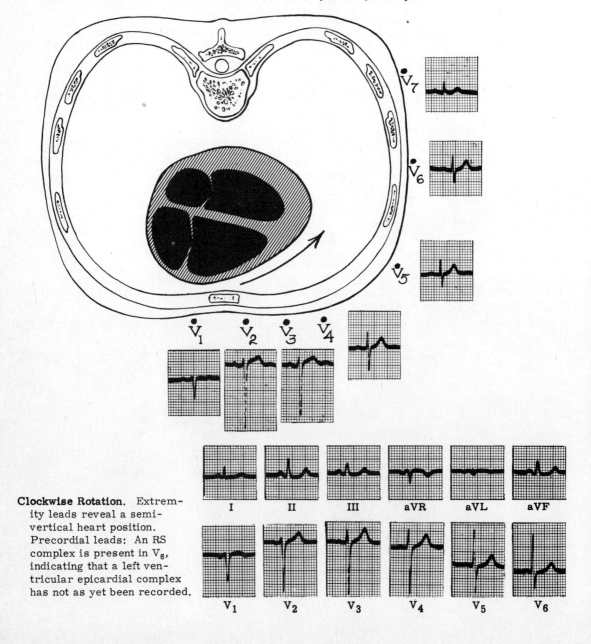

Clockwise Rotation. Extremity leads reveal a semi-vertical heart position. Precordial leads: An RS complex is present in V_6, indicating that a left ventricular epicardial complex has not as yet been recorded.

Counterclockwise Rotation:

In counterclockwise rotation the transitional zone is displaced to the right, resulting in left ventricular epicardial complexes as early as V_2. The mean QRS vector is oriented more anteriorly. ST segment elevation in V_{2-4} is a common accompaniment of counterclockwise rotation.

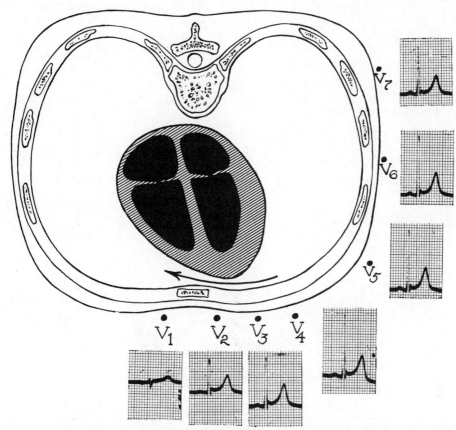

Rotation on Long Axis. Counterclockwise Rotation. A left ventricular epicardial complex is seen in V_2, indicating a transition zone between V_1 and V_2. The ST segments are elevated in V_2 and V_3, a common accompaniment of counterclockwise rotation.

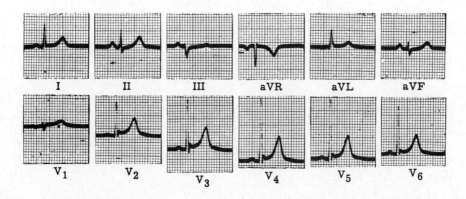

Counterclockwise Rotation. **Standard Leads:** Left axis deviation. **Extremity Leads:** Horizontal heart position. **Precordial Leads:** A left ventricular epicardial complex is seen in V_2, indicating counterclockwise rotation. There is associated ST segment elevation from V_2 through V_6.

ROTATION ON TRANSVERSE AXIS

Forward Rotation:

    This rotation results in a right ventricular epicardial complex being recorded in aVL. Lead aVF reflects a left ventricular epicardial complex and aVR reflects a right ventricular cavity complex. This is a minor variant of the standard vertical heart in that aVL reflects a right ventricular epicardial (due to forward rotation of the apex) instead of a left ventricular cavity complex. This merely indicates that the initial QRS vector is oriented superiorly in the -60 to -120° range, thus producing a small upright deflection (r) in aVL and aVR. The mean QRS vector is as described for a vertical heart.

    Theoretically, a marked degree of forward rotation could cause the "back-of-the-heart" pattern to be reflected in aVF, producing a QR with an inverted T. This pattern has not been described in clinical electrocardiography.

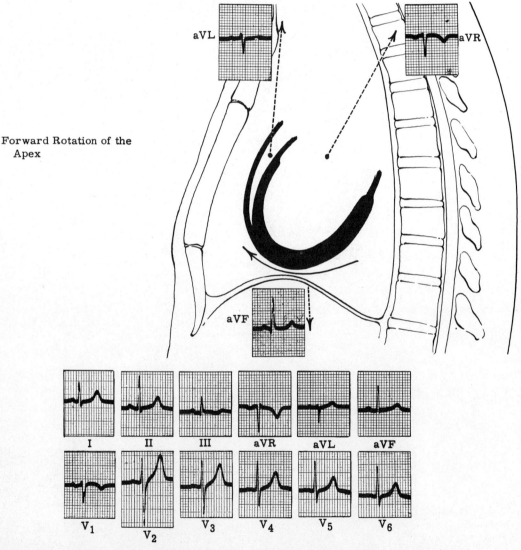

Forward Rotation of the
   Apex

Forward Rotation of the Apex. Standard Leads: Diphasic T in III; this is not abnormal.
  Extremity Leads: Lead aVR records a right ventricular cavity complex; aVF records a left ventricular epicardial complex; lead aVL records a right ventricular epicardial complex, i.e., an upright P, rS, and upright T. The heart position is vertical and the usual left ventricular cavity complex of a vertical heart in aVL has been replaced by a right ventricular epicardial complex due to forward rotation of the apex. **Precordial Leads:** Clockwise rotation.

Backward Rotation:

In this position it is assumed that the left ventricle is displaced posteriorly and superiorly. Thus the posterior aspect (back of the heart) reflects itself into aVR and aVL, resulting in a ''back-of-the-heart'' complex, namely an inverted P, QR, and inverted T in both these leads. Lead aVF will record a right ventricular epicardial pattern, resulting in an rS complex with upright, flat, or inverted T. By vector analysis the first half of the QRS vector is oriented inferiorly in the +60 to +120° range, resulting in a q wave in aVR and aVL and an r wave in aVF. The second half of the QRS vector is oriented superiorly in the -60 to -120° range, producing an r wave in aVR and aVL and an S wave in aVF.

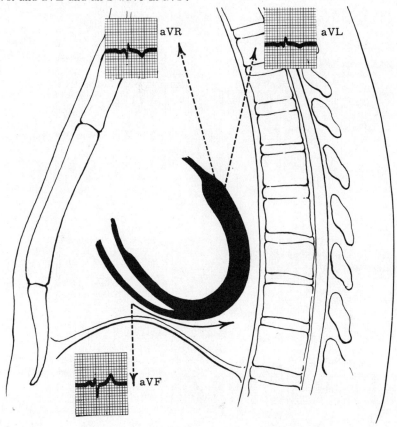

Rotation on Transverse Axis. Backward Rotation of Apex. This rotation results in a right ventricular epicardial complex being recorded in aVF and a back-of-the-heart pattern recorded in both aVR and aVL.

Backward Rotation of the Apex. Both aVR and aVL record similar patterns: inverted P waves, QR complexes, and inverted T waves. Lead aVF reflects a right ventricular epicardial complex.

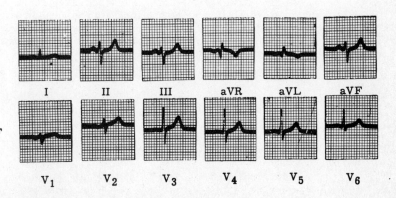

EFFECT OF DEEP RESPIRATION ON THE ROTATIONAL PATTERNS

Deep inspiration and expiration can appreciably alter the appearance of the individual electrocardiographic leads. With deep inspiration the heart position becomes more vertical and there is greater clockwise rotation. With deep expiration the heart becomes more horizontal and there is greater counterclockwise rotation. Variations in right and left heart stroke volume during inspiration and expiration also play a role in these electrocardiographic changes.

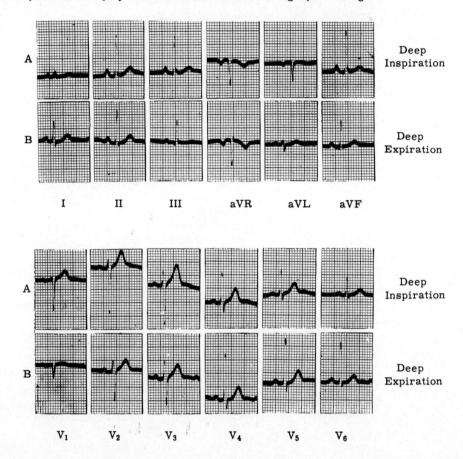

Effect of Deep Respiration on the Electrocardiogram. (A) Deep Inspiration. **(B)** Deep Expiration. In deep inspiration the frontal heart position is vertical; this becomes semi-vertical in deep expiration. In the latter phase the voltage increases in I, V_4, V_5, and V_6 and decreases in aVF.

In the interpretation of the electrocardiogram one should routinely determine the electrical axes along with the determination of the heart rate and rhythm. One then studies the tracing for evidence of abnormalities which are indicative of disturbances in the myocardium.

Chapter 7

THE ELECTROCARDIOGRAM IN INFANTS AND CHILDREN; NORMAL VARIANTS OF THE ADULT ELECTROCARDIOGRAM

FETAL ELECTROCARDIOGRAPHY

By using a standard electrocardiograph equipped with a preamplifier capable of amplifying an input signal 50 times and recording in a frequency range of 12 to 20 cycles per second, it is possible to record maternal and fetal QRS complexes. After voiding, the patient lies down. One electrode of a bipolar lead is placed in the midline of the abdomen at the level of the uterine fundus; the other is placed just above the symphysis pubis.

Fetal electrocardiography is of value (1) in determining fetal life during the second and third trimesters of pregnancy; (2) in the early diagnosis of multiple pregnancy; (3) in detecting fetal arrhythmia; (4) in monitoring the fetal heart rate during labor; and (5) in determining fetal position. If the mother's QRS vector is normal (inferiorly directed, and therefore giving an upright QRS complex), the fetal QRS vector in a vertex presentation will be directed superiorly, producing an inverted QRS complex. In a breech presentation the QRS vector will be directed inferiorly, producing an upright QRS complex.

Comparison of Vertex and Breech Presentations.
Upper tracing is a vertex presentation showing fetal QRS in opposite direction from the maternal. Lower tracing is a breech showing fetal QRS in same direction as the maternal. (Reproduced, with permission, from T. M. Buxton et al.: Fetal electrocardiography. J. A. M. A. 185:441-4, 1963.)

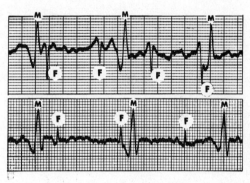

NORMAL ELECTROCARDIOGRAPHIC PATTERNS IN INFANTS AND CHILDREN

Normal Electrocardiogram in Infants: (See tracing on p. 82, top.)
In the fetus the right ventricle performs more work than the left ventricle. Therefore at birth or in infancy there is a relative hypertrophy of the right ventricle. This will result in an electrocardiographic pattern which will simulate that of right ventricular hypertrophy in the adult, i.e., tall R waves in the right precordial leads. However, an initial q wave will never be seen in V_1, and the V. A. T. is not prolonged (see p. 109). Within the first two to four days of life the T waves are upright in leads V_2 through V_6 and may be upright or inverted in V_1. After this period of time the T waves normally become inverted in leads V_1 through V_4.

Normal Electrocardiogram in Children: (See tracing on p. 82, center.)
The tall R waves in right precordial leads usually disappear after the age of five, but inverted T waves in the right precordial leads frequently persist into the second decade.

Juvenile Pattern: (See tracing on p. 82, bottom.)
In Negroes, this "juvenile pattern" of T wave inversion (as in the child) in precordial leads V_{1-4} may persist into the third decade of life.

Normal Electrocardiogram in an Infant (Age Three Days). Standard Leads: Right axis deviation.
Extremity Leads: Vertical heart
position; tall R in aVR. **Precordial Leads:** A tall R is present
in V_1; V. A. T. in V_1 = 0.02 sec.
The T waves are upright in leads
V_{2-6} .

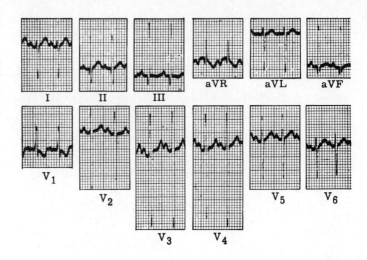

**Normal Electrocardiogram in Eight-
Year-Old Child.** The T waves
are inverted in V_{1-3}. This would
be abnormal in an adult white individual, but is the normal pattern
in a child.

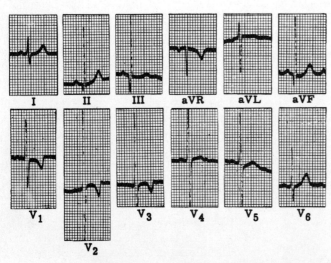

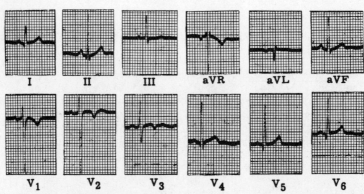

Negro Male, Age 24, With No Clinical Evidence of Heart Disease. Standard Leads: No unusual
axis deviation. **Extremity Leads:** Vertical heart position. **Precordial Leads:** The T waves
are deeply inverted in V_1, V_2, and V_3. This would be abnormal in an adult white individual,
but can be normal in a young Negro. The cardiac diagnosis must depend on the result of the
clinical examination. If no other abnormalities exist, this tracing can be considered to be within normal limits.

DEXTROCARDIA

Dextroversion:

   Dextroversion is a congenital anomaly in which the heart is displaced to the right and the ventricles are rotated in a counterclockwise rotation. The ventricles and atria are not transposed, the left ventricle facing to the left and the right ventricle to the right. The aorta is in a normal position. The P vector remains normal. The mean QRS vector is oriented more anteriorly (counterclockwise rotation). The mean T vector may be oriented to the right and thus result in a negative T wave in lead I. *

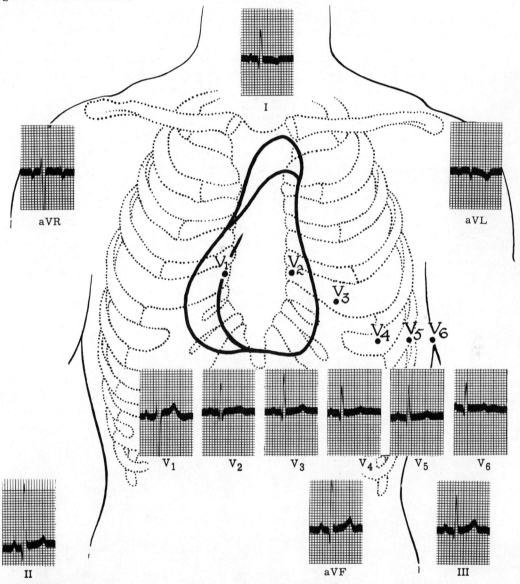

Pattern of Dextroversion. The pattern in precordial leads is that of counterclockwise rotation. Note that the T wave in lead I is inverted. **Clinical Findings:** Heart displaced to the right; bronchiectasis; sinusitis.

---

*This is practically always an abnormal finding. However, in this instance, because of the unusual degree of rotation, the T in aVL (normal left ventricular cavity potential) is deeper than the T in aVR (normal right ventricular potential), resulting in an inverted T in lead I (I = VL-VR) which may not indicate abnormality.

True Dextrocardia:

This is a congenital anomaly in which there is complete transposition of both ventricles and atria. The aortic knob is also to the right. Thus the P vector is oriented to the **right**, inferiorly, and anteriorly, producing an inverted P wave in lead I and an upright P in aVR. The mean QRS vector is directed to the **right**, inferiorly, and slightly posteriorly. The T vector is also oriented to the **right**, inferiorly and anteriorly. This alters the electrocardiogram in the following fashion:

Lead I: A complete reversal of the normal pattern. The P and T are inverted and the "R" wave is downward.

Lead II of the dextrocardia = Lead III of a normal pattern.

Lead III of the dextrocardia = Lead II of a normal pattern.

Lead aVR of the dextrocardia = Lead aVL of a normal pattern.

Lead aVL of the dextrocardia = Lead aVR of a normal pattern.

Precordial leads V_{1-6} will reflect right ventricular epicardial and "back-of-the-heart" complexes. However, if the precordial leads are taken over the right chest, left ventricular epicardial patterns will result.

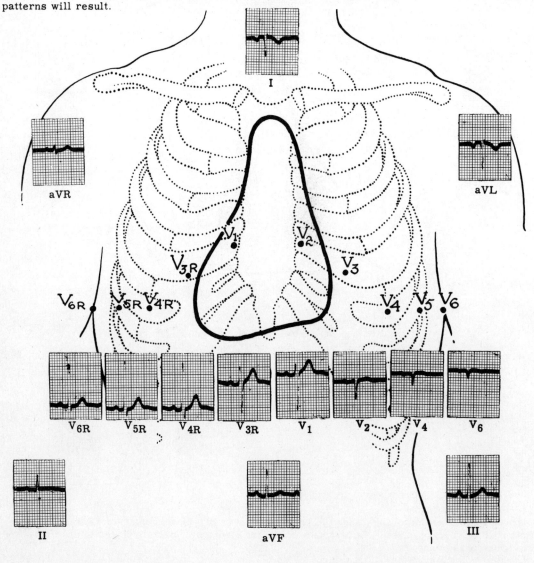

Dextrocardia. Lead I complexes are inverted; the patterns in II-III and aVR-aVL are the reverse of the normal. Left precordial leads record a right ventricular epicardial complex; right precordial leads record a left ventricular epicardial complex. **Clinical Diagnosis:** 30-year-old male with dextrocardia and situs inversus; no evidence of heart disease.

TECHNICAL DEXTROCARDIA

Occasionally a technician will inadvertently interchange the right and left arm electrodes. This will produce a pattern of dextrocardia in the standard and the extremity leads but will not alter the normal pattern in precordial leads.

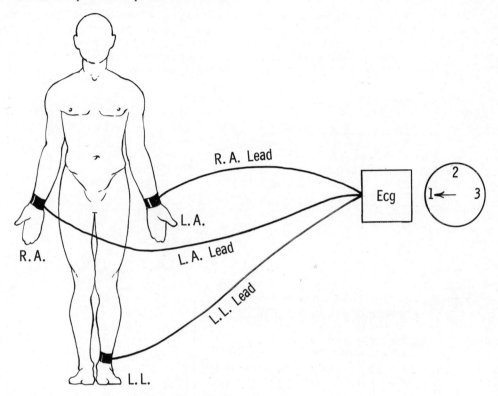

Incorrect Position of Arm Leads Which Produces Electrocardiogram Showing Technical Dextrocardia.

Technical Dextrocardia (from interchange of right and left arm electrodes). The pattern in the standard and extremity leads (A) is that of dextrocardia, i.e., lead I is completely inverted, leads II and III and leads aVR and aVL are transposed. In (B), standard and extremity leads are taken correctly. However, the precordial leads (C) are entirely normal, indicating that this is not a true dextrocardia.

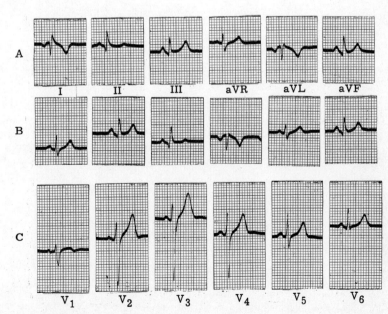

UNUSUAL NORMAL VARIANTS

ST SEGMENT ELEVATION IN PRECORDIAL LEADS

On page 26 it was stated that the ST segment may normally be elevated up to 2 mm. in the precordial leads. Recently a pattern has been described in which up to 4 mm. ST elevation can occur in left precordial leads. The ST segment has an upward concavity, and the T is upright. This has been seen more commonly in young adult Negroes. Following exercise, the ST segments return to the iso-electric line. The explanation for this phenomenon is unknown.

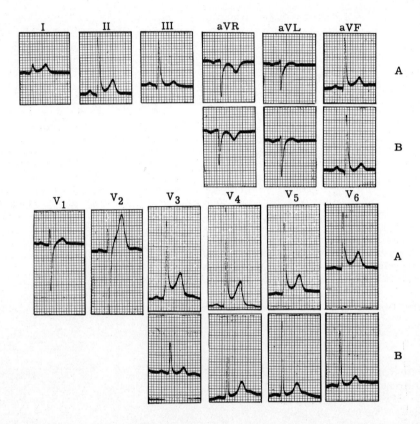

Unusual ST Segment Elevation as a Normal Variant. Note the marked ST segment elevation in leads V_{3-5}. This is 4 mm. in V_3 and V_4 **(A)**. This record was taken on a 24-year-old male Negro. There was no clinical evidence of organic heart disease. Following exercise **(B)**, the ST segments became iso-electric. (From M. J. Goldman, Am. Heart J. **46**:817, 1953.)

ST SEGMENT ELEVATION AND T WAVE INVERSION

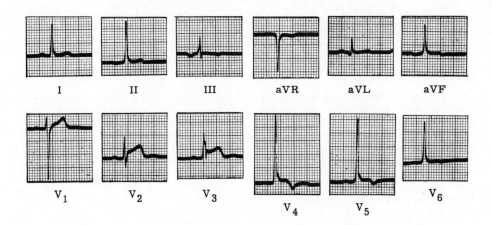

Unusual ST Segment Elevation and T Wave Inversion as a Normal Variant. Note the elevated ST segments from V_2 through V_4. The T waves are inverted in V_{4-5} and diphasic in V_6 and aVF. This record was taken on a 23-year-old Negro male. There was no clinical evidence of heart disease, and this electrocardiographic pattern has remained unchanged for three years. Because of the electrocardiographic finding alone this patient had been subjected to exploratory thoracotomy and pericardial biopsy with normal findings. These ST and T variations are not altered by rest, exercise, hyperventilation, and vagal blocking drugs. (From M. J. Goldman, Am. Heart J. **59**:71, 1960.)

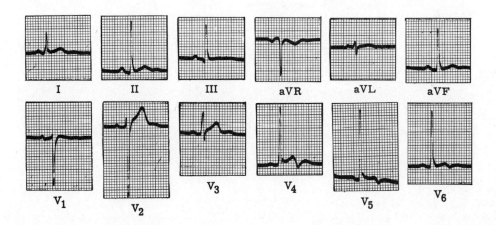

Tracing of a 24-year-old Negro Male. The frontal plane leads are within normal limits. Precordial leads reveal ST segment elevation from V_2 through V_5. There is late T wave inversion in leads V_{4-6}. The voltage of $S_{V_1} + R_{V_5} = 42$ mm. There was no clinical evidence of heart disease. This electrocardiographic pattern has remained stationary over a two-year period of observation and is unchanged by basal conditions, exercise, hyperventilation, or vagal blocking drugs.

ANXIETY REACTION

In patients with supposedly normal hearts who suffer from anxiety and hyperventilation, the following electrocardiographic abnormalities have been described:

1. Prolongation of the P-R interval.
2. Sinus tachycardia; less commonly, arrhythmias of various types.
3. ST segment depression and T wave inversion in left ventricular epicardial leads.

This pattern may simulate coronary insufficiency (see p. 143). Although these findings are described in "healthy" individuals, one wonders if there may not be unsuspected underlying coronary artery disease. The authors who describe these abnormalities ascribe them to imbalance of the autonomic nervous system. Such drugs as ergotamine and atropine can cause the electrocardiogram to revert to normal. Caution is required, however, since it is dangerous to administer ergotamine to a patient with coronary artery disease.

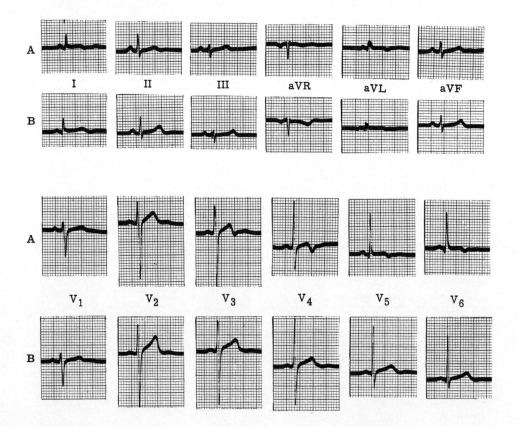

Anxiety Reaction. The above tracings were taken on a 26-year-old Caucasian male with no clinical evidence of heart disease. A: Representative of repeatedly "abnormal" electrocardiograms as evidenced by inverted T waves in leads V_{4-6}. B: After atropine; the T waves in the above-mentioned leads are now normal.

BIPOLAR VS. UNIPOLAR CHEST LEADS

The difference between these leads has been discussed above (see p. 4). In a vertical heart, due to the relatively high voltage in aVF, the potential of the foot lead (aVF) can appreciably alter the chest potential as recorded in a CF lead. An example of this is seen below. This patient was diagnosed as having organic heart disease on the basis of the CF leads. There was no good clinical evidence of heart disease. Subsequent V leads (taken several years later) were normal. Repeated CF leads still showed the "abnormal" pattern. Unfortunately, the patient has become an incurable cardiac invalid (iatrogenic) in the interval. This illustrates not only the inaccuracy of bipolar chest leads, but also the fallacy of diagnosing organic heart disease purely on the basis of "nonspecific" electrocardiographic findings.

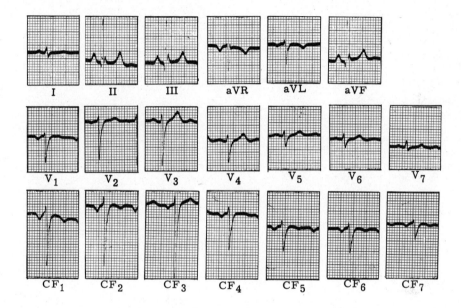

Difference Between CF and V Precordial Leads. CF leads reveal inversion of the T waves in precordial leads through CF$_7$. V leads show normally upright T waves. The "abnormality" in the CF leads is a result of the influence of the potential in aVF, i.e., the T in aVF being taller than the T in V$_{5-7}$ results in inverted T waves in CF$_{5-7}$.

Chapter 8

HYPERTROPHY PATTERNS

ATRIAL HYPERTROPHY

Etiology and Pathology:

Atrial hypertrophy may arise under the following pathologic conditions (in order of incidence):

A. As the result of A-V valvular stenosis, e.g., left atrial hypertrophy associated with mitral stenosis.

B. Secondary to pulmonary hypertension, e.g., right atrial hypertrophy resulting from chronic diffuse pulmonary disease.

C. In association with various congenital heart lesions, e.g., right atrial hypertrophy associated with an interatrial septal defect.

D. Secondary to ventricular hypertrophy, e.g., left atrial hypertrophy secondary to left ventricular hypertrophy of hypertensive cardiovascular disease.

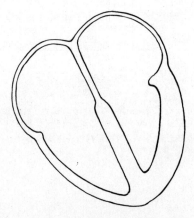

The Normal Heart. Diagrammatic illustration of the four cardiac chambers. Both atria are thin-walled; the normal left ventricle is considerably thicker than the right.

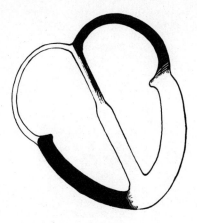

Hypertrophy of the Left Atrium and Right Ventricle (Mitral Stenosis)

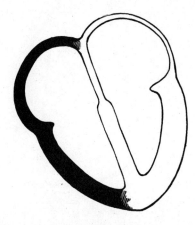

Hypertrophy of the Right Atrium and Right Ventricle (Chronic Pulmonary Disease)

Incidence:
　　From the standpoint of electrocardiographic diagnosis, atrial hypertrophy can frequently be diagnosed in mitral stenosis, chronic pulmonary disease producing pulmonary hypertension, and certain congenital lesions. It is less commonly diagnosed when associated with left ventricular hypertrophy.

Electrocardiographic Criteria:
　　The normal P wave is not over 0.11 sec. in width and 2.5 mm. in height. Any increase in these values is suggestive of atrial hypertrophy. Although it is not always possible to differentiate electrocardiographically between left and right atrial hypertrophy, the criteria given on pages 92 and 93 are helpful.

Clinical Significance:
　　This will depend on the etiology and course of the underlying heart disease.

A. Left Atrial Hypertrophy (as seen in mitral stenosis): This is manifested by broad, notched P waves (''P mitrale''), usually best seen in leads I and II. Lead V_1 characteristically has a wide, slurred, diphasic P wave in which the downward component of the wave is most prominent. The second notch of the P (upright in I and inverted in V_1) is the result of delayed activation of the hypertrophied left atrium.

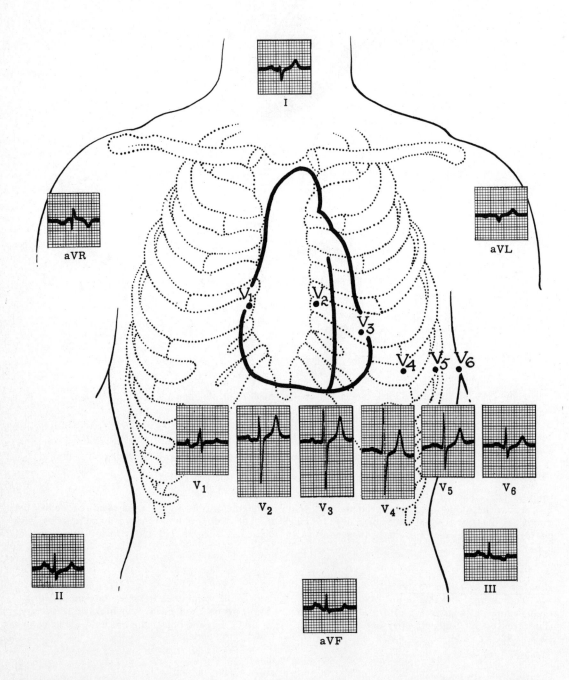

Left Atrial Hypertrophy. Note the broad, notched P waves in standard and extremity leads and V_{4-6}. The characteristic diphasic P with a wide negative component is seen in V_1. **Clinical Diagnosis:** Mitral stenosis.

B. **Right Atrial Hypertrophy (as seen in chronic pulmonary disease):** This is manifested by tall, slender, peaked P waves in leads II, III, and aVF and prominent peaked, diphasic P waves in V_1.

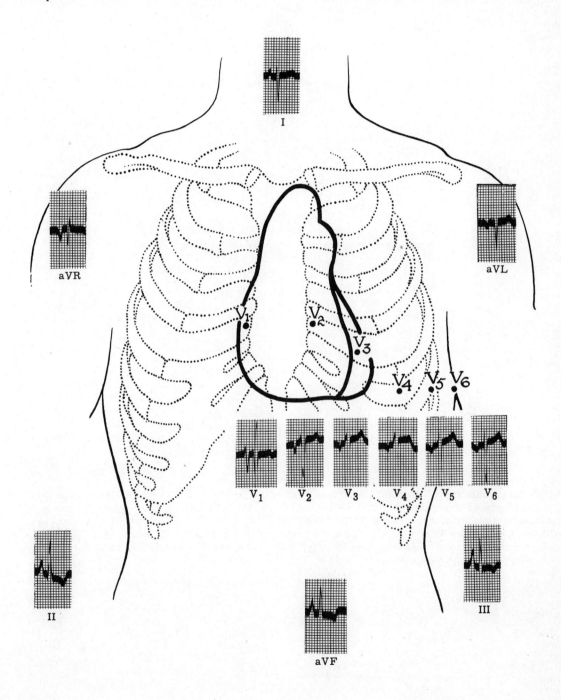

Right Atrial Hypertrophy. There are tall, slender P waves in II, III, and aVF. Note the sharply peaked diphasic P in V_1. **Clinical Diagnosis:** Pulmonary fibrosis with right heart failure.

T_a Waves:

A prominent T_a wave may be seen in atrial hypertrophy. This produces a depression of the PR segment. This finding alone is not diagnostic of atrial hypertrophy.

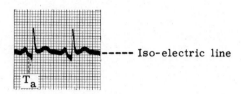

----- Iso-electric line

T_a Wave in Atrial Hypertrophy

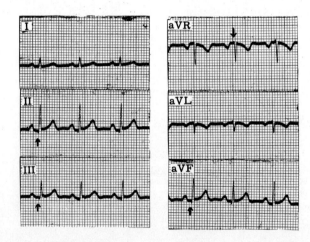

T_a Waves (Simulating ST Segment Elevation). There appears to be ST segment elevation in II, III, and aVF and ST depression in aVR. However, one should compare an ST segment in its relation to the interval between the T and the P. In doing so it is seen that the ST segments are iso-electric. The pattern results from the presence of a prominent T_a wave. Although a visible T_a wave may result from atrial hypertrophy, this finding alone is not sufficient to warrant such an electrocardiographic diagnosis.

VENTRICULAR HYPERTROPHY

Pathology:
    Ventricular hypertrophy results from any pathological process which produces a sufficient load on either ventricle. Myocardial fibrosis of varying degrees may develop later, especially in the subendocardial layer.

Anatomic and Physiologic Abnormalities Which Produce the Electrocardiographic Pattern:
    The electrocardiographic pattern of ventricular hypertrophy is dependent upon the following:
A. Thickness of Muscle Mass: There is a definite correlation between the thickness of the ventricular muscle mass and the height of the R wave. The increased muscle mass resulting from ventricular hypertrophy will therefore increase the electrical potential of ventricular depolarization, resulting in an increased voltage of the R wave.

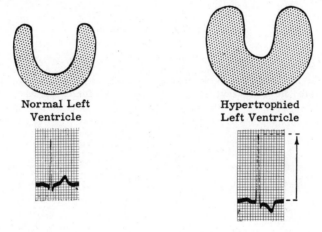

Normal Left
Ventricle

Hypertrophied
Left Ventricle

Height of R Increased by Thickness of Muscle Mass

B. Delay in Conduction: Due to the increased muscle mass there is a delay and alteration of conduction, resulting in an increased width of the QRS complex. Usually this does not exceed 0.12 sec. but may occasionally do so. This also will increase the V.A.T.

Normal

V.A.T.

QRS

Hypertrophy

V.A.T. and QRS Interval Increased

C. Endocardial Changes: ST segment depression may be seen in a lead reflecting epicardial potential. This is probably due to endocardial changes (partly fibrosis).

Normal

Hypertrophy

ST Segment Depressed

D. Changes in Repolarization: Due to changes in repolarization (the reasons for which are not clearly understood), the T wave is inverted. The inversion characteristically begins after a definite ST interval and is asymmetrical. The inversion may be shallow or deep.

Normal

Hypertrophy

T Inverted

Electrocardiographic Criteria:
  A. Epicardial Pattern: The typical pattern which reflects the epicardial surface of a hypertrophied ventricle will be (1) a tall R wave, (2) slight prolongation of the QRS interval, (3) prolongation of the V.A.T., (4) ST segment depression, and (5) an inverted T wave.

  B. A lead reflecting cavity potential or the potential recorded from a lead overlying the opposite nonhypertrophied ventricle will show (1) a deep S wave (or QS complex), (2) an elevated ST segment, and (3) an upright T wave.

It must be realized that not all the above criteria are necessary for making a diagnosis of ventricular hypertrophy.

VENTRICULAR STRAIN

This term is used to describe an electrocardiographic pattern in which the only abnormalities are the ST and T wave changes described above.

Clinically the term is used to describe more acute and possibly reversible changes which affect the ventricular musculature.

The correlation between electrocardiographic and anatomic findings is not too great. Only nonspecific ST and T wave changes may be evident in the electrocardiogram of a patient with definite ventricular hypertrophy. Furthermore, patients who show clinical and anatomic evidence of acute ventricular strain may have abnormally tall R waves. An incomplete (or complete) bundle branch block (see p. 116) may be the electrocardiographic pattern of clinical acute heart strain.

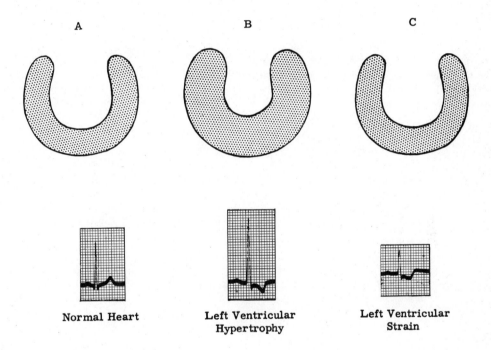

A   B   C

Normal Heart   **Left Ventricular Hypertrophy**   **Left Ventricular Strain**

LEFT VENTRICULAR HYPERTROPHY

Etiology:
    Left ventricular hypertrophy commonly results from the following clinical states:

A. Hypertension: Essential, renal, or hormonal.

B. Aortic Valvular Disease: Aortic stenosis and/or aortic insufficiency.

C. Rheumatic mitral insufficiency.

D. Long-standing coronary artery disease.

E. Nutritional and Idiopathic Hypertrophies: Beri-beri heart disease and the chronic myocarditides and myocardopathies.

F. Congenital Heart Disease: Patent ductus arteriosus; coarctation of the aorta; tricuspid atresia.

Incidence:
    An electrocardiographic diagnosis of left ventricular hypertrophy can be made very commonly when left ventricular hypertrophy is anatomically present. In fact, the electrocardiogram may be diagnostic before any roentgenographic evidence is present.

Electrocardiographic Criteria:
    The criteria discussed under ventricular hypertrophy (see p. 96), when applied to those leads which reflect a left ventricular epicardial complex, will allow for the diagnosis of left ventricular hypertrophy. The specific leads in which the pattern is seen will depend upon the heart position.

Clinical Significance and Prognosis:
    This will depend upon the underlying disease. The electrocardiographic pattern will persist unless the course can be corrected. In left ventricular hypertrophy secondary to hypertension, the electrocardiogram may improve or revert to normal following successful medical or surgical treatment of the hypertension.

    Electrocardiographic evidence of left ventricular hypertrophy in a patient being considered for mitral commissurotomy is an exceedingly important finding. It indicates either functionally significant mitral insufficiency, associated aortic valvular disease, or another disease (e.g., hypertension). It is practically an absolute contraindication to the performance of mitral valve surgery alone.

ELECTROCARDIOGRAPHIC PATTERNS OF LEFT VENTRICULAR HYPERTROPHY

Rotation on the Anteroposterior Axis:

A. Horizontal Heart: This is the most common position in left ventricular hypertrophy.
1. Standard leads - Left axis deviation greater than $-30°$; a tall R in lead I and a deep S in lead III; the voltage of $R_1 + S_3$ is over 26 mm.; ST depression and T wave inversion in leads I and II.
2. Extremity leads - Since a left ventricular epicardial complex is recorded in aVL, a tall R with depressed ST and inverted T will be seen in this lead. In general an R wave of over 13 mm. is consistent with left ventricular hypertrophy.
3. Precordial leads - In the absence of unusual rotation on the long axis, abnormally tall R waves with depressed ST segments and inverted T waves will be seen in leads V_{4-6}. The QRS interval may be over 0.1 sec. and the V.A.T. greater then 0.05 sec. Since the S wave in right precordial leads (e.g., V_1) is a reflection of the greater left ventricular potential, these waves will be abnormally deep. As a general rule the total voltage of $[SV_1 + RV_5]$ or $[SV_1 + RV_6]$ is greater than 35 mm., or an R of over 27 mm. in V_5 or V_6

is indicative of left ventricular hypertrophy. This is only applicable to adults over age 30. Furthermore, fever, anemia, thyrotoxicosis, or other high-output failures can increase this voltage without representing left ventricular hypertrophy. Therefore, an electrocardiographic diagnosis of left ventricular hypertrophy on the basis of voltage alone should be made only if these variables do not exist.

4. Vector analysis - The mean QRS vector is oriented more superiorly (greater than -30° in the frontal plane) and more posteriorly. The magnitude of the QRS vector is increased. The ST and T vectors are oriented approximately 180° from the mean axis of the QRS.

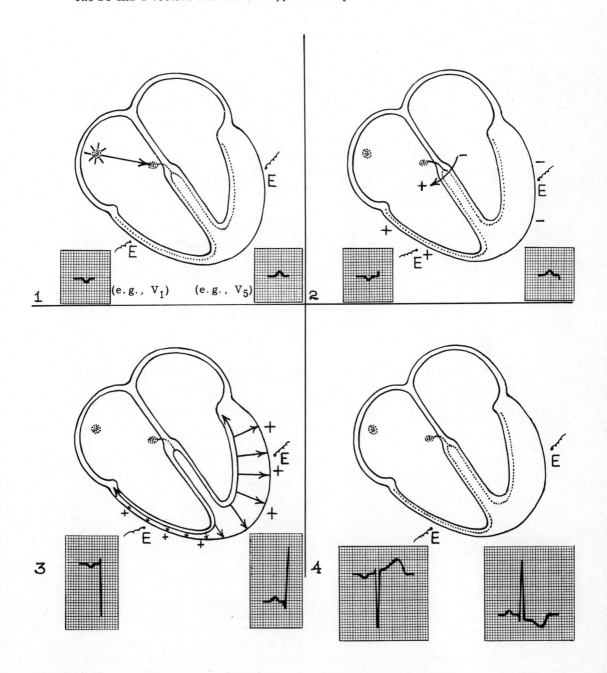

Left Ventricular Hypertrophy. 1. Spread of impulse from S-A to A-V node. 2. Activation of interventricular septum. 3. Activation of both ventricles. 4. Repolarization.

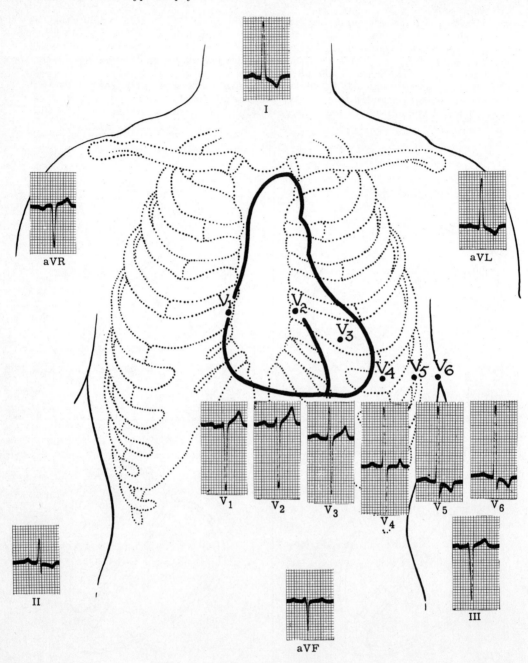

Left Ventricular Hypertrophy, Horizontal Heart. Standard leads: Frontal plane axis = -20°, $R_1 + S_3$ = 38 mm.; the T is inverted in I. **Extremity leads:** Horizontal heart position; the R in aVL measures 18 mm.; the T is inverted in aVL. **Precordial leads:** $SV_1 + RV_5$ = 49 mm. There is ST depression and T wave inversion in V_5 and V_6. **Clinical Diagnosis:** Hypertensive cardiovascular disease.

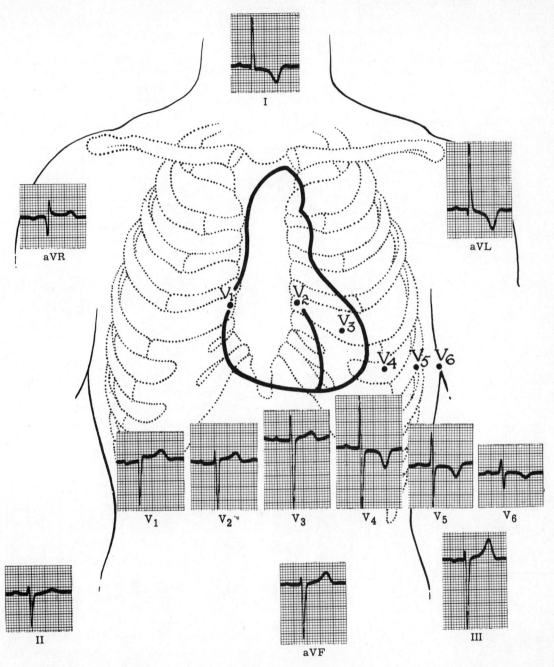

Left Ventricular Hypertrophy. The frontal plane axis = -47°; R = 24 mm. in aVL; ST depression and T wave inversion in I and aVL. The above are indicative of left ventricular hypertrophy. Precordial leads do not have voltage criteria ($SV_1 + RV_5$ or RV_6) for left ventricular hypertrophy. This is in part due to the marked superior (left) axis, as a result of which the lead axes of V_{5-6} are far removed from the mean QRS. The T waves are inverted in leads V_{4-6}, but this itself is not diagnostic of left ventricular hypertrophy. **Autopsy Diagnosis**: Left ventricular hypertrophy due to hypertension; no evidence of myocardial infarction.

B. Vertical Heart:

1. Standard leads - Frontal plane axis between +45° and +90°; tall R waves with depressed ST segments and inverted T waves in leads II and III.

2. Extremity leads - Since a left ventricular complex is recorded in aVF, this lead will show a tall R wave with depressed ST and inverted T. Although some authors state that an R wave of over 20 mm. in aVF is diagnostic of left ventricular hypertrophy, most authorities believe that this in itself is insufficient evidence for such a diagnosis.

3. Precordial leads - In the absence of any unusual rotation on the long axis, the pattern in the precordial leads will be the same as described for a horizontal heart.

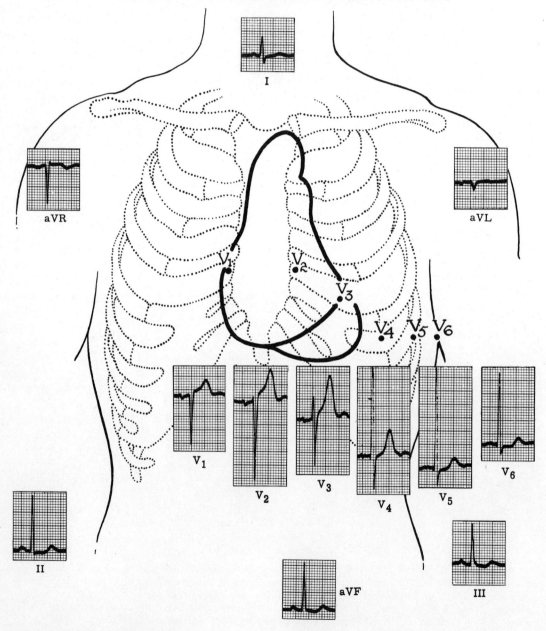

Left Ventricular Hypertrophy, Vertical Heart. The frontal plane axis is +75°; there are tall R waves with depressed ST segments in leads II, III, and aVF. $SV_1 + RV_5 = 55$ mm.; there is ST depression in V_{5-6}. The P waves are notched in all leads. **Clinical and Autopsy Diagnosis:** Left ventricular and left atrial hypertrophy. The patient was not receiving digitalis at the time this tracing was taken.

Clockwise Rotation on the Long Axis:

This may be associated with a vertical or horizontal heart position.

A. Standard and Extremity Leads: The pattern in these leads will mainly be dependent upon the degree of rotation in the frontal plane. Marked clockwise rotation can produce a tall R in aVR.

B. Precordial Leads: The transitional zone is shifted to the left, so that a typical left ventricular hypertrophy pattern may not be seen until leads V_{7-9} are taken.

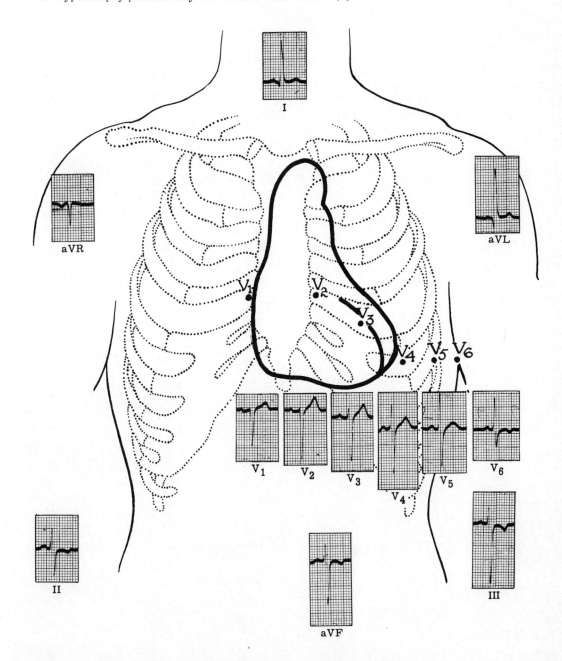

Left Ventricular Hypertrophy, Clockwise Rotation. The heart position is horizontal. The frontal plane axis is -37°. The tall R in aVL (17 mm.) is indicative of left ventricular hypertrophy. Precordial leads show marked clockwise rotation (persistent S in V_6) and a diphasic T in V_6. **Clinical Diagnosis:** Hypertensive cardiovascular disease.

Counterclockwise Rotation on the Long Axis:

This is more commonly associated with a horizontal heart position.

A. Standard and Extremity Leads: The pattern will be dependent upon the degree of rotation on the anteroposterior axis.

B. Precordial Leads: Since the transitional zone is shifted to the right, a left ventricular hypertrophy pattern may be seen in leads as far to the right as V_2 or V_3.

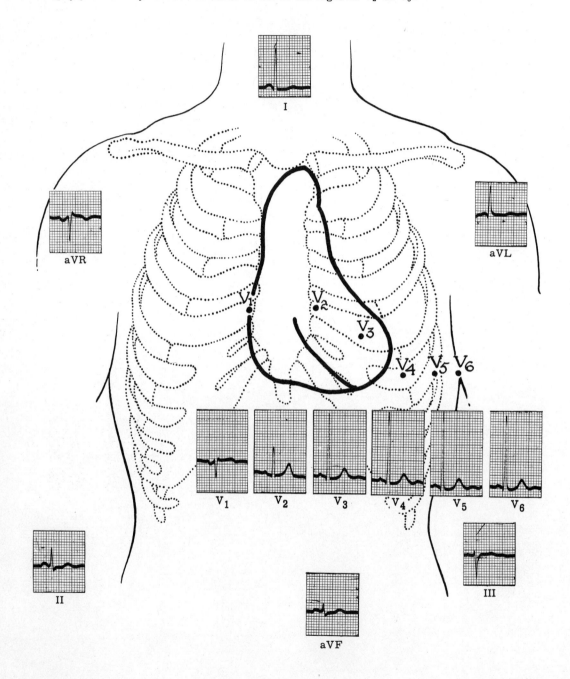

Left Ventricular Hypertrophy, Counterclockwise Rotation. The heart position is semi-horizontal; the frontal plane axis is -1°; the T is flat in aVL. Precordial leads reveal a left ventricular epicardial complex in V_2. Tall R waves are seen in V_{3-6}. R = 28 mm. in V_5. **Clinical Diagnosis:** Hypertensive cardiovascular disease.

Backward Rotation on the Transverse Axis:

This is a rather uncommon event. It can be diagnosed only by the pattern in the frontal plane leads and is an expression of marked left axis deviation. Because of the marked superior orientation of the QRS vector, leads aVR and aVL will show tall R waves. In such an instance, the tall R waves in aVR should not be interpreted as a manifestation of right ventricular hypertrophy (see p. 108).

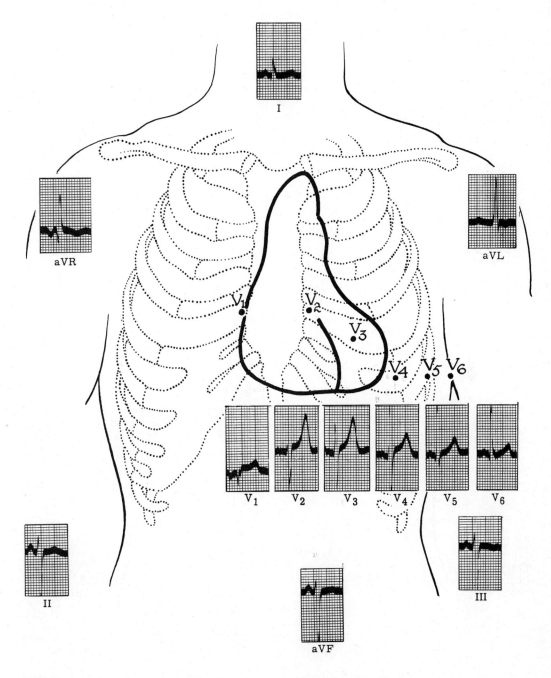

Left Ventricular Hypertrophy, Backward Rotation. Note the tall R waves in aVR and aVL. The frontal plane axis = -75°. This markedly superior QRS vector produces the tall R waves in aVR and aVL. Precordial leads are normal. **Clinical and Autopsy Diagnosis:** Hypertensive cardiovascular disease.

LEFT VENTRICULAR STRAIN

The electrocardiographic pattern of left ventricular strain is that of ST segment depression and T wave inversion in those leads which record a left ventricular epicardial complex. There are no abnormally tall R waves and no prolongation of the QRS interval or V. A. T. Since these ST-T changes are "nonspecific" and can be produced by many other conditions (see p. 267 to 291), a positive electrocardiographic diagnosis cannot be made. Proper electrocardiographic interpretation will depend upon correlation with the clinical findings.

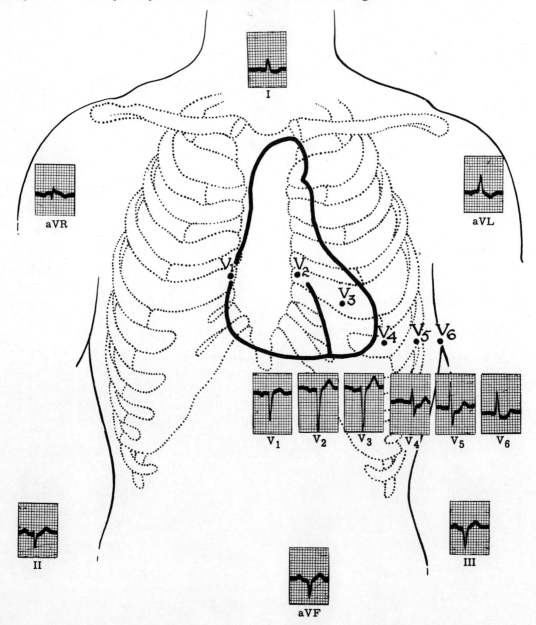

Left Ventricular Strain. ST segment depression is seen in I, aVL, and V_{4-6}; the T is inverted in aVL. The changes are not diagnostic of left ventricular strain. **Clinical Diagnosis:** Hypertensive cardiovascular disease. The patient was not receiving digitalis and there was no clinical evidence of angina, infarction, or electrolyte disturbance. **Autopsy Diagnosis:** Left ventricular hypertrophy.

SUMMARY OF ELECTROCARDIOGRAPHIC CRITERIA
OF LEFT VENTRICULAR HYPERTROPHY

A. Precordial Leads: These are the best leads
   for diagnosis.
   1. Voltage - R waves in V_5 or V_6 over 27
      mm. S in V_1 + R in V_5 or V_6 over 35 mm.
   2. V.A.T. over 0.05 sec. in V_{5-6}.
   3. QRS interval - May be prolonged over
      0.1 sec. in V_{5-6}.
   4. ST segment depression and T wave in-
      version in V_{5-6}.

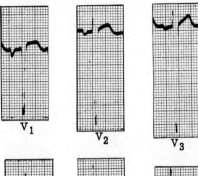

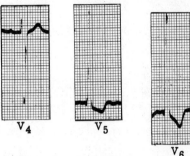

B. Extremity Leads:
   1. Horizontal heart - R wave of 13 mm. or
      more in aVL; V.A.T., QRS interval, ST-
      T changes as described for precordial
      leads.

   2. Vertical heart - R wave of over 20 mm.
      in aVF; V.A.T., QRS interval, ST-T
      changes as described for precordial leads.
      Unless confirmed by precordial leads,
      this pattern in aVF is not diagnostic of
      left ventricular hypertrophy (since right
      ventricular hypertrophy can give a
      similar pattern in aVF).

C. Standard Leads: These reflect the same
   pattern of the extremity leads.

      Horizontal heart - Left axis deviation
   (-30° or more); R_1 + S_3 over 26 mm.;
   pattern in I similar to aVL.

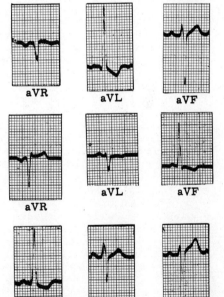

<hr />

Minimal Criteria:
   R in aVL >13 mm.; or R in V_{5-6} >27 mm.; or S in V_1 + R in V_{5-6} >35 mm. (if other variables
mentioned on p. 99 do not exist).

Equivocal Criteria:
   ST depression and T wave inversion in left precordial leads in the absence of definite voltage
criteria.

RIGHT VENTRICULAR HYPERTROPHY

Etiology:
  A. Mitral stenosis.
  B. Chronic diffuse pulmonary disease (e. g., emphysema, bronchiectasis, tuberculosis).
  C. Congenital heart disease (e. g., tetralogy of Fallot, pulmonic stenosis, Eisenmenger's syndrome; reverse patent ductus arteriosus).
  D. Nutritional and idiopathic, usually in association with left ventricular hypertrophy.

Incidence:
    An electrocardiographic diagnosis of right ventricular hypertrophy can be made less frequently in the above-mentioned diseases than can the electrocardiographic diagnosis of left ventricular hypertrophy in the presence of a pathologically hypertrophied left ventricle. The incidence of correct electrocardiographic diagnosis is highest in the congenital heart group; diagnosis is less accurate in those patients with mitral stenosis and chronic pulmonary disease.

Electrocardiographic Criteria:
    The criteria mentioned for the diagnosis of ventricular hypertrophy (see p. 93) are applicable to the leads recording a right ventricular complex (most commonly aVR, V_3R, and V_1).

Clinical Significance and Prognosis:
    A definite electrocardiographic diagnosis of right ventricular hypertrophy is as a general rule a more ominous sign than is left ventricular hypertrophy. The prognosis will of course depend upon the underlying disease. The electrocardiographic pattern can improve or revert to normal following successful surgical correction of the congenital lesions and mitral stenosis.

Electrocardiographic Patterns:
  A. Standard Leads: There may be no unusual axis deviation or there may be right axis deviation. Axis deviation of greater than +110° in an adult, in the absence of an I-V conduction defect, is good presumptive evidence of right ventricular hypertrophy. Tall R waves with depressed ST segments and inverted T waves are seen in leads II and III. This is the identical pattern that may be seen in standard leads in left ventricular hypertrophy with a vertical heart. Therefore, one cannot always differentiate electrocardiographically left and right ventricular hypertrophy by the standard leads, in the absence of an abnormal frontal plane axis.
  B. Extremity Leads: The pattern will vary with the degree of rotation in the frontal plane. The most common heart position is vertical.
      Lead aVR will frequently show a tall R wave, either as a QR, qR or R complex. However, a QR complex can occur in a normal heart with marked clockwise rotation or backward rotation of the apex. Therefore, although aVR may suggest right ventricular hypertrophy, confirmatory evidence should be present in right precordial leads to make such a diagnosis.
      Occasionally the hypertrophied right ventricle will overlie the left diaphragm and thereby reflect its pattern in aVF. Thus, one will see a small q, tall R, depressed ST and inverted T in aVF. Such a pattern, as mentioned above under standard leads, is identical with that seen in left ventricular hypertrophy in a vertical heart. Here again, the proper diagnosis of right ventricular hypertrophy will depend upon the findings in right precordial leads.
  C. Precordial Leads: Right precordial leads will typically show tall R waves; the V. A. T. is increased to over 0. 03 sec.; the QRS interval may be widened, but rarely up to 0. 12 sec.; the ST segments are depressed and the T waves inverted. At times these criteria will not be seen even in V_1 and will be seen in V_3R or V_4R. Therefore, these latter leads should always be taken when one clinically suspects right ventricular hypertrophy.
      Instead of an initial tall R wave in V_1 (or V_3R), one may see a small q preceding the R. This is probably the result of a slight delay in activation of the right ventricle, resulting from hypertrophy.
      Although voltage criteria have been assigned to the height of the R waves in right precordial leads as an index of right ventricular hypertrophy, a better criterion is the progressive changes from right to left precordial leads. In right precordial leads one sees R waves of greater voltage than the S. The R/S ratio is usually greater than 1/1 in V_1 or V_3R. As leads are taken progressively to the left, the R decreases and the S increases in amplitude. This latter finding of prominent S waves in V_6 or further laterally is a result of clockwise rotation plus the delayed spread of excitation through the hypertrophied right ventricle.
  D. Vector Analysis: The mean QRS vector is oriented to the right (110° or more), anteriorly, and either inferiorly or superiorly.

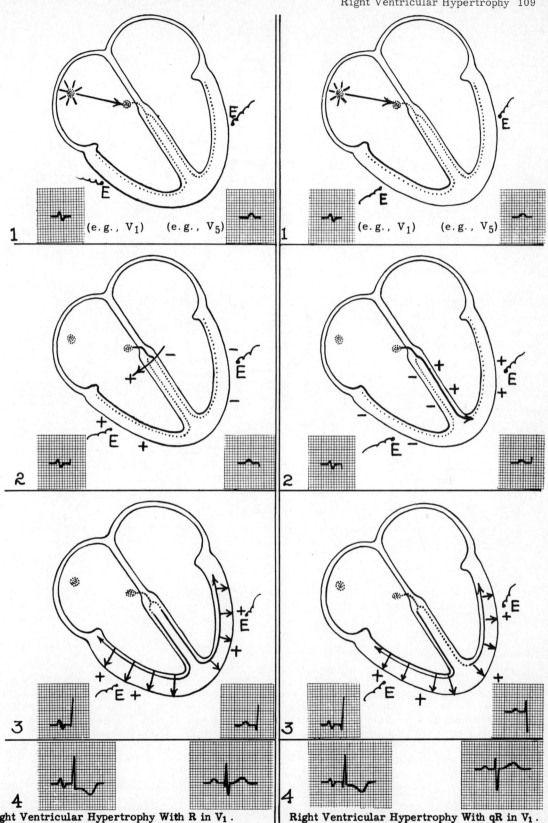

Right Ventricular Hypertrophy With R in V₁.
1. Atrial activation.
2. Normal interventricular septal activation.
3. Activation of both ventricles.
4. Repolarization.

Right Ventricular Hypertrophy With qR in V₁.
1. Atrial activation.
2. Delay in activation of hypertrophied rt. vent.
3. Activation of both ventricles.
4. Repolarization.

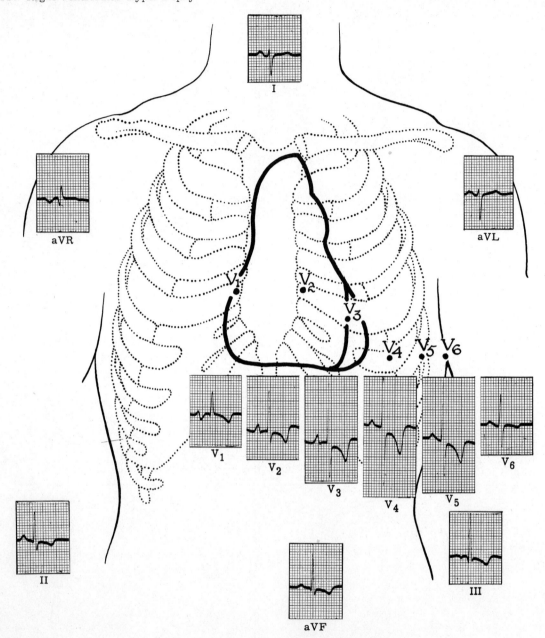

Right Ventricular Hypertrophy.   The frontal plane axis is +115°.   A qR is seen in V_1.   The R becomes progressively smaller and the S progressively larger from V_2 to V_6.   The T waves are inverted from V_1 through V_6 and the ST segments depressed from V_2 through V_5.   Lead aVF records a right ventricular epicardial complex similar to V_1.   **Clinical Diagnosis:** Mitral stenosis.

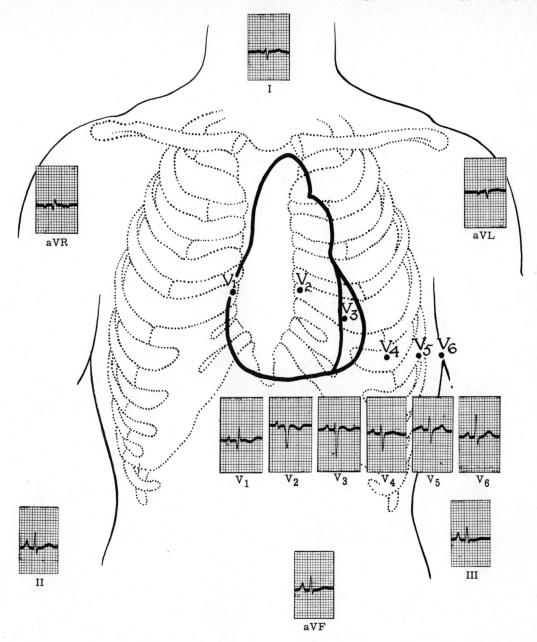

Right Ventricular Hypertrophy. The diagnosis is made from the pattern in V_1: QR, V.A.T. = 0.05 sec. In addition the T waves are inverted in V_{1-3}. The frontal plane axis is +105°.
Clinical Diagnosis: Pulmonary emphysema with right heart failure. **Autopsy Diagnosis:** Right ventricular hypertrophy.

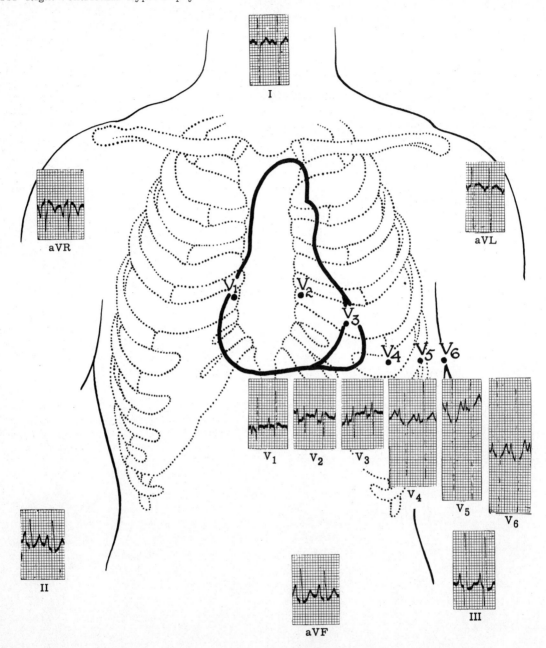

Right Ventricular Hypertrophy, Congenital Heart Disease (Four-month-old Infant). The heart rate is 177. The slight variation in rate in the various leads is due to sinus arrhythmia. This rapid rate in an infant is an indication of sinus tachycardia and does not indicate a paroxysmal atrial tachycardia. Prominent P waves are seen in II, III, and aVF, suggesting right atrial hypertrophy. A qR pattern is seen in V_1. The V. A. T. is 0.03 sec. The tall R wave could be a normal finding in an infant. However, an initial q wave is never normally present in infancy. This pattern is therefore indicative of right ventricular hypertrophy. **Clinical Findings:** Cyanotic infant with cardiac enlargement. **Clinical Diagnosis:** Tetralogy of Fallot.

RIGHT VENTRICULAR STRAIN
(Acute Cor Pulmonale)

Right ventricular strain is the electrocardiographic term which is used to describe a pattern in which only the ST segment and T wave changes described on p. 97 are seen in right ventricular leads. Such a pattern not uncommonly occurs in acute pulmonary infarction and during acute exacerbations of chronic pulmonary disease. The following patterns may be seen in precordial leads. The standard and extremity leads will not be discussed since they do not contribute materially.

ST segment depression with inverted T waves is seen in right precordial leads. The R waves are not abnormal. There frequently is clockwise rotation. Electrocardiographically such a pattern is consistent with but not absolutely diagnostic of right ventricular strain, since other conditions can give a similar pattern (e.g., coronary artery disease; normal pattern in children and some adult Negroes).

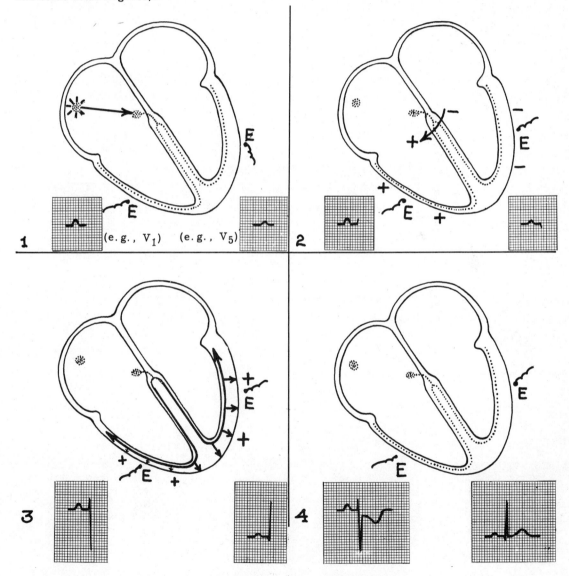

Right Ventricular Strain. (1) Atrial activation. (3) Activation of both ventricles.
(2) Interventricular septal activation. (4) Repolarization.

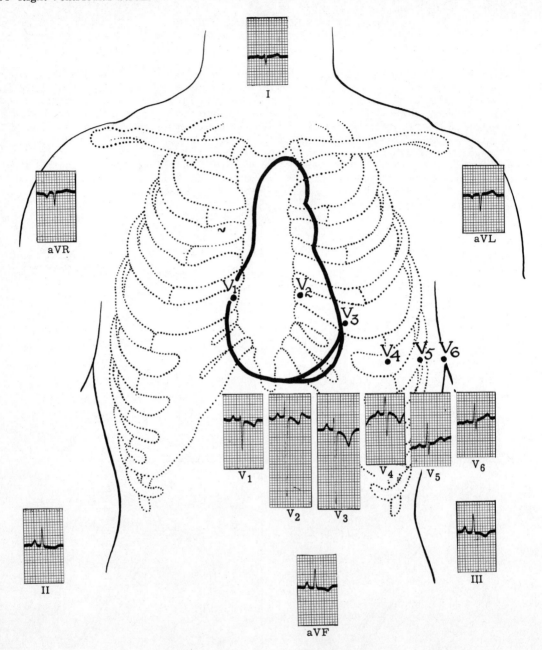

Right Ventricular Strain. Right axis deviation (+100°); vertical heart position; inverted T waves in II, III, and aVF; normal R waves in precordial leads; inverted T waves and depressed ST segments in V_{1-4}. **Clinical Diagnosis:** Pulmonary sarcoidosis, before therapy. See illustration on p. 115 for change after therapy.

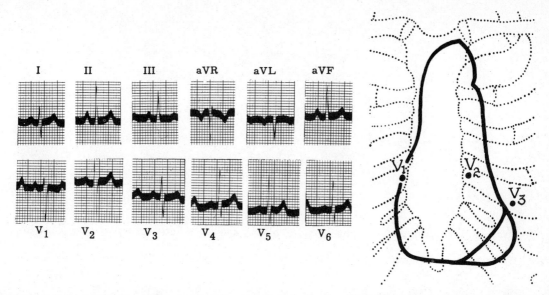

Right Ventricular Strain or Hypertrophy. Reversal to normal. **Clinical Diagnosis:** Pulmonary sarcoidosis after therapy with cortisone, which resulted in clearing of the lung lesions and disappearance of right heart failure. For electrocardiogram before therapy see preceding page.

Miscellaneous Right Ventricular Hypertrophy Patterns:

   A. Questionable Right Ventricular Hypertrophy: Prominent P waves suggestive of atrial hypertrophy may be indirect evidence of associated right ventricular strain or hypertrophy.

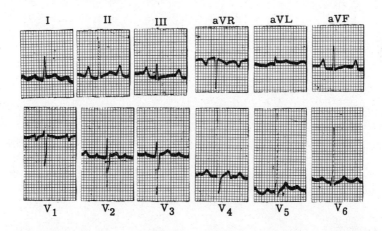

Questionable Right Ventricular Hypertrophy. There are no criteria in the QRS-T complexes to suggest right ventricular hypertrophy. Tall P waves in II, III, and aVF are consistent with right atrial hypertrophy. Clinically, the patient had diffuse pulmonary fibrosis and early signs of right heart failure. Only in combination with the clinical findings is one justified in making a diagnosis of right ventricular hypertrophy.

   B. Suggestive Right Ventricular Hypertrophy: Marked clockwise rotation may be the only electrocardiographic finding. However, a diagnosis must not be made on this basis alone. When combined with evidence of atrial hypertrophy, the diagnosis becomes more likely but still is not absolute. When marked clockwise rotation is combined with a frontal plane axis of +110° or more, the diagnosis becomes more certain.

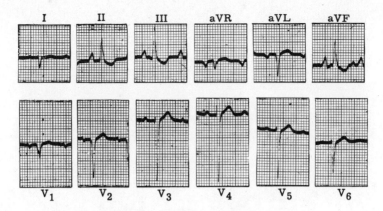

Suggestive Right Ventricular Hypertrophy. Tall P waves in II, III, and aVF are consistent with right atrial hypertrophy. The frontal plane axis is +115°. There is marked clockwise rotation. The combination of these three findings is strongly suggestive of right ventricular hypertrophy. **Clinical Diagnosis:** Pulmonary emphysema and bronchiectasis with right heart failure.

C. An incomplete (or complete) right bundle branch block may be a manifestation of right ventricular strain (see pp. 121 to 130).

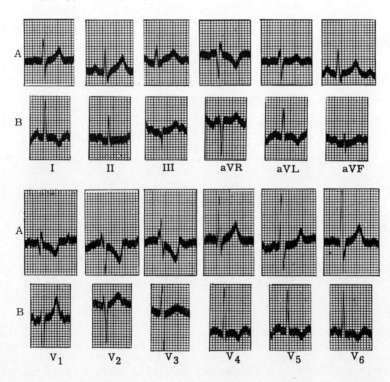

Incomplete Right Bundle Branch Block as Manifestation of Acute Right Ventricular Strain. A: The pattern is that of an incomplete bundle branch block (rsr' complexes with depressed ST segments and inverted T waves in V_{1-3}). **B:** Five days after A: There has been a marked change. The incomplete right bundle branch block is no longer present. In the interval the T waves have become inverted in leads I, aVL, and V_{4-6}. **Clinical Status:** At (A) the patient had an episode of acute pulmonary infarction. Five days later he had markedly improved. The electrocardiogram in (A) was a reflection of acute right ventricular strain. The pulmonary hypertension had clinically subsided by (B), and the second electrocardiogram demonstrated the abnormalities associated with the basic heart disease, beri-beri.

Clinical Significance and Prognosis of the Foregoing Patterns:

All of the above patterns can be seen in association with true pathologic right ventricular hypertrophy. Therefore one cannot differentiate, in a single electrocardiographic record, between strain and hypertrophy. The clinical findings and serial electrocardiographic changes (such as reversal to normal) are necessary for proper interpretation.

The prognosis will depend upon the nature of the underlying disease.

SUMMARY OF ELECTROCARDIOGRAPHIC CRITERIA
OF RIGHT VENTRICULAR HYPERTROPHY

A. Precordial Leads: These are the best leads for diagnosis.
   1. R wave of greater voltage than S in V_1 or V_{3R}.
   2. qR pattern in V_1 or V_{3R}.
   3. V.A.T. over 0.03 sec. in V_1 or V_{3R}.
   4. Persistent S waves in V_{5-6}.
   5. ST segment depression and T wave inversion in V_1 or V_{3R}.

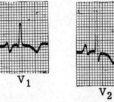 V_1

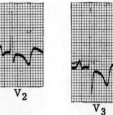 V_2

V_3

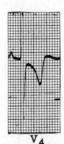 V_4

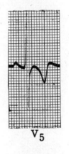 V_5

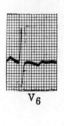 V_6

B. Extremity Leads:
   1. Tall R in aVR; unless accompanied by the criteria in A, this alone is not indicative of right ventricular hypertrophy.
   2. Tall R with depressed ST and inverted T in aVF; unless confirmed by precordial leads this pattern in itself is in no way diagnostic of right ventricular hypertrophy.

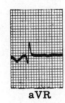 aVR

 aVL

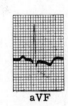 aVF

C. Standard Leads: Right axis deviation (+110° or more); depressed ST and inverted T in II and III.

 I

 II

 III

Minimal Criteria:

Rs or qR complex in V_1 or V_{3R} with V.A.T. >0.03 sec. Right axis deviation.

Equivocal Criteria:

Abnormally tall or notched P waves and clockwise rotation; or ST depression with T wave inversion in V_{3R} and V_{1-3} in the absence of a tall R in these leads; or incomplete or complete right bundle branch block.

COMBINED RIGHT AND LEFT VENTRICULAR HYPERTROPHY

The electrocardiographic diagnosis of ventricular hypertrophy is far from perfect. Correlation of the electrocardiogram with autopsy findings has furnished the following results: A correct electrocardiographic diagnosis of left ventricular hypertrophy (proved at autopsy) can be made in 85% of cases using the criteria discussed above. However, using the same criteria a false-positive diagnosis has been made in 10 to 15% of cases. The electrocardiographic diagnosis of autopsy-proved right ventricular hypertrophy is less reliable. The correlation has ranged from 23 to 100%, the latter figure only occurring in analysis of patients with congenital heart disease. Combined right and left ventricular hypertrophy commonly is not diagnosed electrocardiographically. The autopsy correlation is only 8 to 26%. In the author's opinion the most reliable criteria are the presence of signs of left ventricular hypertrophy in precordial leads plus a frontal plane axis of more than +90°. This is especially valid if serial electrocardiograms demonstrate a progressive change of frontal plane axis to the right of +90° in the presence of precordial lead criteria of left ventricular hypertrophy.

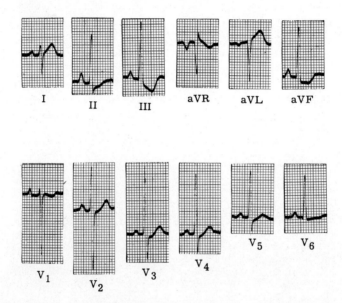

I II III aVR aVL aVF

V_1 V_2 V_3 V_4 V_5 V_6

Combined Right and Left Ventricular Hypertrophy. The mean frontal plane axis is +105°; there is ST depression in leads II, III, aVF, V_5, and V_6; the T is flat in II and V_6, inverted in III and aVF. $SV_1 + RV_5 = 39$ mm. **Clinical and Autopsy Diagnosis:** Right and left ventricular hypertrophy, idiopathic.

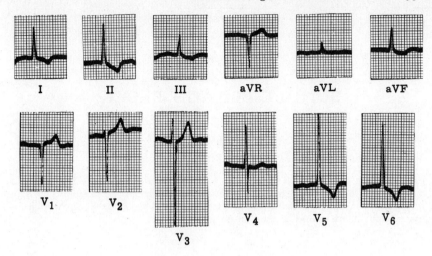

Left Ventricular Hypertrophy. The rhythm is atrial fibrillation. The frontal plane axis is +50°. $SV_1 + RV_5 = 42$ mm.; there is ST depression and T wave inversion in I, II, III, aVF, and V_{5-6}. Some of the ST-T changes are the result of digitalis therapy. **Clinical Diagnosis**: Hypertensive cardiovascular disease.

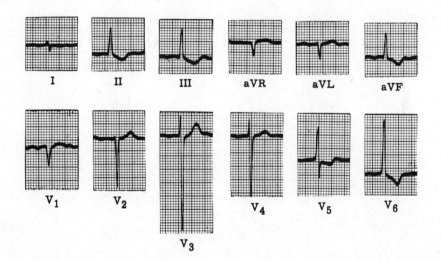

Combined Right and Left Ventricular Hypertrophy. This electrocardiogram was taken on the same patient 6 years after the above tracing. In the interval the patient had developed progressive right heart failure. The frontal plane axis has changed to +100°. Voltage criteria (SV_1 + RV_5 or RV_6) are no longer present for the diagnosis of left ventricular hypertrophy. The ST-T abnormalities in II, III, aVF, and V_{5-6} are the result of digitalis therapy plus left ventricular hypertrophy.

Chapter 9

BUNDLE BRANCH BLOCK

Pathology:

Bundle branch block occurs most commonly when there is a lesion, either pathological or physiological, involving either the right or the left bundle branch. Occasionally a similar electrocardiographic pattern can result from a pathologic process (hypertrophy) involving one or the other ventricle without involvement of the bundle itself.

Classification:

A. Complete: Right or left. In electrocardiographic interpretation the term "bundle branch block" implies the complete type.

B. Incomplete: Right or left.

Electrocardiographic Criteria:

A. Complete:

1. Delay of excitation and abnormal spread of excitation through the ventricle whose bundle is "blocked," resulting in an abnormal QRS configuration. (The term "QRS" is used because it is the traditional electrocardiographic identification of ventricular depolarization. The actual pattern discussed here is not QRS but rSR'.)

2. Prolongation of the QRS interval to 0.12 sec. or longer.

3. V.A.T. (measured to the peak of the R') is prolonged.

4. The ST segments are depressed and the T waves inverted in leads which record the abnormal R' waves.

B. Incomplete: An incomplete bundle branch block is an arbitrary subclassification of the above in which the same abnormalities are present except that the QRS interval is less than 0.12 sec. and the V.A.T. is less than that seen in a complete bundle branch block.

RIGHT BUNDLE BRANCH BLOCK

Etiology:
  A right bundle branch block may be present in almost any type of heart disease, including:
A. Coronary artery disease.

B. Hypertensive cardiovascular disease.

C. The same diseases which produce right ventricular hypertrophy.

D. Congenital lesions involving the septum.

  A right bundle branch block may also be found in normal individuals, i.e., those with no clinical evidence of heart disease and even in those in whom no apparent cardiac lesion is found at autopsy.

Incidence:
  Right bundle branch block is a fairly common electrocardiographic finding. In itself it is in no way diagnostic of heart disease per se or of any type of heart disease.

Mechanism:
  The spread of excitation from the S-A node to the A-V node and through the main bundle of His occurs in a normal fashion. Septal activation occurs normally from left to right.

A. Right Ventricular Epicardial Complex (e.g., V_1):

  1. As a result of the normal septal activation, which is oriented to the right and anteriorly, a small initial r will be recorded.

  2. Since the right bundle is "blocked" the excitation wave will next spread down the left bundle and through the left ventricular myocardium, resulting in an S wave.

  3. The impulse will then pass around the "blocked" right bundle into the right ventricular myocardium, producing a wide R' wave. Thus a typical pattern will be an rSR' complex.

  4. Occasionally the s wave is small, resulting in an rsR' complex.

B. Left Ventricular Epicardial Complex (e.g., V_5):

   1. An initial small q will be seen as a result of septal activation.

   2. This will be followed by an R resulting from left ventricular activation.

   3. There will follow a wide S wave resulting from delayed activation of the right ventricle. The ST segment is usually iso-electric and the T upright.

C. Left Ventricular Cavity Complex (e.g., aVL in a vertical heart): A QS complex will be present as under normal conditions, but will be wide. The ST segment is iso-electric and the T wave is inverted.

D. Right Ventricular Cavity Complex (e.g., aVR): An initial r may be recorded as occurs normally. This will be followed by an S resulting from the spread of the excitation through the left ventricle (as in a normal heart). A late, wide R wave may follow as a result of the late activation of the right side of the interventricular septum. The ST segment is isoelectric or elevated; the T is inverted.

The Electrocardiographic Pattern of Right Bundle Branch Block:
    The characteristic feature of a right bundle branch block is the late and delayed electrical force of right ventricular depolarization oriented to the right and anteriorly. This late right vector force produces the wide S wave in leads I, V_{4-6} (left ventricular epicardial complex) and the wide R or R̂ in aVR. The anterior component of this late force will produce the wide R waves in right precordial leads, V_3R, V_1, and V_2 (right ventricular epicardial complex). This same late force may be directed superiorly or inferiorly. If superior it will produce a wide S in aVF; if inferior, a wide R̂ in aVF. The ST segment and the T wave are opposite in direction to this late force of ventricular depolarization, resulting in ST depression and T wave inversion in right precordial leads. The QRS interval is 0.12 sec. or greater.

    The pattern of septal and left ventricular depolarization in an uncomplicated right bundle branch block will be normal. Therefore, these will vary with heart position within the range of normal. In a right bundle branch block it will be of little significance to determine the mean frontal plane axis of the entire QRS. Instead one should evaluate the initial 0.04-0.06 sec. of the QRS (representing normal septal and left ventricular depolarization) in frontal plane leads and determine the frontal plane axis therefrom (see p. 35).
  A. Vertical Heart: The mean of the forces resulting from septal and left ventricular depolarization will be oriented between +45° and +110° in the frontal plane (including semi-vertical heart position). Thus this portion of the QRS complex in an uncomplicated right bundle branch block will be the same as in any normal vertical (or semi-vertical) heart. The factors which produce the right bundle branch block are as given above.

[B. See p. 125.]

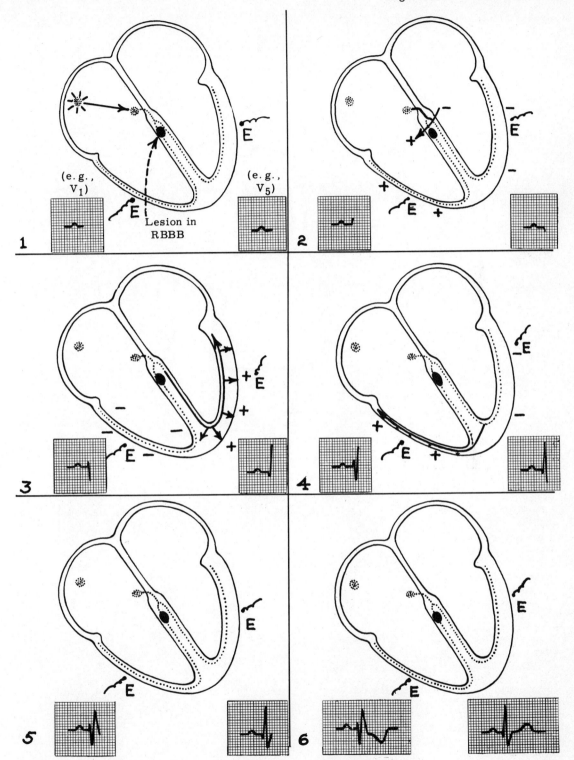

Development of Right and Left Ventricular Epicardial Complexes in Right Bundle Branch Block.

1. Atrial activation.
2. Normal interventricular septal activation.
3. Right bundle branch blocked; therefore the left ventricle is activated first.
4. Delayed activation of the right ventricle "around" the block.
5. Depolarization complete.
6. Repolarization complete.

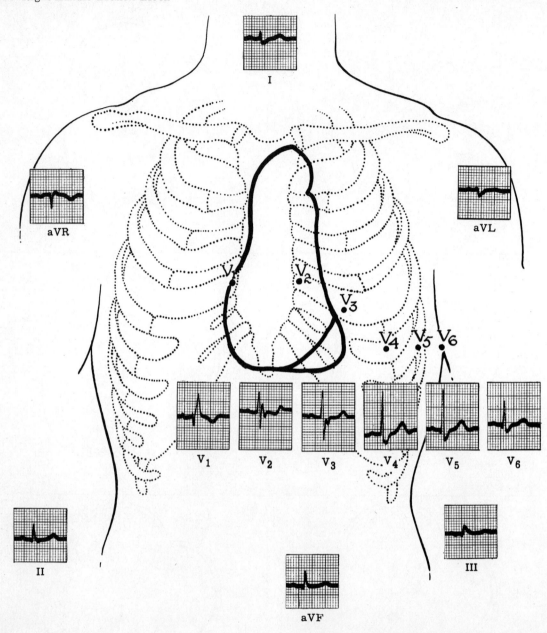

Complete Right Bundle Branch Block, Vertical Heart. The mean frontal plane axis of the initial 0.04 sec. of the QRS (determined by measuring r I and qr III, disregarding the wide s I and wide r III) = + 60°. The QRS interval = 0.14 sec. The wide s waves in I, V_{4-6} and the R′ waves in V_{1-2} are typical of right bundle branch block.

B. Horizontal Heart: The mean of the forces resulting from septal and left ventricular depolarization will be oriented between +15° and -30° in the frontal plane (including semi-horizontal
heart position). Thus this portion (the initial 0.04-0.06 sec.) of the QRS complex in an uncomplicated right bundle branch block will be the same as in any normal horizontal (or semi-
horizontal) heart. The factors which produce the right bundle branch block are as stated on
p. 122.

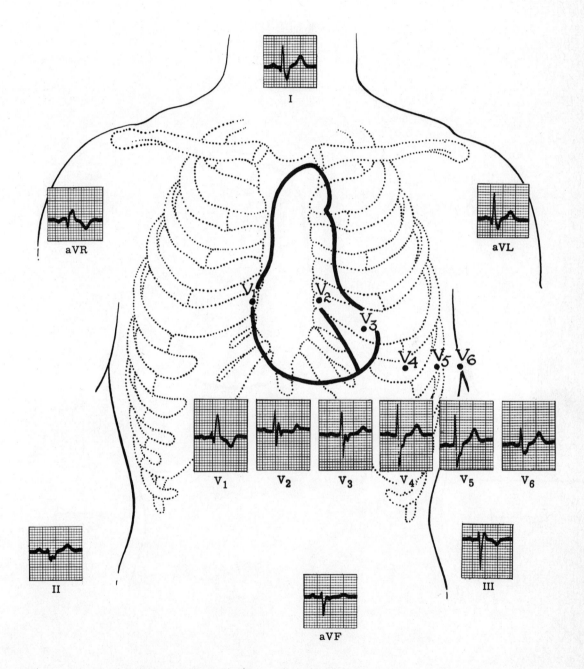

Right Bundle Branch Block, Horizontal Heart. The mean frontal plane axis of the initial 0.04
sec. of the QRS (determined by measuring q and R in I and r and S in III, disregarding the wide
S I and wide r III) = -40° and therefore, by definition (see p. 34), is left axis deviation and is
abnormal. The QRS interval = 0.14 sec. The wide S waves in I, II, aVL, and V_{4-6}, the wide
r in III and aVR, and the wide R in V_1 and V_2 are typical of right bundle branch block.

Right Bundle Branch Block With Left Ventricular Hypertrophy:

In this situation the tracing may show, in addition to the right bundle branch block pattern, the typical characteristics of left ventricular hypertrophy in leads I, aVL and V_{4-6}. Thus, these leads will show abnormally tall R waves and ST-T changes. The heart position is usually horizontal, resulting in left axis deviation and an abnormally tall R wave in aVL.

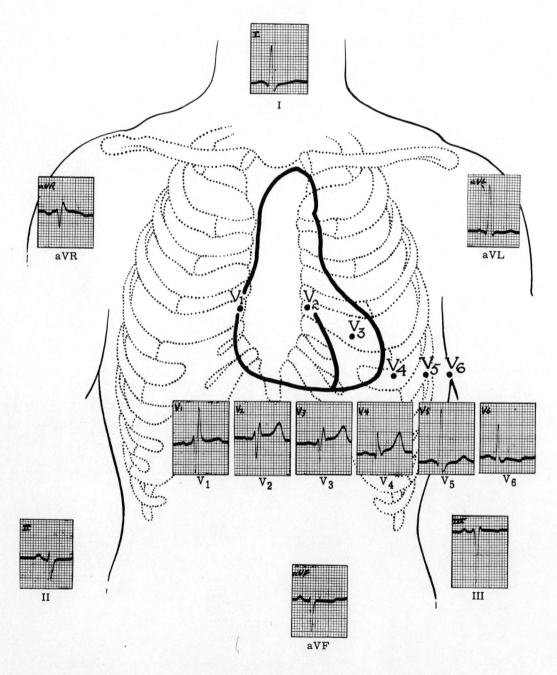

Right Bundle Branch Block and Left Ventricular Hypertrophy. Precordial leads show the typical pattern of a right bundle branch block. The R in aVL = 17 mm. This is indicative of left ventricular hypertrophy. The inverted T in V_6 is probably also a manifestation of this latter diagnosis. **Clinical Diagnosis:** Hypertensive cardiovascular disease.

Incomplete Right Bundle Branch Block:

The pattern is similar to that of a complete right bundle branch block with the following exceptions: the QRS interval is under 0.12 sec. and the V. A. T. is under 0.06 sec. An incomplete right bundle branch block may occur as a result of right ventricular hypertrophy or strain (see pp. 116 and 129).

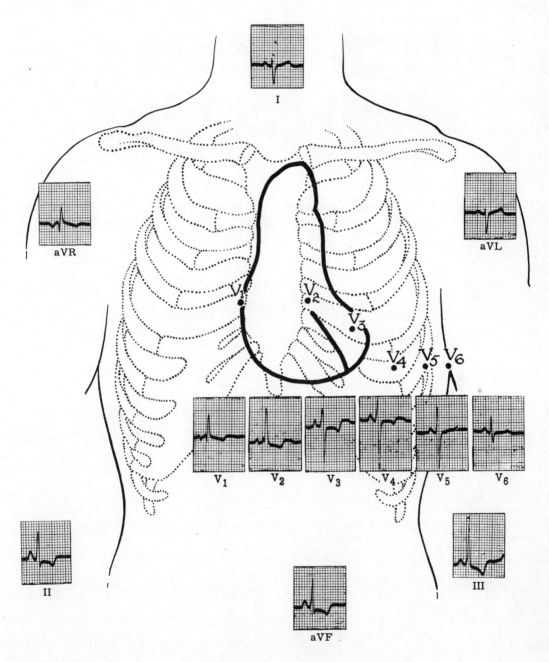

Incomplete Right Bundle Branch Block. The pattern is similar to that of a right bundle branch block except that the QRS interval = 0.08-0.1 sec. The right axis deviation, +110°, and the rR complex in V_2 indicate associated right ventricular hypertrophy. **Clinical Diagnosis:** Pulmonary sarcoidosis with right heart failure.

Normal rSr' Pattern in V_1:

The pattern of an incomplete right bundle branch block can resemble the normal pattern in which an rSr' is seen in V_1. However, in the latter the r' in V_1 is narrow whereas in an incomplete right bundle branch block the r' in V_1 appears widened. At times it is impossible to differentiate these two patterns.

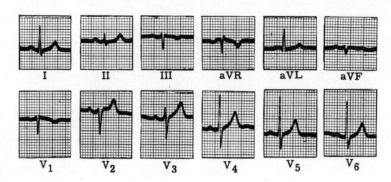

Normal rsr' in V_1. An rsr' pattern is seen in V_1. The r' is small and narrow. This pattern is a normal variant (see p. 45). The small r' in V_1, the s in I and V_6, and the late r in aVR are all the result of the normal small late QRS vector, which is oriented to the right, anteriorly, and superiorly (see p. 61).

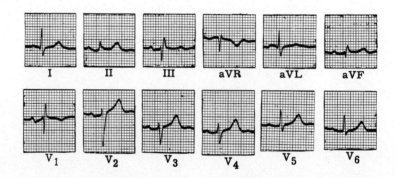

Incomplete Right Bundle Branch Block or a Normal Tracing. An rSR' complex is seen in V_1 and aVF. The R' is narrow in V_1 but wide in aVF. This tracing could be interpreted as normal or as an incomplete right bundle branch block. The latter electrocardiographic diagnosis does not necessarily indicate organic heart disease.

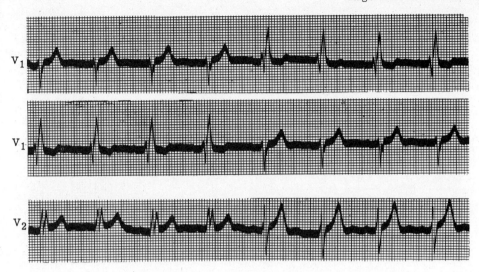

Intermittent **Right Bundle Branch Block.** Leads V_1 and V_2 illustrated. The pattern is changing from a normal complex to that of a right bundle branch block. **Clinical Diagnosis:** Arteriosclerotic heart disease. Two months later the pattern became that of a permanent right bundle branch block.

Differential Diagnosis of Right Bundle Branch Block and Right Ventricular Hypertrophy:

A complete or incomplete right bundle branch block may be a manifestation of right ventricular hypertrophy. However, it may be impossible to diagnose right ventricular hypertrophy in the presence of a right bundle branch block from the electrocardiogram alone.

Typically the following points are of differential value:

A. In right bundle branch block, the QRS interval is 0.12 sec. or longer; in right ventricular hypertrophy the QRS interval is under 0.12 sec.

B. In right bundle branch block a right precordial lead (such as V_1) shows an rSR´ complex. In right ventricular hypertrophy only an R wave, qR complex, or rR complex is seen.

C. In right bundle branch block the V.A.T. in a right precordial lead (V_1) is 0.06 sec. or more. In right ventricular hypertrophy the V.A.T. is between 0.03 and 0.05 sec.

Clinical Significance:

Right bundle branch block does not necessarily imply organic heart disease; it may occur in a normal individual. The pattern may be permanent or transient (in serial tracings or in the same tracing), depending upon the etiology. Pulmonary embolism or an acute exacerbation of some chronic pulmonary disease can produce a transient right bundle branch block.

A complete or incomplete right bundle branch block is a typical finding in the patient with an interatrial septal defect. In the presence of this congenital anomaly left axis deviation of the initial 0.04-0.06 sec. of the QRS is strongly suggestive of an ostium primum defect. A normal frontal plane axis of the initial 0.04-0.06 sec. QRS favors the presence of an ostium secundum.

SUMMARY OF ELECTROCARDIOGRAPHIC CRITERIA OF
RIGHT BUNDLE BRANCH BLOCK

A. Precordial Leads:
    1. RSR´ or rsR´ complexes in V_{3R}, V_{1-2}. An initial q wave is never present in these leads unless there is associated infarction or marked right ventricular hypertrophy or dilatation.
    2. Wide S waves in V_{5-6}.
    3. QRS interval = 0.12 sec. or more.
    4. V.A.T. = 0.06 sec. or more in V_{3R}, V_{1-2}.
    5. ST depression and T wave inversion in V_{1-3}; these findings are common, but are not essential for the diagnosis.

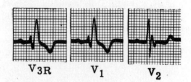

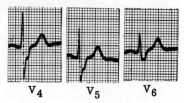

B. Extremity Leads:
    1. Wide rSr´ complex in aVR.
    2. Patterns in aVL and aVF will depend on heart position.

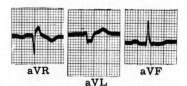

C. Standard Leads: A wide S wave is invariably present in lead I.

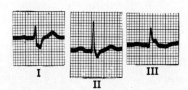

Minimal Criteria:
    rsR´ complex in a right precordial lead (V_{3R}, V_1, V_2) with QRS interval > 0.12 sec. A wide S wave in lead I.

LEFT BUNDLE BRANCH BLOCK

Etiology and Incidence:
   Left bundle branch block may occur in almost any form of heart disease, including the following:
   1. Coronary artery disease.
   2. Any of the diseases which produce left ventricular hypertrophy.
   3. Congenital lesions involving the septum.
   Left bundle branch block is a common finding in coronary artery disease. It may be seen as an electrocardiographic finding in those diseases which produce left ventricular hypertrophy, such as hypertension and aortic valvular disease. It is a rare finding in rheumatic heart disease with isolated mitral **valvulitis**. It is a much less common finding in congenital heart disease than is right bundle branch block. Rarely is it seen in an individual with no clinical evidence of organic heart disease.

Mechanism:
   The spread of excitation from the S-A to the A-V node and the bundle of His occurs in a normal fashion. However, septal activation occurs from right to left. This is the opposite of usual septal activation.
   A. Left Ventricular Epicardial Complex (e.g., V_5):
      1. As a result of septal activation from right to left, a small initial r wave will be recorded.

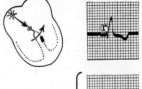

      2. Since the left bundle is "blocked" the excitation wave will next spread down the right bundle and through the right ventricular myocardium, resulting in an s wave.

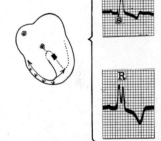

      3. Because of the relative thinness of the right ventricle, this s wave may not go below the iso-electric line but merely produce a notch in the R wave.

      4. The impulse then passes around the "blocked" left bundle into the left ventricular myocardium, producing a wide R´ wave.

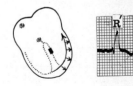

      5. Thus a typical pattern will be an rsR´ or notched or slurred widened R.

         The V.A.T. is prolonged to 0.09 sec. or longer; the QRS interval is 0.12+ sec.; usually the ST segments are depressed and the T waves inverted.

   B. Right Ventricular Epicardial Complex (e.g., V_1):
      1. An initial small q wave results from septal activation (right to left).

2. This is followed by a small r wave resulting from the normal activation of the right ventricle.

3. The impulse then passes around the "blocked" left bundle
and into the left ventricular myocardium, producing a deep,
wide S wave.

4. Occasionally either the small initial q or r may not be recorded.
   The patterns are therefore either qrS (B. 1., 2., 3.), rS or
QS complexes. The ST segment may be elevated, and the T is
upright.

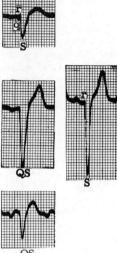

C. Right Ventricular Cavity Complex: Since septal activation is
from right to left, the cavity will be negative throughout ventricular depolarization, producing a wide QS complex. The
ST segment may be elevated, and the T is upright.

D. Left Ventricular Cavity Complex: Experimental data indicate that the left ventricular cavity
depolarization pattern is a wide upright deflection. This would not be expected from the
classic theory of abnormal (right to left) septal depolarization followed by delayed mural depolarization. This pattern in human left bundle branch block remains to be elucidated.

Clinical Significance and Prognosis:
   A left bundle branch block may be permanent or transient in the same tracing or in serial
tracings. Transient left bundle branch block may occur in the course of myocardial infarction,
heart failure, acute myocarditis, and as the result of quinidine or digitalis therapy. Permanent
left bundle branch block is practically always the result of organic heart disease. The prognosis
will depend on the nature of the underlying heart disease. In the rare instance in which a left
bundle branch block is found in a "normal" person, it has been assumed that a congenital lesion
of the left bundle branch exists.

The Electrocardiographic Pattern of Left Bundle Branch Block:
   The patterns in standard leads and unipolar extremity leads will vary with heart positions.
The pattern in the precordial leads will vary much less with change in heart position.
A. Horizontal Heart: This is the most common heart position.
   1. Standard leads - Left axis deviation; QRS interval = 0.12+ sec.; wide and slurred R waves
      in I and II; depressed ST segments and inverted T waves in I and II.
   2. Extremity leads - Lead aVL records a left ventricular epicardial complex, producing an
      rsR' or wide slurred R; the ST is depressed and the T inverted. Lead aVF records a right
      ventricular epicardial complex, producing a qrS, QS, or rS complex with an elevated or
      iso-electric ST segment and upright T wave.
   3. Precordial leads - Left precordial leads (V_{4-6}) will show the typical left ventricular epi-
      cardial pattern of a wide notched R wave or rsR' complex. The V.A.T. is prolonged to
      more than 0.09 sec. The ST segments are depressed and the T waves inverted. Right
      precordial leads reflect a right ventricular epicardial complex.
   4. Vector analysis - The normal initial QRS vector (directed to the right and anteriorly) is
      absent. Instead the initial QRS vector is directed to the left and posteriorly, which ex-
      plains the absence of a normal septal q wave in lead I and left precordial leads. Conduction
      delay is present through the last half of the QRS vector, producing the broad and slurred R
      waves in left precordial leads. The ST and T vectors are oriented to the right and
      anteriorly.

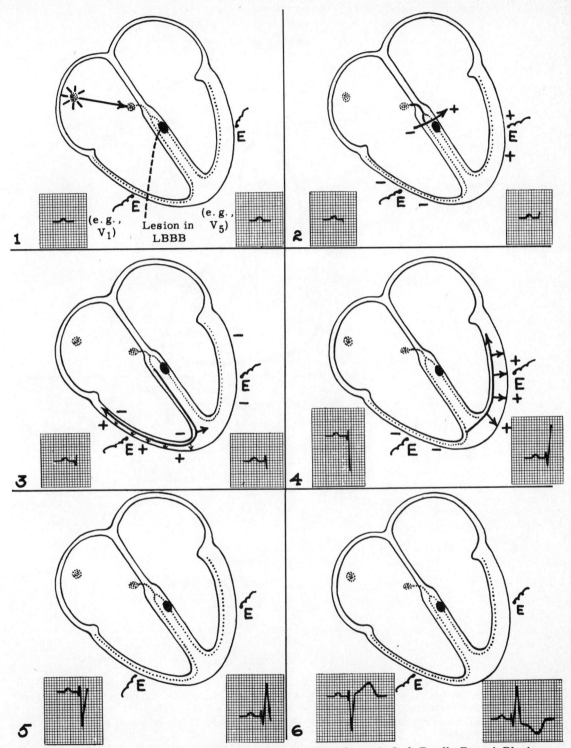

Development of Left and Right Ventricular Epicardial Complexes in Left Bundle Branch Block.

1. Atrial activation.
2. Interventricular septal activation from right to left.
3. Left bundle branch blocked; therefore right ventricle activated first.
4. Delayed activation of the left ventricle "around" the blocked bundle.
5. Depolarization complete.
6. Repolarization complete.

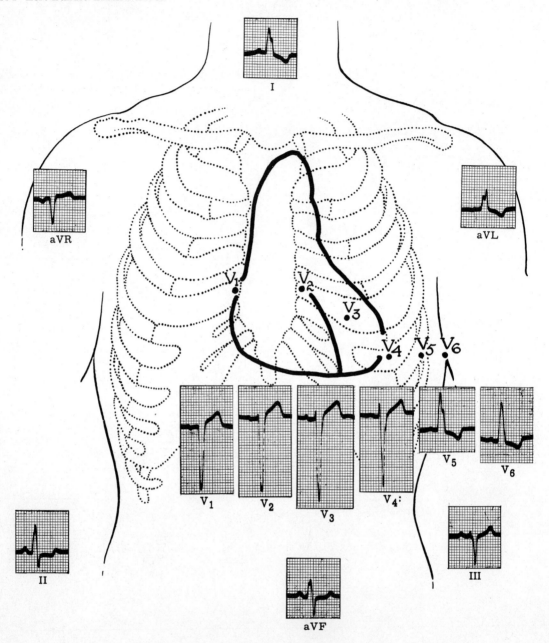

Left Bundle Branch Block, Horizontal Heart Position. Precordial leads show the typical pattern of left bundle branch block. A wide, notched R wave with depressed ST and inverted T is seen in V_{5-6}; QRS interval = 0.12 sec.; V. A. T. = 0.1 sec. Lead aVL records a left ventricular epicardial complex and resembles V_5 and V_6. **Clinical Diagnosis:** Hypertensive and arteriosclerotic heart disease.

Vertical Heart:

1. Standard leads - Normal frontal plane axis; wide, slurred R waves with depressed ST and inverted T in I, II, and III.

2. Extremity leads - The typical left ventricular epicardial complex is recorded in aVF.

3. Precordial leads - The same as stated for a horizontal heart. As in right bundle branch block, the diagnosis of a left bundle branch block is best made from a study of the precordial leads.

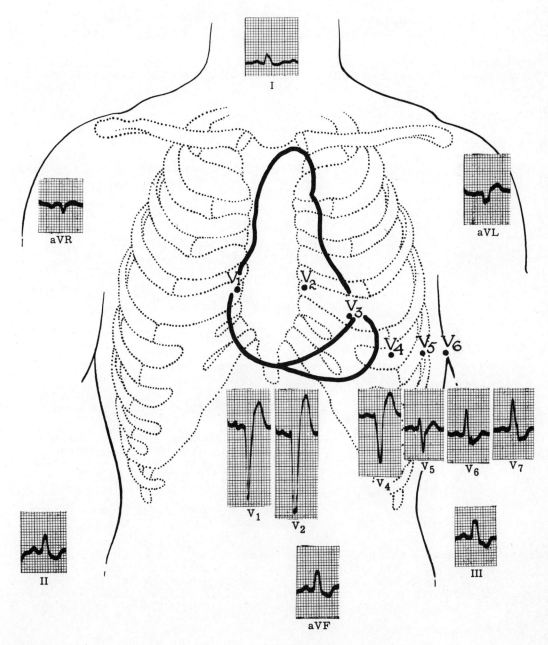

Left Bundle Branch Block, Vertical Heart. The pattern in precordial leads is that of a left bundle branch block. Lead aVF records a left ventricular epicardial complex and resembles V_7.
  Clinical and Autopsy Diagnosis: Hypertensive and arteriosclerotic heart disease; no evidence of myocardial infarction.

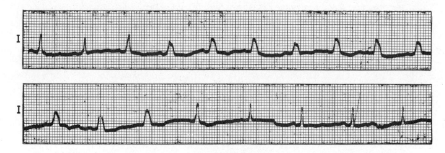

Intermittent Left Bundle Branch Block. Lead I. The pattern abruptly shifts from normal QRS complexes to those of a left bundle branch block. **Clinical Diagnosis:** Arteriosclerotic heart disease.

Effect of Deep Respiration:
    Deep inspiration and expiration, by altering the heart position, can greatly modify the electrocardiographic pattern, especially in the extremity leads.

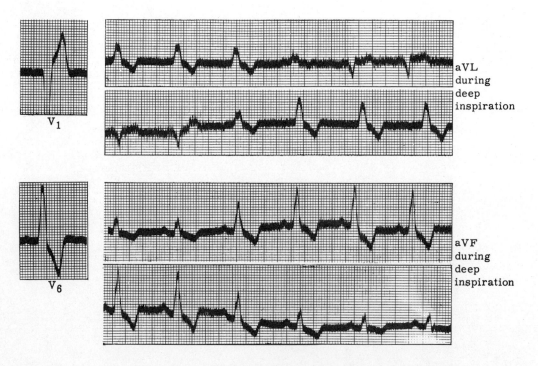

Change in Left Bundle Branch Block With Deep Inspiration. aVL: As a result of deep inspiration the typical left ventricular epicardial complex is converted into a right ventricular epicardial complex. This results from a change from horizontal to vertical position. **aVF:** As a result of the same change, lead aVF records a more typical left ventricular epicardial complex during deep inspiration. Leads V_1 and V_6 indicate the presence of the left bundle branch block.

Incomplete Left Bundle Branch Block:
    The pattern is similar to that of a complete left bundle branch block except that the QRS interval is under 0.12 sec. and the V.A.T. is under 0.09 sec.

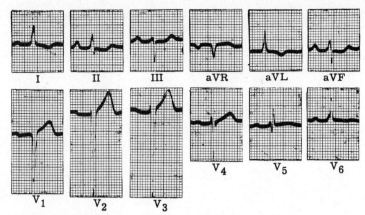

Incomplete Left Bundle Branch Block. Standard Leads: P-R = 0.25 sec., indicating a first degree A-V block; QRS = 0.07 sec.; left axis deviation; inverted T in I. **Extremity Leads:** Horizontal heart; inverted T in aVL. **Precordial Leads:** rsR′ complex in V_5; slurred R in V_6; absent initial q waves in V_{5-6} (also I and aVL); the T is flat in V_{5-6}. **Clinical Diagnosis:** Hypertensive cardiovascular disease.

Differential Diagnosis of Left Bundle Branch Block and Left Ventricular Hypertrophy:

A left bundle branch block may be seen in the same clinical conditions which produce left ventricular hypertrophy. The important point in the differential diagnosis of the above two conditions is the absence of a q wave in leads which definitely record septal activity in the right-left axis (i.e., I, V_{5-6}). The presence of a q wave in leads I and V_{5-6} negates the diagnosis of left bundle branch block or indicates associated infarction. Recent unpublished data of the author indicate that voltage criteria for the diagnosis of left ventricular hypertrophy remain valid in the presence of a left bundle branch block.

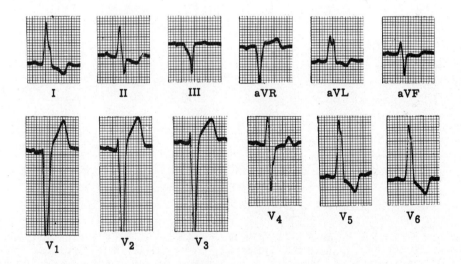

Left Bundle Branch Block. The heart position is horizontal; QRS interval = 0.15 sec.; absent q waves with wide, slurred R waves, depressed ST segments, and inverted T waves in leads I, aVL, V_{5-6}. $SV_1 + RV_5$ = 51 mm. **Clinical Diagnosis:** Syphilitic aortic insufficiency. **Autopsy Diagnosis:** Syphilis of the aorta; left ventricular hypertrophy.

138

SUMMARY OF ELECTROCARDIOGRAPHIC CRITERIA
OF LEFT BUNDLE BRANCH BLOCK

A. Precordial Leads: These are the best leads for diagnosis.
   1. Wide, slurred R waves or rsR' or RsR' complexes in V_{4-6}; absent q waves in these leads, with the possible exception of one lead (e.g., V_4) which borders on the transitional zone.
   2. QRS interval = 0.12+ sec.
   3. V.A.T. = 0.09+ sec. in V_{4-6}.
   4. ST depression and T wave inversion in V_{4-6}; these findings are common, but are not essential for the diagnosis.

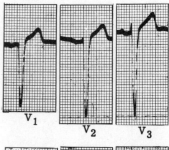

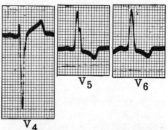

B. Extremity Leads: Pattern similar to that seen in V_{4-6} is present in aVL if heart is horizontal (more common); in aVF if heart is vertical (less common).

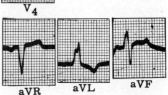

C. Standard Leads: These reflect the same pattern as in extremity leads. Absent q wave; wide and abnormal R wave (or rsR' complex); ST depression and T wave inversion in lead I.

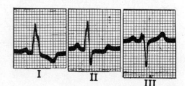

Minimal Criteria:
   rsR' complex or wide, notched R wave in left precordial leads (V_{4-7}) and lead I; absence of q waves in these leads; QRS interval > 0.12 sec.

LEFT INTRAVENTRICULAR BLOCK
(PARIETAL BLOCK): See p. 291.

Chapter 10

CORONARY ARTERY DISEASE:
MYOCARDIAL ANOXIA

The common clinical and electrocardiographic manifestations of coronary artery disease are myocardial anoxia and myocardial infarction.

Myocardial anoxia (i.e., coronary insufficiency) refers to changes in the myocardium resulting from a temporarily insufficient blood supply. These changes are commonly seen during spontaneous angina and induced coronary insufficiency (exercise test).

Etiology and Incidence:
Arteriosclerosis of the coronary arteries is the most frequent cause of myocardial anoxia. Patients with marked left ventricular hypertrophy may develop angina with exertion since the coronary vessels, even though not seriously diseased, cannot supply enough oxygen to the hypertrophied myocardium during periods of stress. Aortic stenosis with its low cardiac output reduces the coronary blood flow and therefore can produce myocardial anoxia. Syphilitic aortitis, by encroaching upon the orifices of the coronary arteries, can result in angina. Pulmonary hypertension, such as results from mitral stenosis and chronic diffuse pulmonary disease, reduces the left ventricular cardiac output and can produce angina. Polycythemia, by increasing the viscosity of the blood and slowing its circulation, can produce myocardial anoxia. Rarely, other arteritides such as Buerger's disease, rheumatic fever, and the other collagen diseases involve the coronary arteries and result in coronary insufficiency. Diabetes mellitus and myxedema, by increasing the degree of arteriosclerosis, are commonly associated with coronary artery disease. Other pathologic conditions which can induce coronary insufficiency are anemia, hyperthyroidism, and rapid paroxysmal arrhythmias.

Differential Diagnosis of the Electrocardiogram:
Since the electrocardiographic findings of coronary insufficiency are ST segment and T wave changes, a single electrocardiogram is not pathognomonic of coronary insufficiency. Similar changes can be produced by a variety of conditions, e.g., left ventricular hypertrophy (see p. 96), drug effect, hypokalemia, pericarditis, and myocarditis (see pp. 267 to 291). The diagnosis is dependent upon the clinical evaluation of the patient and electrocardiographic changes during spontaneous angina or coronary insufficiency induced by exercise tests.

Clinical Significance:
The diagnosis of myocardial anoxia (angina, coronary insufficiency) must never depend entirely upon the electrocardiogram. A normal resting record and even a normal exercise tracing does not exclude the diagnosis. A careful history is frequently of more value in diagnosis than the electrocardiogram.

Prognosis:
Although a patient with angina is subject to sudden death, he must not be made a permanent invalid since most patients can lead useful and productive lives for many years under sensible management.

A sudden appearance of angina in a previously asymptomatic individual or a sudden increase in the severity of symptoms is an indication of impending myocardial infarction. It is wise to treat such patients as one would a definite case of myocardial infarction.

Mechanism of the Electrocardiographic Pattern:
The electrocardiographic changes resulting
from myocardial anoxia are transitory ST segment deviations and T wave changes.

A. ST Segment Changes:* It is believed that
currents of injury produce the ST segment
deviation.   Two theories have been proposed as explanations of this phenomenon.

1. Injury current of rest - "Injured"
muscle (as occurs in myocardial anoxia
and myocardial infarction) is electrically negative in relation to normal
resting muscle.

a. This can be illustrated by observation of the events which occur in an
injured muscle strip. The pattern
overlying the injured area (right side
of diagram) will be considered first.
Diagram (1) represents a normal
resting muscle; E. is an electrode,
and the straight and dotted line represents the base line of the electrocardiogram. Diagram (2) represents a muscle the right end of which
has been injured. This area is now
electrically negative. The overlying
electrode will therefore record a depressed base line during the resting
period. In (3) the left end of the
muscle strip has been stimulated,
initiating an advancing negative
charge in front of which is a positive
charge (see p. 20). The electrode
therefore records a positive deflection. At (4) the stimulus has reached
the injured area. At this point there
is no longer any difference of electrical potential between the two ends of
the muscle strip, so the tracing returns to the base line as in a normal
resting muscle (1). This produces
the appearance of ST segment elevation. The tracing remains at this
level until the uninjured portion of
the muscle returns to the resting
state (5), at which time a difference
of potential again exists (as in 2) and
the tracing returns to the lower base
line.

b. The reverse occurs when the electrode faces the uninjured side of the
muscle strip (see complexes on left
side of diagram). At (2) the electrode is facing a positive charge, and
the base line is therefore elevated.
At (3) the electrode is facing a negative charge resulting from the
muscle stimulation, producing a
downward deflection. At (4) there is
again no difference in electrical
potential, so the tracing returns to

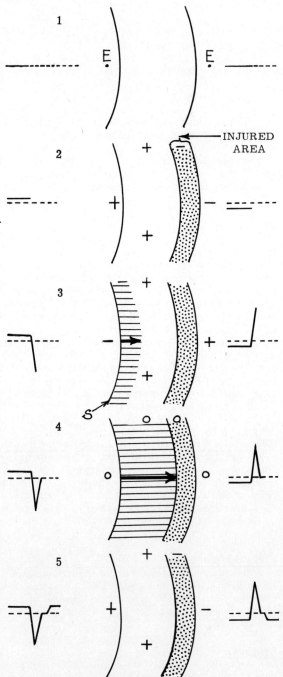

Theory of Injury Current of Rest. (The muscle
strips are curved to simulate the wall of the
myocardium.)

*See note on next page.

the base line corresponding to normal
resting muscle.   At (5) the electrical
difference again occurs, and the
tracing returns to the elevated base
line.   Thus a pattern of ST depression results.

2. Injury current of activity - This theory
assumes that injured muscle does not
become as electrically negative as normal muscle when stimulated.   Thus the
injured muscle during stimulation will
have a lesser negative charge and
hence a greater positive charge than
normal stimulated muscle.   An electrode directly overlying the injured end
of the muscle will face this positive
charge and result in an elevation of the
ST segment.   An electrode overlying
the uninjured end will face a negative
charge during stimulation and will
therefore record an ST segment depression.

As a practical rule, an electrocardiographic tracing taken directly over injured muscle will record ST segment elevation.   If normal muscle lies between the
injured muscle and the electrode, ST segment depression will result.

B. T Wave Changes: As a result of ST segment depression the T wave may be
"dragged" downward, producing the appearance of T wave inversion.   In addition,
true T wave inversion may occur in those
leads which record ST segment depression.   This T wave inversion is usually of
slight to moderate degree.   Occasionally
one may see very deep T wave inversion
simulating that seen in myocardial infarction.

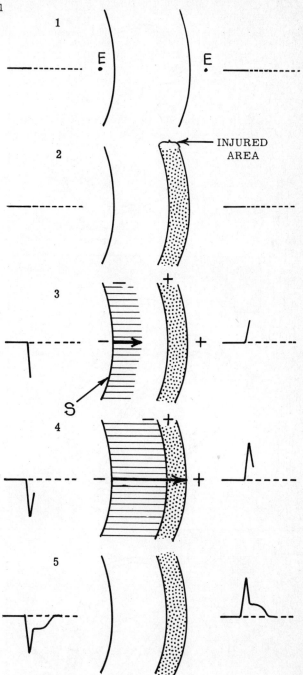

Theory of Injury Current of Activity. (The
muscle strips are curved to simulate the
wall of the myocardium.)

---

*There is increasing evidence (Prinzmetal, et al.) that the mechanism for ST segment depression,
at least in relation to myocardial anoxia, may not be as described above. By use of intramural
leads it has been shown that ST segment deviation produced by reduction in coronary blood flow
occurs only in the epicardial half of the myocardium.   Moderate myocardial anoxia produces ST
segment depression in an epicardial lead, and major myocardial anoxia produces ST segment
elevation.

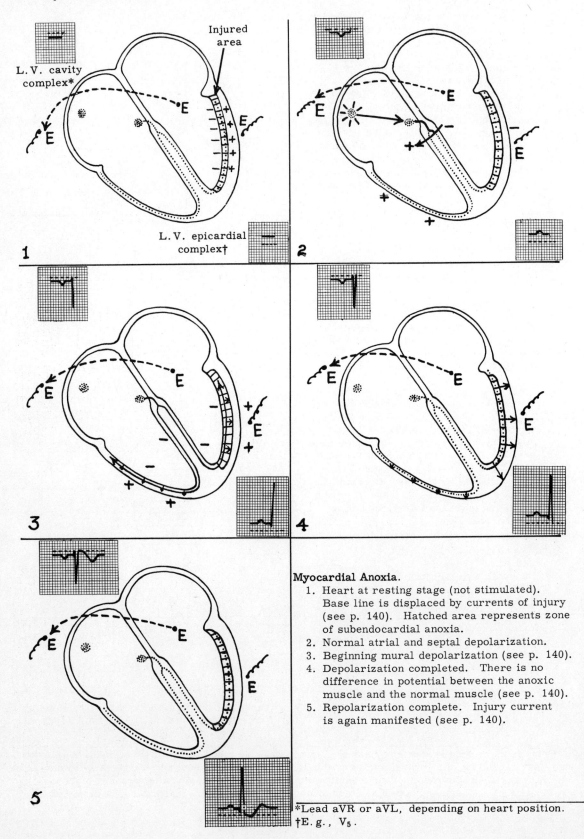

L.V. cavity
complex*

Injured
area

L.V. epicardial
complex†

Myocardial Anoxia.
1. Heart at resting stage (not stimulated).
   Base line is displaced by currents of injury
   (see p. 140). Hatched area represents zone
   of subendocardial anoxia.
2. Normal atrial and septal depolarization.
3. Beginning mural depolarization (see p. 140).
4. Depolarization completed. There is no
   difference in potential between the anoxic
   muscle and the normal muscle (see p. 140).
5. Repolarization complete. Injury current
   is again manifested (see p. 140).

*Lead aVR or aVL, depending on heart position.
†E.g., V_5.

ELECTROCARDIOGRAPHIC PATTERNS RESULTING
FROM MYOCARDIAL ANOXIA

<u>Spontaneous Angina Pectoris</u> (Acute Coronary Insufficiency):

    Frequently the electrocardiogram is normal in patients who suffer with angina. However, if a tracing is taken during an attack of pain one may see the pattern of myocardial anoxia. Typically this produces ST segment depression and, at times, associated T wave inversion in leads which reflect the left ventricular epicardial potential. These are usually the left precordial leads V_{4-6} and, occasionally, leads aVL or aVF, depending upon the heart position. These changes are thought to be due to subendocardial currents of injury. As in the muscle strip illustrations, a left precordial lead electrode records ST segment depression. A cavity lead (such as aVR or aVL, again depending upon heart position) directly faces the muscle area (subendocardial) which has the current of injury and records an ST segment elevation.

    In the above circumstances, the electrocardiogram returns to normal in a matter of minutes after the anginal episode subsides.

Spontaneous Angina (Coronary Insuf-
    ficiency, Myocardial Anoxia).
  A. Taken when patient was free
     of pain. Tracing is within
     normal limits.
  B. Taken during attack of an-
     gina. ST segment depres-
     sion is most marked in leads
     II, aVF, V_4, and V_6. De-
     pression is 2 mm. in aVF
     and V_4. Slight ST elevation
     in aVR.

<u>Clinical Diagnosis:</u> Arterio-
    sclerotic heart disease,
    anginal syndrome.

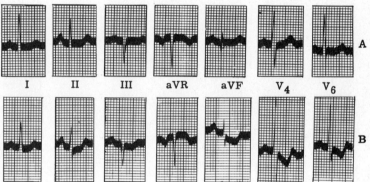

    Spontaneous angina (coronary insufficiency) with T wave changes: If T wave changes do occur, the more common event is inversion of previously upright T waves in left precordial leads and corresponding frontal plane leads (I, aVL). Inverted T waves occasionally become upright during coronary insufficiency. This sudden change is just as indicative of further coronary insufficiency as the former pattern, even though the tracing has a more "normal" appearance.

Spontaneous Angina (Coronary
    Insufficiency).
  A. Taken when patient was free
     of pain. T waves are in-
     verted in V_{3-6}; indicative of
     anterior wall damage; clin-
     ically, the result of an old
     anterior wall infarction.
  B. During episode of angina.
     ST segments are now de-
     pressed, but T waves are
     upright in V_{2-6}. This ab-
     rupt change from an in-
     verted to an upright T is
     just as diagnostic of coro-
     nary insufficiency as the
     more usual reverse pattern.
     The pattern reverted to that
     seen in (A) a few minutes
     after the pain subsided.

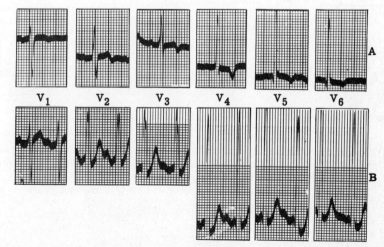

Spontaneous angina with ST elevation: ST segment depression is the most typical pattern in left precordial leads. On rare occasions one may see ST segment elevation during angina. It is thought that the epicardial rather than the subendocardial surface of the heart carries the current of injury or that - as has been suggested by recent experimental work (Prinzmetal) - the ST segment elevation results from severe myocardial anoxia (in contrast to the more usual ST segment depression associated with angina resulting from a lesser degree of myocardial anoxia). In this situation a cavity lead and epicardial leads 180° from the area of myocardial anoxia will show reciprocal ST segment depression.

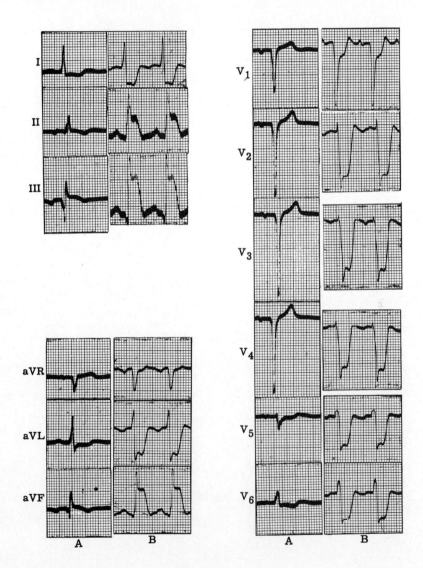

Spontaneous Angina.
  A. Tracing of a patient with old anterior and inferior wall infarction. The rhythm is A-V nodal. *
  B. This tracing was taken during an episode of substernal pain. There is very marked ST segment elevation in II, III (12 mm.), and aVF. This is most consistent with early inferior wall infarction. However, 12 hours after this tracing, the electrocardiogram was the same as (A) and remained so for several weeks. Therefore these marked changes were the result of myocardial anoxia of the inferior wall. Marked reciprocal ST depression is seen in I, aVL, and all precordial leads (16 mm. in V₃). The rhythm is now regular sinus. (Alternating current interference is present in II and III.)

*A-V nodal rhythm is discussed on p. 233.

EXERCISE TESTS

Since the electrocardiogram is normal in 25 to 40% of patients with angina, exercise tests have been devised to produce myocardial anoxia. It is to be emphasized that the electrocardiographic findings must be used in conjunction with the clinical findings for proper evaluation of the patient.

Master's Test:

One of the commonly used tests is the "two-step" exercise test devised by Master. Two steps are used, each nine inches high, eight to ten inches deep, and 18 to 27 inches wide. A resting electrocardiogram is taken first. One trip consists of ascent up one side of the steps and descent down the other. The patient is then instructed to walk up and down the steps for a definite number of trips in one and one-half minutes. The number of trips is determined by Master's tables, the variables being the patient's age, sex, and weight (see p. 147). An electrocardiogram is **rapidly** taken immediately after the exercise and, if abnormal, may be repeated at intervals of several minutes to determine the duration of the abnormality. Master's criteria for a positive (i.e., abnormal) two-step test are: (1) ST segment depression of more than 0.5 mm. (the isoelectric line is taken to be the level of the PR segment and not the TP level); (2) the change from an upright T to a flat or inverted T in any lead except lead III or the change from an inverted T to a flat or upright T; and (3) the appearance of cardiac arrhythmias which were not present in the pre-exercise tracing.

Since the electrocardiogram may remain normal in a patient with angina after the two-step test, Master has devised the double two-step test. This should only be done if the single two-step electrocardiogram is normal. It should not be done within one hour of the single two-step test. The patient performs this test by walking double the number of trips of the single test in three minutes. The criteria for a positive double two-step test are the same as for the single test.

Other Tests:

Many other authorities feel that it is impossible to standardize a biologic experiment as is done by Master. It is felt that electrocardiographic findings do not depend on age, sex, and weight but on the condition of the coronary arteries. The type and amount of exercise should depend upon the physician's evaluation of the patient. The patient who complains of chest pain on slight exertion may develop electrocardiographic changes by sitting up and lying down a few times. The patient who has pain only with strenuous exertion may require much more effort to produce electrocardiographic changes. The exercise should not be continued until the patient has pain since there is no necessary correlation between the occurrence of chest pain and the degree of electrocardiographic changes. It is therefore wise to have the patient first perform mild exercise; if the electrocardiogram is normal, more strenuous exercise is then permitted. Standardized treadmill tests, in which speed and inclination can be controlled, are becoming increasingly popular.

All of these exercise tests routinely record the electrocardiogram immediately after exercise and at various intervals thereafter. Some authorities advise the recording of the electrocardiogram during exercise, claiming a higher yield of positive response. However, current data do not provide conclusive evidence for the diagnostic superiority of this latter technic.

Author's Criteria:

Since some normal individuals show changes after exercise (see p. 149), one must be exceedingly cautious in the clinical interpretation of the results. The most significant criterion for a positive test is ST depression of 1 mm. or more in any precordial lead (V_{3-6}) or aVL or aVF. (The author prefers to take leads V_{3-6}, aVR, aVL, and aVF, in that sequence, in the post-exercise record. This allows for speed and is sufficient for evaluation.) The ST depression must have a duration of 0.06-0.08 sec. or more and be inscribed horizontally or obliquely downward. Of lesser diagnostic significance is a change from an upright to a flat or inverted T wave, or the reverse, in any lead. The appearance of an arrhythmia is of questionable diagnostic significance.

Indications for the Exercise Test:
  A. The major indication for the exercise test is a situation wherein the physician is uncertain of the diagnosis of coronary artery disease and the resting electrocardiogram is normal.
  B. It has also been used in the military service and in industry as a screening test for coronary artery disease.

Contraindications to the Exercise Test:
  An exercise test should not be done in the following circumstances:
  A. When acute myocardial infarction is suspected.
  B. When there is unequivocal evidence of organic heart disease in the presence of a normal rest-

STANDARD NUMBER OF ASCENTS FOR MALES*

Weight (lb.)	Age in Years												
	5–9	10–14	15–19	20–24	25–29	30–34	35–39	40–44	45–49	50–54	55–59	60–64	65–69
40–49	35	36											
50–59	33	35	32										
60–69	31	33	31										
70–79	28	32	30										
80–89	26	30	29	29	29	28	27	27	26	25	25	24	23
90–99	24	29	28	28	28	27	27	26	25	25	24	23	22
100–109	22	27	27	28	28	27	26	25	25	24	23	22	22
110–119	20	26	26	27	27	26	25	25	24	23	23	22	21
120–129	18	24	25	26	27	26	25	24	23	23	22	21	20
130–139	16	23	24	25	26	25	24	23	23	22	21	20	20
140–149		21	23	24	25	24	24	23	22	21	20	20	19
150–159		20	22	24	25	24	23	22	21	20	20	19	18
160–169		18	21	23	24	23	22	22	21	20	19	18	18
170–179			20	22	23	23	22	21	20	19	18	18	17
180–189			19	21	23	22	21	20	19	19	18	17	16
190–199			18	20	22	21	21	20	19	18	17	16	15
200–209				19	21	21	20	19	18	17	16	16	15
210–219				18	21	20	19	18	17	17	16	15	14
220–229				17	20	20	19	18	17	16	15	14	13

STANDARD NUMBER OF ASCENTS FOR FEMALES*

Weight (lb.)	Age in Years												
	5–9	10–14	15–19	20–24	25–29	30–24	35–39	40–44	45–49	50–54	55–59	60–64	65–69
40–49	35	35	33										
50–59	33	33	32										
60–69	31	32	30										
70–79	28	30	29										
80–89	26	28	28	28	28	27	26	24	23	22	21	21	20
90–99	24	27	26	27	26	25	24	23	22	22	21	20	19
100–109	22	25	25	26	26	25	24	23	22	21	20	19	18
110–119	20	23	23	25	25	24	23	22	21	20	19	18	18
120–129	18	22	22	24	24	23	22	21	20	19	19	18	17
130–139	16	20	20	23	23	22	21	20	19	19	18	17	16
140–149		18	19	22	22	21	20	19	19	18	17	16	16
150–159		17	17	21	20	20	19	19	18	17	16	16	15
160–169		15	16	20	19	19	18	18	17	16	16	15	14
170–179		13	14	19	18	18	17	17	16	16	15	14	13
180–189			13	18	17	17	17	16	16	15	14	14	13
190–199			12	17	16	16	16	15	15	14	13	13	12
200–209				16	15	15	15	14	14	13	13	12	11
210–219				15	14	14	14	13	13	13	12	11	11
220–229				14	13	13	13	13	12	12	11	11	10

*From A. M. Master: Exercise Tests (Am. Heart J. **10**:497, 1935).   Reproduced with permission.

ing electrocardiogram.   Valid exception to this may be the evaluation of the patient for cardiac surgery or for rehabilitation.

C. When the resting electrocardiogram is abnormal.   An additional exception to those under B. above occurs when the clinical evaluation suggests that the "abnormality" does not indicate heart disease.

D. When the patient is on digitalis therapy or is hypokalemic.   Under these conditions the appearance of the ST changes after exercise described above are not necessarily indicative of myocardial anoxia.

E. When the electrocardiogram demonstrates ventricular hypertrophy.   Diagnostic changes may appear that indicate myocardial anoxia but do not prove the existence of coronary artery disease.

F. When a W-P-W rhythm is present (see p. 258).   Clinically normal individuals with this electrocardiographic finding may develop, after exercise, significant ST depression that is not indicative of myocardial ischemia.

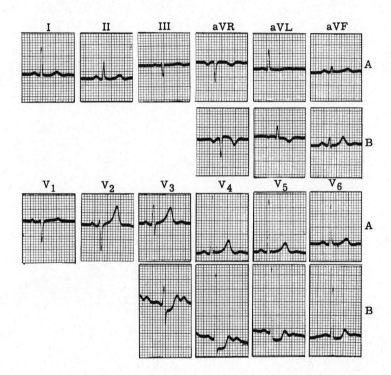

Effect of Exercise (Induced Myocardial Anoxia).

A. Taken when patient was free of pain.   The only suggestive abnormality is a flat T wave in aVL.

B. Taken after a standard Master's exercise test.   (It is the author's policy to omit standard leads and V_{1-2} in the post-exercise tracing.)   There is minimal ST elevation in aVR, and slight ST depression with T wave inversion in aVL.   The most striking changes are seen in the precordial leads: there is 2 mm. ST depression in V_3 and V_5; 3.5 mm. in V_4; 1 mm. in V_6.   **Clinical Diagnosis:** Arteriosclerotic heart disease; anginal syndrome.

ANEMIA

Any anemia (pernicious anemia, anemia resulting from gastrointestinal hemorrhage, etc.) can result in an electrocardiographic pattern of myocardial anoxia, but this usually does not occur in a "normal" heart subjected to anemia. When it is seen in the absence of clinical evidence of heart disease, it usually indicates that there is some degree of subclinical heart disease. In such instances the electrocardiogram becomes normal when the anemia is corrected.

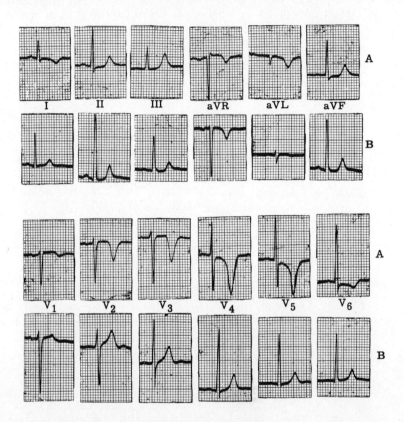

Anemia.
  A. Tracing of a 55-year-old male with pernicious anemia; RBC = 1.0 million. Note the very deep and symmetrically inverted T waves in the precordial leads with a lesser degree of T wave inversion in leads I and aVL. This pattern is quite consistent with myocardial infarction (? subendocardial). Clinically, however, this patient had no evidence of heart disease.
  B. Taken ten days after A. The patient had received blood transfusions and vitamin B_{12}; RBC = 4.0 million. The present tracing is within normal limits. Several subsequent tracings remained normal.

The above pattern in (A) is an extreme and unusual pattern of myocardial anoxia. Actual myocardial infarction was initially suspected, but the lack of clinical evidence of heart disease and the reversal to a normal pattern in ten days favor a diagnosis of myocardial anoxia.

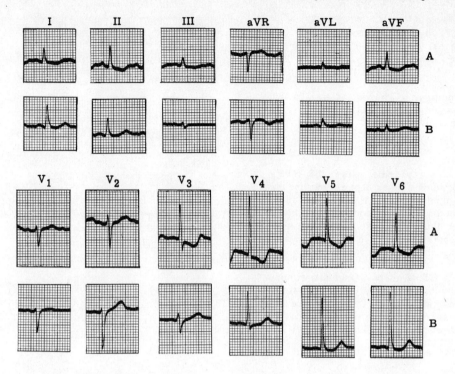

Anemia.

A. Tracing of a 50-year-old male with massive gastrointestinal hemorrhage from a bleeding duodenal ulcer. RBC = 1.2 million. There is ST depression in leads aVF and V_{3-6}. Such a pattern is consistent with but by no means diagnostic of myocardial anoxia, since other conditions can produce a similar pattern. Clinically there was no evidence of heart disease. The patient was not in shock at the time of this record.

B. Taken three days after A; patient had received blood transfusions; RBC = 3.5 million. Slight ST depression persists in V_{4-6}, but marked improvement has occurred.

PSEUDODEPRESSION VS. CORONARY ST DEPRESSION

Some normal individuals will show ST segment depression in either a resting or post-exercise electrocardiogram. This is usually associated with tachycardia or anxiety (see p. 88). The presence of a prominent T_a wave explains this electrocardiographic finding. The T_a wave persists through ventricular depolarization and is still evident after the QRS complex, thereby producing pseudodepression of the ST segment. This latter pattern can be distinguished from true ST segment depression by the contour of the ST segment. In pseudodepression associated with tachycardia and an exaggerated T_a wave, the ST segment displays a continuous ascent with upward concavity. In true ST segment depression associated with myocardial anoxia the ST segment assumes a horizontal or sagging depression.

Pseudodepression vs. Coronary Type of ST Segment Depression.

A. Normal tracing; rate = 92; ST segment iso-electric.

B. Prominent T_a waves; rate = 100; ST segment is iso-electric, being on the same level as the T-P segment.

C. Sinus tachycardia; rate = 168; ST segments appear depressed, but the ST segment displays a continuous ascent with upward concavity. This is typical of the pseudodepression associated with tachycardia and an exaggerated T_a wave.

D. True ST segment depression associated with myocardial anoxia (post-exercise record); the contour of the ST segment is that of horizontal depression.

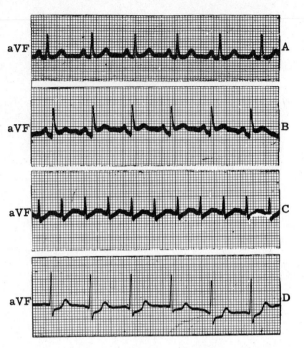

SUMMARY OF ELECTROCARDIOGRAPHIC CRITERIA OF MYOCARDIAL ANOXIA
(E.g., Coronary Insufficiency, Angina)

A. Precordial Leads: ST segment depression and/or T wave inversion in left precordial leads (V_{4-6}).

B. Extremity Leads: Changes similar to those described in precordial leads are seen in aVL or aVF (depending upon the direction of the frontal plane vector).
   Reciprocal ST segment elevation may be seen in aVR.

C. Standard Leads (Not Shown): These will reflect the pattern present in the extremity leads. If the changes mentioned above are seen in aVL, they will be present in I; if seen in aVF, they will be present in III.

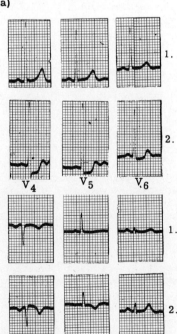

The above changes seen in any single electrocardiogram are not diagnostic of coronary insufficiency. The sudden change from a normal tracing to the above pattern, or the reverse, in association with clinical evidence of angina, is necessary for correct evaluation.

1. Resting electrocardiogram.
2. During spontaneous angina or after exercise.

Chapter 11

CORONARY ARTERY DISEASE:
MYOCARDIAL INFARCTION

Myocardial infarction is characterized by the necrosis of a portion of the myocardium resulting from a lack of sufficient blood supply to keep the muscle viable.

Etiology and Incidence:

The same conditions which produce coronary insufficiency (myocardial anoxia) can produce myocardial infarction. The most common cause is complete occlusion of a coronary artery by arteriosclerotic coronary thrombosis. However, infarction may result from incomplete occlusion of a coronary artery if this latter process sufficiently reduces the blood supply to that portion of the myocardium and if collateral circulation is insufficient. Furthermore, complete thrombosis of a coronary artery can occur without myocardial infarction if a sufficient collateral circulation already exists. Hence the terms myocardial infarction and coronary thrombosis are not synonymous. The left ventricle is involved in practically all instances of myocardial infarction. Uncommonly, the right ventricle may become infarcted in association with left ventricular infarction. Isolated right ventricular infarction is extremely rare.

Differential Diagnosis:

The electrocardiographic differential diagnosis is discussed on pp. 190 to 196. Clinically, the diagnosis of myocardial infarction must be differentiated from many disease processes which occur within the thorax and abdomen, e.g., pulmonary embolism, hiatus hernia, dissecting aneurysm, thoracic radiculitis, and diseases of the biliary tract, upper gastrointestinal tract, and pancreas.

Clinical Significance:

The diagnosis of myocardial infarction must never rest solely upon electrocardiographic findings. The electrocardiogram may actually be normal in myocardial infarction or may merely show nonspecific changes which are not diagnostic of infarction. It is frequently necessary to take serial electrocardiograms to show progressive changes. More than the usual 12 leads may be necessary to demonstrate the pattern.

Of the greatest importance is the fact that the electrocardiogram must be used in conjunction with the clinical findings. If the history, physical examination, and other laboratory data (white blood cell count, sedimentation rate, serum transaminase) strongly indicate myocardial infarction, the diagnosis must not be discarded merely because the infarct cannot be diagnosed by the electrocardiogram.

Prognosis:

In general an uncomplicated inferior (or posterior) wall infarction has a less serious immediate prognosis than an anterior wall infarction. However, the location and "size" of the infarct as interpreted from the electrocardiogram must not be used alone in evaluating the immediate prognosis. A "small" infarct can be fatal, and a patient with a "large" infarct may have an entirely uneventful course.

In the long-term follow-up of the patient, the electrocardiogram should not be relied upon as the sole method of evaluation. Naturally a stable electrocardiogram is a favorable sign. However, even if the electrocardiogram reverts to normal, neither the physician nor the patient should be lulled into believing that the heart is "normal."

151

A sudden change of previously inverted T waves to more ''normally'' upright T waves usually means further coronary insufficiency rather than improvement.

MECHANISM OF THE ELECTROCARDIOGRAPHIC PATTERN

THE ABNORMAL Q WAVE AND THE QS COMPLEX

The most characteristic electrocardiographic finding in infarction is an abnormal Q (negative) wave. In order to understand the genesis of this Q wave, one must understand the normal depolarization patterns of the left ventricular cavity and the left ventricular epicardium, and the left ventricular intramural potentials at varying depths. The patterns of the left ventricle will be illustrated, since the great majority of infarctions involve the left ventricle rather than the right.

The normal left ventricular cavity and left ventricular epicardial complexes have already been discussed. The former produces a QS complex and the latter a qR complex. Intramural complexes have only recently been described. Ventricular depolarization throughout the endocardial half of the myocardium produces QS complexes which are exactly like normal cavity complexes. These QS complexes are believed to result from rapid activation of this inner layer of the myocardium at a speed too rapid to be recorded by the electrocardiogram. Activation of the outer (epicardial) half of the myocardium occurs at a slower rate, producing a gradually increasing R wave as the epicardial surface is approached.

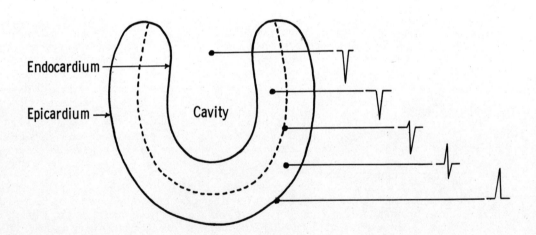

Normal depolarization complexes of the left ventricular myocardium from the cavity through the myocardium to the epicardial surface. These records are obtained by needle electrodes.

QRS PATTERNS OF INFARCTION

Infarction of the Endocardial Layer:

Infarction occurring only in the endocardial half the left ventricle will not produce an abnormal Q wave in an overlying epicardial lead. This is apparent since this portion of the myocardium is "electrocardiographically silent" even under normal circumstances. Because the epicardial half is not involved, a normal epicardial complex will be found (see p. 182).

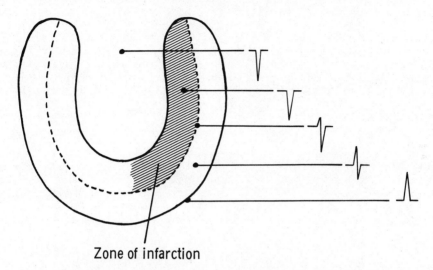

Zone of infarction

Infarction of the Endocardial Half of the Myocardium. The complexes are the same as normally seen, since this area is "electrocardiographically silent."

Infarction of the Epicardial Layer:

If the entire epicardial half of the myocardium is completely infarcted it cannot produce any electrical activity. Therefore the normal negative cavity and endocardial potentials (QS) will be transmitted to the surface and an epicardial lead will record a QS.

Clinically this is a rare occurrence.

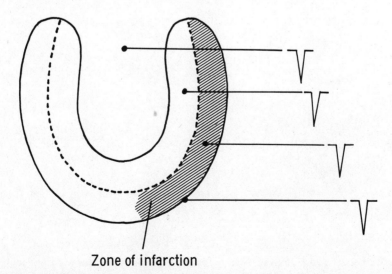

Zone of infarction

Infarction of Epicardial Half of Myocardium. Similar QS complexes are present in cavity, intramural, and epicardial leads.

Complete Transmural Infarction:

If the entire thickness of the myocardium is infarcted, an epicardial lead will record a QS (negative) complex, as in epicardial infarction.

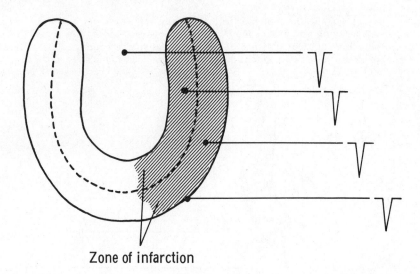

Zone of infarction

Transmural Infarction. QS complexes are present in cavity, intramural and epicardial leads.

"Incomplete" Transmural or Epicardial Infarction:

If some viable muscle fibers remain in the area of infarction, the QS complex can be altered. Depending upon the amount of living (and hence electrically active) muscle remaining, epicardial leads may record notched or slurred QS complexes, and as more living muscle is present the pattern may become a Qr, QR, rS or only an r.   These areas of living muscle must be within the epicardial half of the myocardium to be recorded, since their presence within the "silent" endocardial half would have no effect upon the electrocardiogram.

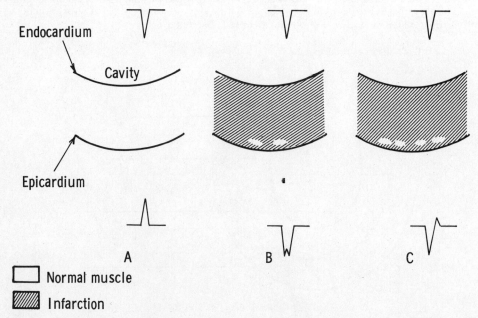

Normal muscle

Infarction

Alterations in the Epicardial Complex With Increasing Amounts of Remaining Viable Muscle.
A: Normal; B-E: Increasing amounts of viable muscle in epicardial area. (D and E are shown on next page.)

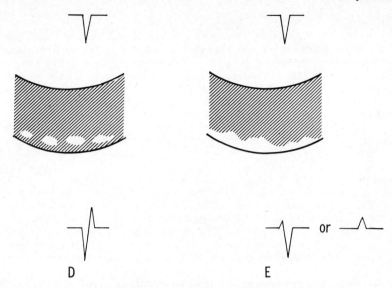

D   E

Alterations in the Epicardial Complex With Increasing Amounts of Remaining Viable Muscle.
(Cont'd. from previous page.) Note that no abnormal Q wave is seen when the epicardial musculature is intact.

Pattern Bordering an Area of Transmural (or Epicardial) Infarction:
As mentioned earlier, any lead in routine electrocardiographic practice is taken at some distance from the heart. It does not record the potential from any one point of the heart but records all of the events of the cardiac cycle as viewed from that lead site. Therefore, any such lead taken near an area of infarction can record a "summation" of the infarction pattern and the pattern of the remaining noninfarcted muscle. Such complexes may be Qr, QR, or qR.

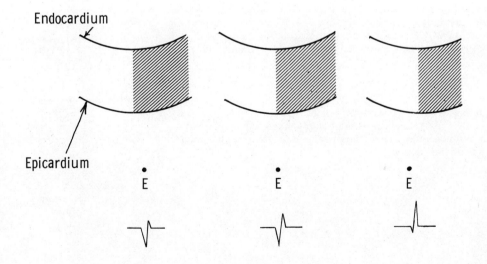

Summation of Infarction and Normal Patterns

Summary:

From the foregoing discussion it can be seen that subendocardial infarction does not produce an abnormal Q wave or QS complex (see p. 182, note). Epicardial infarction per se is probably a rare clinical entity. Transmural infarction, if complete, will produce a QS complex. If viable muscle is present the QS may be notched or slurred, or Qr or qR complexes may be seen. These Q (or q) waves will be abnormal. The important criterion of an abnormal Q wave is that its duration must be 0.04 sec. or greater. Of slightly less significance is its depth, 25% or more of the R wave in the same complex (provided the R wave itself exceeds 5 mm.) being considered abnormal. If enough viable muscle is present in the epicardial layer, no abnormal Q waves will be seen. Instead the R wave will be of reduced voltage, producing an rS complex or r wave.

Vector Analysis:

The alterations in the QRS vector resulting from transmural infarction are as follows:

A. The QRS vector, and especially the initial 0.04 sec., is abnormally directed, pointing away from the zone of infarction. Thus in anterior wall infarction the vector is directed posteriorly; in posterior wall infarction it is directed anteriorly; in inferior wall infarction it is directed superiorly; and in lateral (left) wall infarction it is directed to the right. This produces the abnormal Q wave or QS complex in the electrocardiogram.

B. This abnormally directed QRS vector is at least 0.04 sec. in duration; for this reason the abnormal Q wave is similarly at least 0.04 sec. in duration.

THE ST SEGMENT CHANGES

A. Most frequently the first electrocardiographic finding in myocardial infarction is ST segment elevation in a lead overlying the area of infarction. The ST segment characteristically has a convex upward curvature.

**Epicardial Lead
Directly Over
Infarct**

B. Cavity leads and leads which are placed approximately 180° from the area of infarction show reciprocal ST segment depression. These changes are analogous to those described for injury currents in the isolated muscle strip. (See p. 140.)

Cavity Lead

It is believed that completely dead muscle cannot produce ST segment changes. Therefore the occurrence of these changes early in infarction indicates the presence of some viable muscle in the epicardial region.

**Epicardial Lead
180° From
Infarct**

THE T WAVE CHANGES

A. After a period of hours or days (up to two weeks), the ST segment returns to the iso-electric line and T wave changes occur. The T wave changes may begin to develop while the ST segments are still deviated. The T waves begin to invert in those leads which showed ST segment elevation.

Over infarct

B. The typical infarction T wave is abnormally symmetrical, i.e., the peak of the T is midway between the beginning and the end.

Over infarct

C. In leads which showed ST segment depression, the T waves become tall and are likewise symmetrical.

180° from infarct

D. The "coronary T" or "Pardee T" refers to an inverted T wave in which the ST segment is iso-electric but shows an upward convexity.

E. The "cove-plane T" refers to an elevated ST segment with upward convexity followed by an inverted T

The T waves may remain inverted for the remainder of the patient's life, or after many months the T waves may gradually revert to normal.

The abnormal Q waves may appear very early or late. They are usually not seen within the first few hours following an infarction. They may appear at any time thereafter, being seen while the ST segment changes are present or appearing after the ST segment has become iso-electric. They usually appear before marked T wave changes occur, but this is not invariable. As stated above, abnormal Q waves may never appear; instead there may be reduced voltage of the R wave.

LOCALIZATION OF MYOCARDIAL INFARCTION BY ELECTROCARDIOGRAPHIC PATTERNS

By observing the above infarct patterns in specific leads of the electrocardiogram, one can localize anatomically the site of the infarction. In order to have a clearer understanding of this it will be wise to review briefly the anatomy of the coronary circulation.

The blood supply to the heart is derived from the left and right coronary arteries, which arise from the left and right aortic sinuses, respectively. Shortly after its origin, the left coronary artery divides into the left anterior descending and the left circumflex arteries. The former supplies the anterior surface of the left ventricle, the medial portion of the anterior surface of the right ventricle, and the lower third of the posterior surface of the right ventricle. The remainder of the right ventricle is supplied by the right coronary artery. The left circumflex artery supplies the lateral wall and the lower (apical) half of the posterior wall of the left ventricle. The upper (basal) half of the posterior wall of the left ventricle is supplied by the right coronary artery.

The S-A node is supplied by the right coronary artery in 60 to 75% of individuals. The A-V node is supplied by a branch of the right coronary artery in 90%. Both bundle branches are supplied by branches from both coronary arteries.

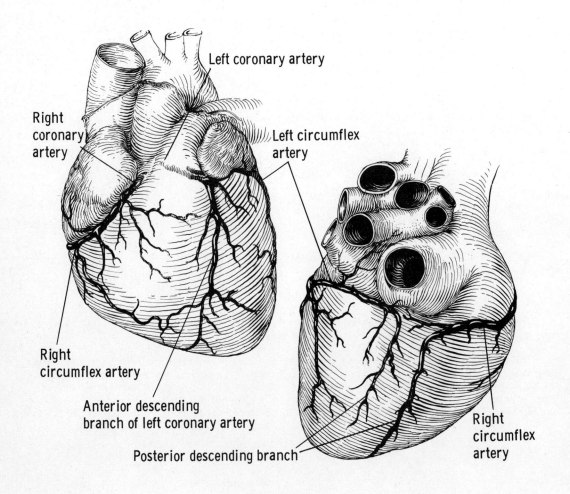

Coronary Circulation

ANTERIOR WALL INFARCTION

Diagrammatic Illustration of Serial Electrocardiographic Patterns in Anterior Infarction:

A. Normal tracing.

B. Very Early Pattern (Hours After Infarction): ST segment elevation in I, aVL, and V_{3-6}; reciprocal ST depression in II, III, and aVF.

C. Later Pattern (Many Hours to a Few Days): Q waves have appeared in I, aVL, and V_{5-6}. QS complexes are present in V_{3-4}. This indicates that the major transmural infarction is underlying the area recorded by V_{3-4}; ST segment changes persist, but are of lesser degree, and the T waves are beginning to invert in those leads in which tne ST segments are elevated.

D. Late Established Pattern (Many Days to Weeks): The Q waves and QS complexes persist; the ST segments are iso-electric; the T waves are symmetrical, and deeply inverted in leads which had ST elevation and tall in leads which had ST depression. This pattern may persist for the remainder of the patient's life.

E. Very Late Pattern: This may occur many months to years after the infarct. The abnormal Q waves and QS complexes persist. The T waves have gradually returned to normal.

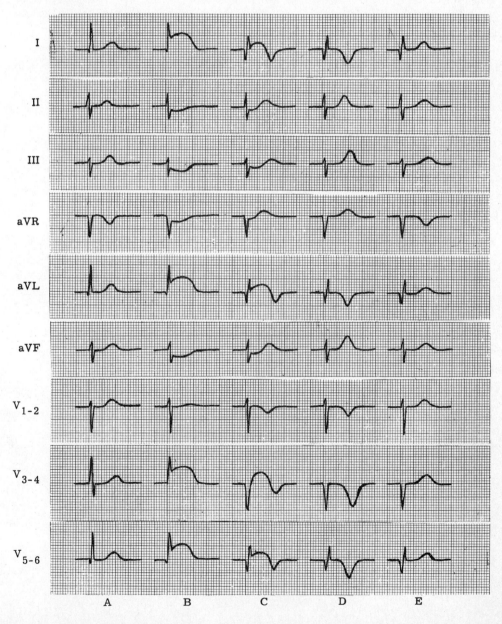

ANTERIOR WALL INFARCTION

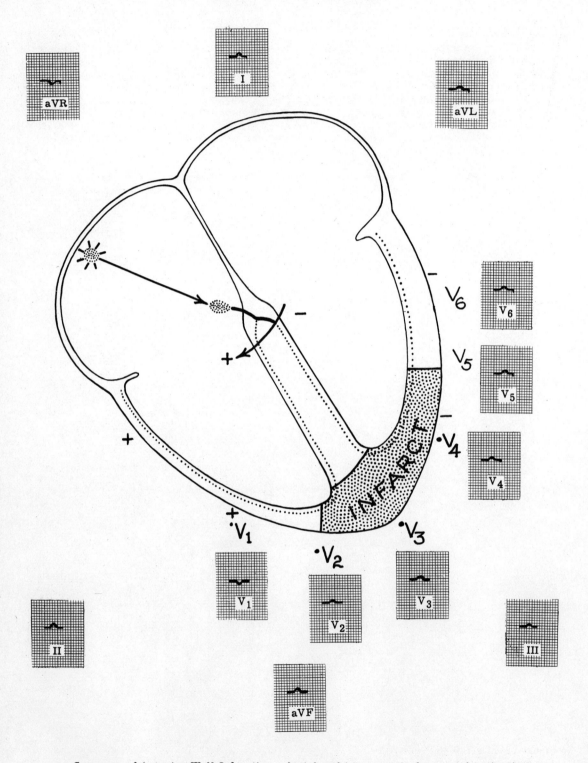

Sequence of Anterior Wall Infarction. Atrial and interventricular septal activation.

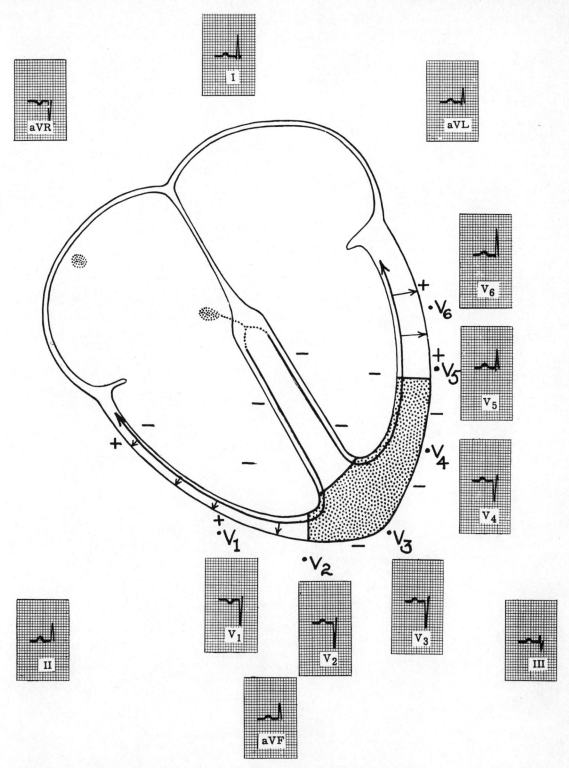

Sequence of Anterior Wall Infarction. Ventricular depolarization. The pattern as illustrated demonstrates an infarct of several days' duration, thus accounting for abnormal Q waves and ST segment and T wave changes. The initial 0.04 sec. QRS vector is oriented posteriorly (as a result of the anterior wall infarct), producing the abnormal Q waves in V_{2-4}.

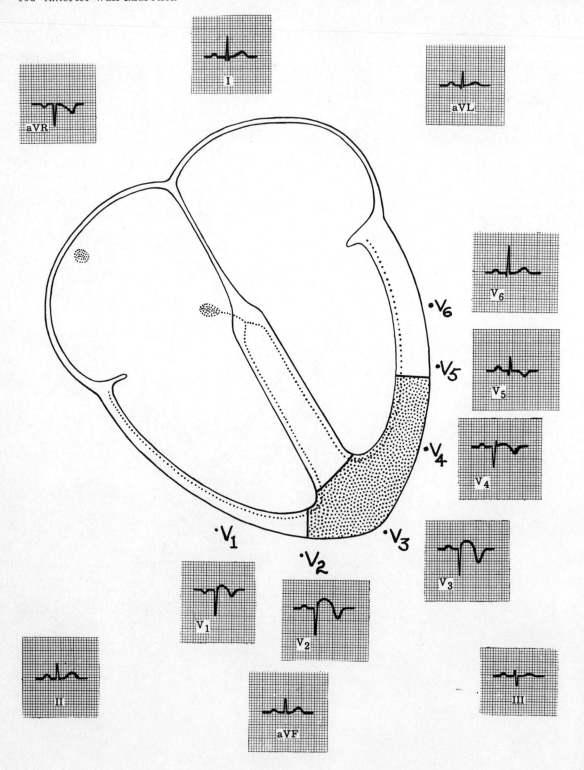

Sequence of Anterior Wall Infarction. Ventricular repolarization.

Early and Late Anterior Wall Infarction:

The precordial leads best reflect infarction of the anterior wall. In frontal plane leads, I and aVL will usually show the infarction pattern. The characteristic findings in transmural infarction involving the entire thickness of the anterior wall will be:

A. Standard Leads: Epicardial infarction pattern (ST elevation → abnormal Q wave and T wave inversion) in I. Lead III may show reciprocal change, most characteristically ST depression.

B. Extremity Leads: The heart position is usually horizontal, and the left ventricular epicardial pattern will therefore be seen in aVL. Lead aVF may show reciprocal ST segment depression and, later, tall T waves.

C. Precordial Leads: Depending upon the extent of the anterior wall infarct, precordial leads from V_1 to V_7 will show the infarct.

D. Vector Analysis: The initial 0.04 sec. QRS vector is directed posteriorly, resulting in abnormal Q waves or QS complexes in precordial leads. If this initial vector is oriented to the right, an abnormal Q wave will be seen in lead I. In the early stage of infarction the ST vector is oriented anteriorly (and to the left), resulting in ST segment elevation in left precordial leads (and lead I). In the later stage the T vector is oriented posteriorly (and to the right), producing inverted T waves in left precordial leads (and lead I).

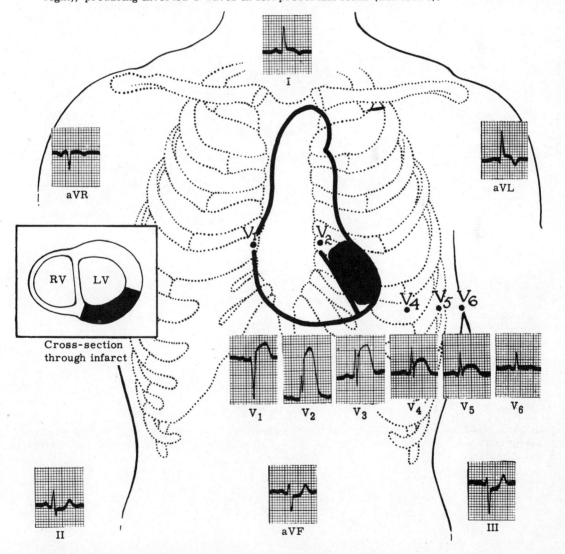

Early Anterior Wall Infarction. Note the marked convex ST segment elevation in leads V_{2-5}; the lesser degree of ST elevation with T wave inversion in I and aVL; the reciprocal ST depression in II, III, and aVF. **Clinical Diagnosis:** Recent (6 hours) myocardial infarction.

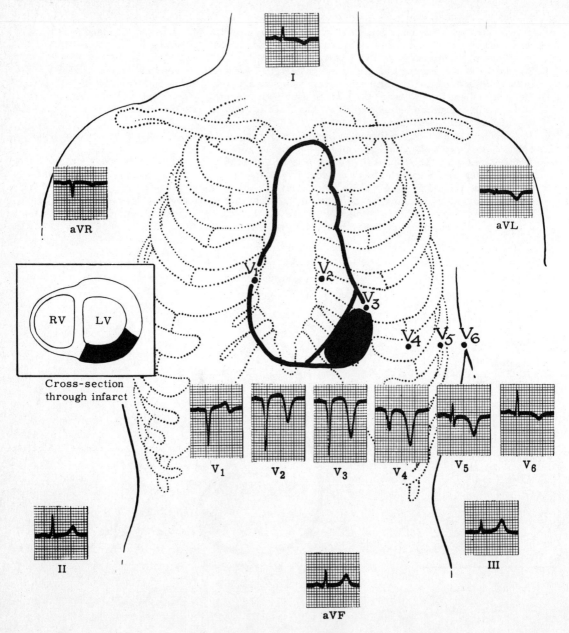

Late Pattern of Anterior Wall Infarction. QS complexes are present in V_{1-4}. The T waves are deeply and symmetrically inverted in I, aVL, V_{2-6}. **Clinical Diagnosis:** Myocardial infarction, six months old.

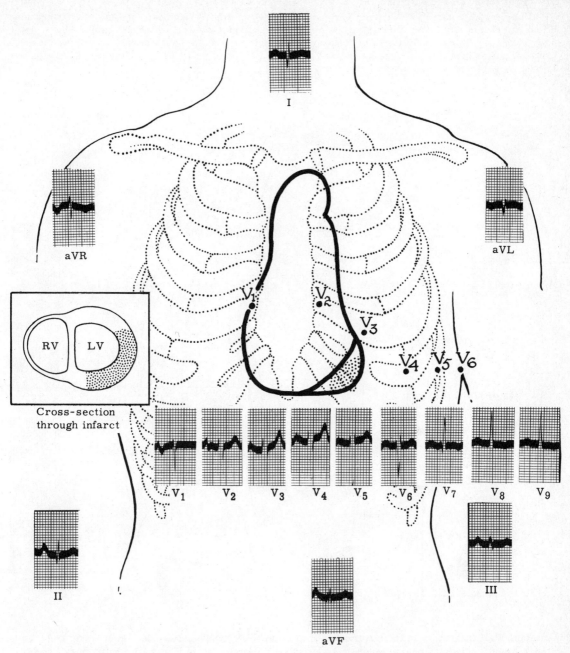

Cross-section
through infarct

Late Pattern of Anterior Wall Infarction. There are no abnormal Q waves in this tracing. Small initial r waves with rsr′ complexes are seen in I, aVL, and V_{5-7}. This record is not diagnostic of infarction. The patient had had a myocardial infarct three years previously. Autopsy revealed extensive old transmural infarction. The initial r waves resulted from small areas of viable muscle in the epicardial layer.

Rarely with anterior wall infarction and a true vertical heart position, the infarct pattern may be reflected into aVF. This will give the appearance of inferior wall infarction (see below). In such an instance one cannot exclude the possibility of both anterior and inferior wall infarction. However, if esophageal leads do not reveal an infarct pattern, one can then consider such a pattern to be only anterior wall infarction.

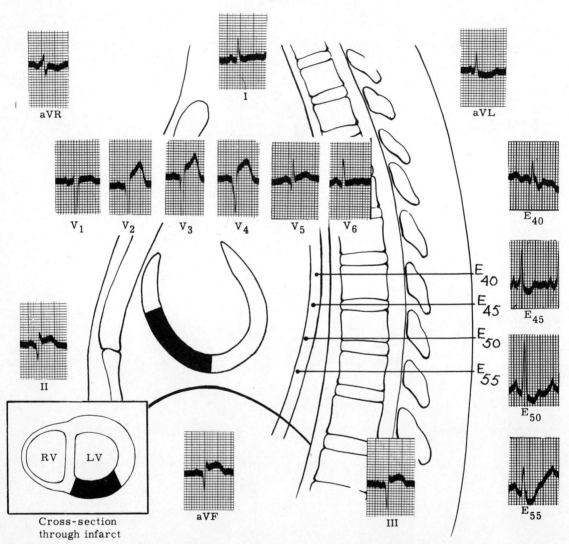

Cross-section through infarct

Anterior Wall Infarction Pattern Reflected into Lead aVF. Standard Leads: There are deep, wide Q waves (producing Qr complexes) with elevated ST segments in II and III. **Extremity Leads:** Deep, wide Q with elevated ST in aVF. The pattern in standard and extremity leads is typical of recent inferior wall infarction. **Precordial Leads:** Normal r in V_1; small r in V_2; QS complexes in V_3 and V_4; qR pattern in V_5. The ST segments are elevated in V_{2-5}. The T waves in these leads are still upright. This pattern definitely indicates recent anterior wall infarction. The above tracing indicates early infarction of the anterior and inferior walls of the left ventricle. **Esophageal Leads:** To further investigate the latter diagnosis, esophageal leads were done. Leads E_{40} through E_{55} show no abnormal Q waves. This definitely indicates the absence of true posterior wall infarction and makes inferior wall infarction unlikely. **Clinical Diagnosis:** Recent myocardial infarction (two days old). **Autopsy Diagnosis:** Recent infarction of anteroseptal and anteroapical surfaces of left ventricle; occlusion of left anterior descending coronary artery; no infarction present on inferior or posterior walls. Thus the patterns in leads II, III, and aVF are a reflection of the anterior wall infarct, probably due to backward displacement of the apex allowing the anterior wall to overlie the left diaphragm.

Anterior Wall Infarction Involving Limited Areas:

Anterior wall infarction can be further subdivided into the following categories:

A. Anteroseptal Infarction: The infarct pattern will be seen in precordial leads V_{1-3}. Since the infarction does not extend to the lateral wall of the left ventricle it will not be reflected into lead aVL; hence the extremity leads and standard leads will not show the infarct pattern.

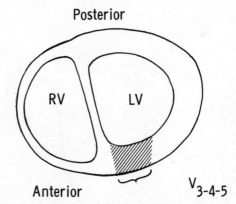

Anteroseptal Infarction

B. Anteroapical Infarction: Precordial leads V_{3-5} will show the infarct pattern. Again this may not be seen in extremity and standard leads.

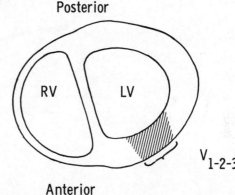

Anteroapical Infarction

C. Anterolateral Infarction: The pattern is seen in precordial leads V_{4-7}. It is reflected into leads aVL and I.

In high anterolateral wall infarction, the usual precordial leads may not show the typical patterns. However, lead aVL usually will reflect the infarct pattern. In such an instance it is necessary to take higher precordial leads (such as third interspace leads) to confirm the pattern seen in aVL.

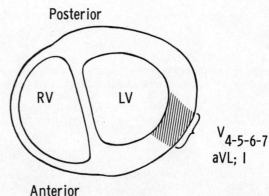

Anterolateral Infarction

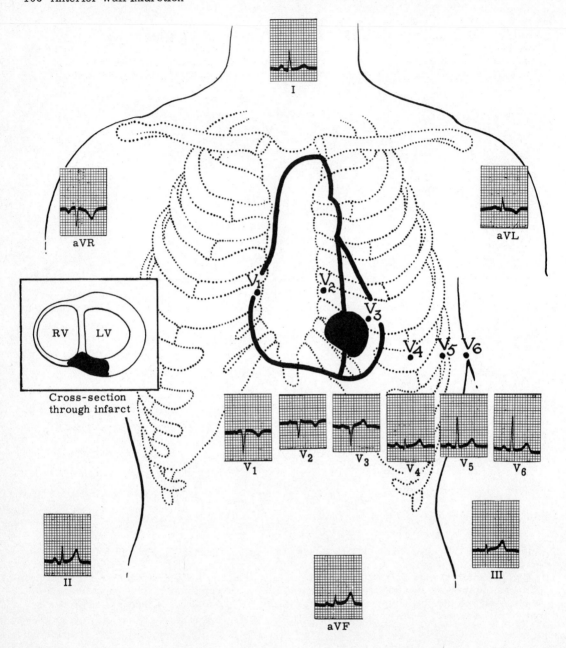

Anteroseptal Infarction (Late Pattern). QS complexes are present in V_{2-3}. The T is inverted in V_{1-2} and aVL. **Clinical and Autopsy Diagnosis:** Anteroseptal infarction, six months old.

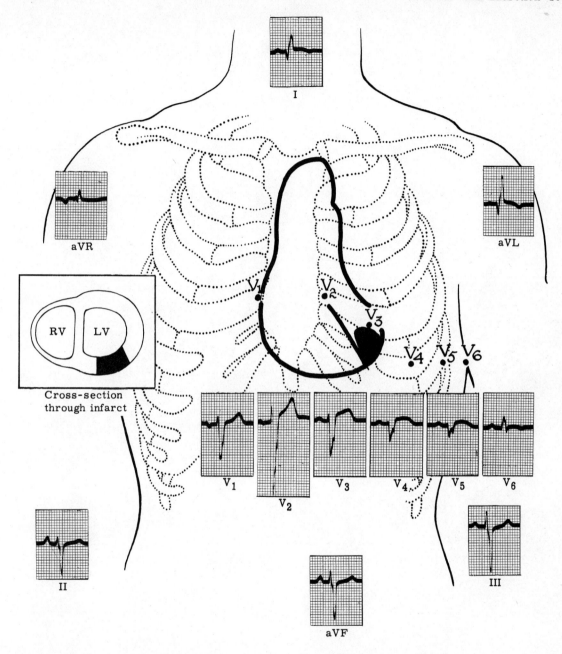

I

aVR

aVL

V₁ V₂ V₃ V₄ V₅ V₆

RV LV

Cross-section
through infarct

V₁ V₂ V₃ V₄ V₅ V₆

II

aVF

III

Anteroapical Myocardial Infarction. Wide Q waves are present in I and aVL; minute r waves are seen in V_{4-5}; the T waves are inverted in I, aVL, and V_6; the ST segments are elevated in I, aVL, and V_{2-5}. **Clinical Diagnosis:** Myocardial infarction, two weeks old.

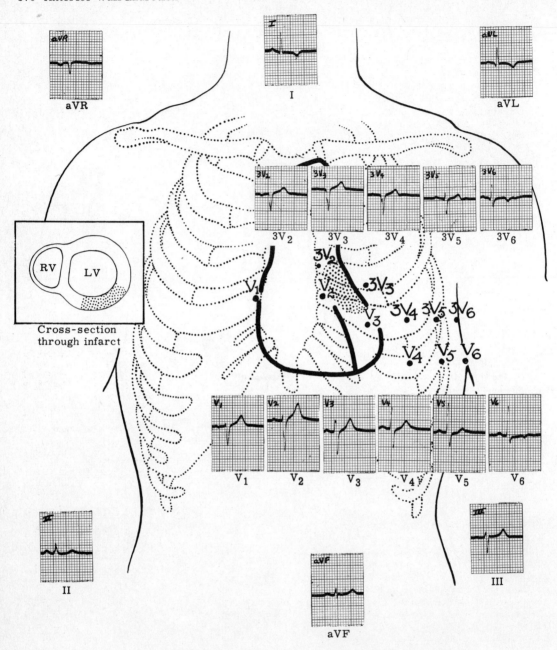

High Anterior and Lateral Wall Infarction. The above illustration shows the value of third inter-space leads. A small, but wide q wave is present in I and aVL. The T waves are inverted in V_6, aVL, and I. The precordial leads are not indicative of infarction. In view of the suspicious pattern in aVL, third interspace leads were taken, revealing QS complexes in $3V_{2-4}$. **Clinical Diagnosis:** Arteriosclerotic heart disease; history of myocardial infarction one year previously.

SUMMARY OF ELECTROCARDIOGRAPHIC CRITERIA
OF ANTERIOR MYOCARDIAL INFARCTION

A. Precordial Leads:
   1. Convex ST segment elevation in more than one lead from V_3 through V_6 (early).
   2. QS complexes or abnormal Q waves (i.e., Q waves of 0.04 sec. or more in width and/or 25% or more of the voltage of the R wave in the same lead) in more than one lead from V_3 through V_6 (late).
   3. T wave inversion (typically deep, symmetrical inversion) in more than one lead from V_3 through V_6 (late).

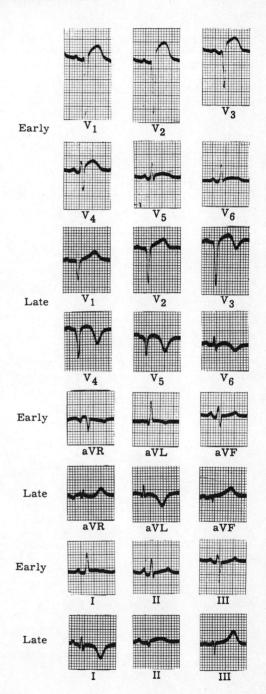

B. Extremity Leads: The pattern described in precordial leads may be seen in aVL if the infarction involves the anterolateral wall (e.g., seen in V_{6-7}).

   A QS complex (vertical heart position) or a QR complex (backward rotation of the heart) may normally be seen in aVL. In these circumstances the P is inverted. The presence of an upright P with a QS or QR complex in aVL, and the presence of normal precordial leads or precordial leads which are not diagnostic of infarction, should make one suspicious of a high anterolateral wall infarction. In this circumstance third interspace precordial leads should be taken.

C. Standard Leads: These reflect the same pattern seen in extremity leads.

POSTERIOR WALL INFARCTION
(And Inferior Wall Infarctions)

In electrocardiography the term posterior wall infarction is used to describe an infarction which anatomically involves the inferior (diaphragmatic) wall and the true posterior wall of the left ventricle.

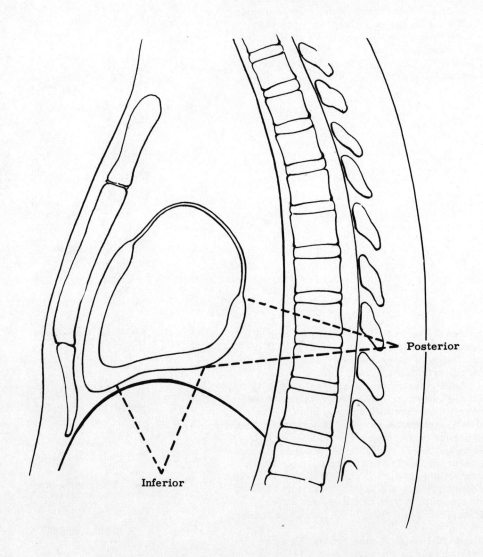

Inferior (Diaphragmatic) and Posterior Locations

Diagrammatic Illustration of Serial Electrocardiographic Pattern in Inferior and Posterior Wall Infarction:

A. Normal tracing.

B. Very Early Pattern (Hours After Infarction): ST segment elevation in II, III, and aVF; ST segment depression in I, aVR, aVL, and all precordial leads.

C. Later Pattern (Many Hours to a Few Days): Abnormal Q waves have appeared in II, III, and aVF. There is less ST segment elevation in these leads and less reciprocal ST segment depression in the leads shown in (B). The T waves are becoming inverted in II, III, and aVF.

D. Late Established Pattern (Many Days to Weeks): The ST segments are now iso-electric. Deep, symmetrically inverted T waves are seen in II, III, and aVF. This is evidence of inferior wall infarction. The T waves are abnormally tall and symmetrical in I, aVL, and precordial leads. These are the reciprocal results of true posterior wall infarction.

E. Very Late Pattern (Many Months to Years): The abnormal Q waves persist, but the T waves have become normal.

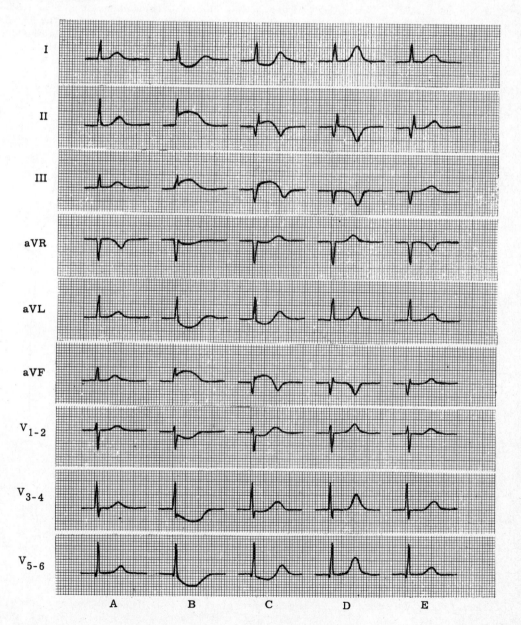

Inferior (Diaphragmatic) Wall Infarction:

   Since this area of infarction overlies the left diaphragm the pattern will be seen in leads aVF, II and III. The characteristic findings of transmural infarction in this area will be:

A. Standard Leads: Infarct pattern in leads II and III. At the time of ST segment elevation in leads II and III, reciprocal ST depression will be seen in lead I. Later, with deep T wave inversion in II and III, the T will become tall in I.

B. Extremity Leads: Infarct pattern in aVF. Similar reciprocal changes in aVL, as seen in lead I.

C. Precordial Leads: Usually the precordial leads are not abnormal. At times they may show reciprocal changes with early ST segment depression and, later, abnormally tall, symmetrical T waves.

D. Vector Analysis: The initial 0.04 sec. QRS vector is directed superiorly, thus producing the abnormal Q wave in leads aVF, II, and III. In the early stage of infarction the ST vector is directed inferiorly, producing ST segment elevation in these leads. In the later stage the T vector is oriented superiorly, resulting in inverted T waves in aVF, II and III.

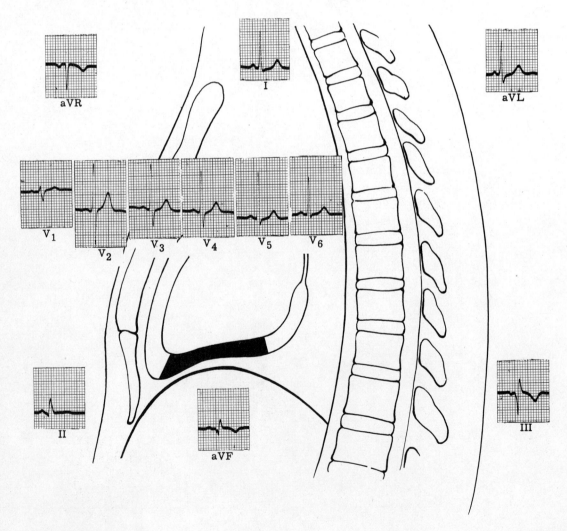

Inferior Wall Infarction. The ST segment is elevated in leads III and aVF; there is reciprocal ST depression in leads I, aVL, and V_{3-5}. Abnormal Q waves are seen in II, III, and aVF. The T wave is inverted in III and aVF. **Clinical Diagnosis:** Myocardial infarction, three weeks old.

(a) Atrial and Interventricular
    Septal Activation

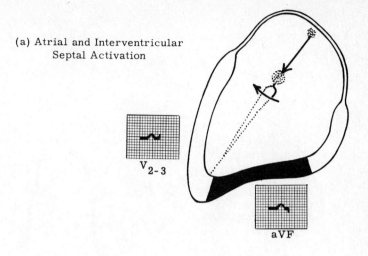

(b) Ventricular De-
    polarization

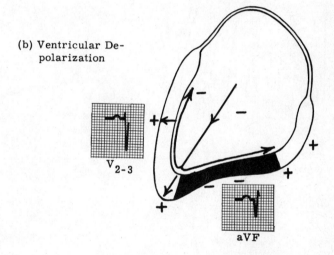

(c) Ventricular Re-
    polarization

Inferior Wall Infarction. The pattern
as illustrated demonstrates an infarct of several days' duration, thus
accounting for the abnormal Q waves
and ST segment and T wave changes.
The initial 0.04 sec. QRS vector is
oriented superiorly (Q in aVF), the
ST vector is oriented inferiorly (ST
elevation in aVF) and posteriorly
(ST depression in V_{2-3}), and the T
vector is oriented superiorly (inverted
T in aVF) and anteriorly (abnormally
tall T in V_{2-3}).

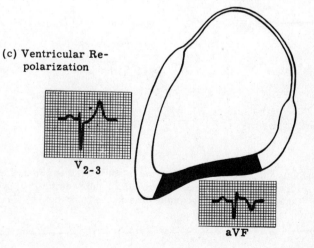

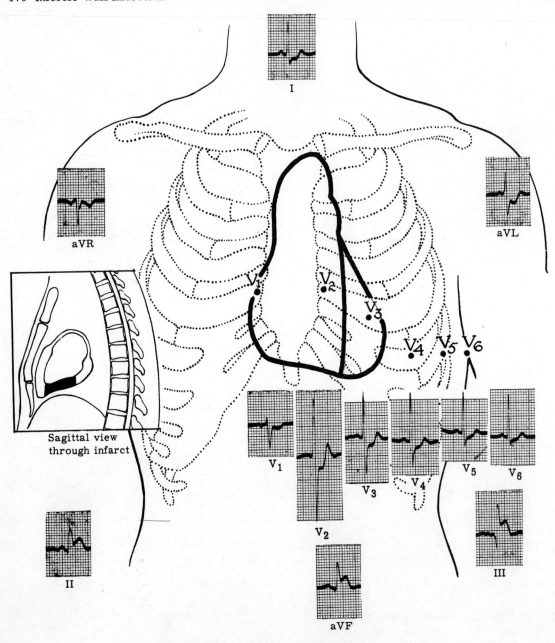

Sagittal view
through infarct

Early Inferior Wall Infarction: Note the ST segment elevation with small but wide q waves in leads II, III, and aVF; the reciprocal ST depression in I, aVL, and precordial leads. **Clinical Diagnosis:** Recent myocardial infarction (four hours).

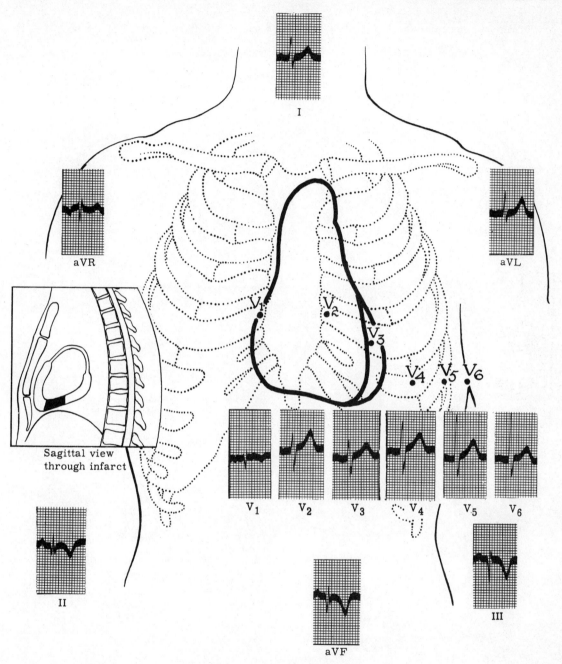

I

aVR

aVL

V$_1$ V$_2$ V$_3$ V$_4$ V$_5$ V$_6$

Sagittal view
through infarct

V$_1$ V$_2$ V$_3$ V$_4$ V$_5$ V$_6$

II

III

aVF

Late Inferior Wall Infarction. Wide Q waves with deeply inverted T waves are present in II, III, and aVF. The precordial leads are normal. The ST segments are iso-electric. **Clinical Diagnosis:** Myocardial infarction, four weeks old.

True Posterior Wall Infarction:

In this instance the infarct is not overlying the diaphragm and hence is not reflected into aVF. Therefore the usual leads (I-III, aVR, aVL, aVF, V_{1-6}) may not show a definite infarct pattern. Posterior chest leads, such as V_{7-9} and $3V_{7-9}$, may reveal the infarct. Esophageal leads will definitely be the most revealing.

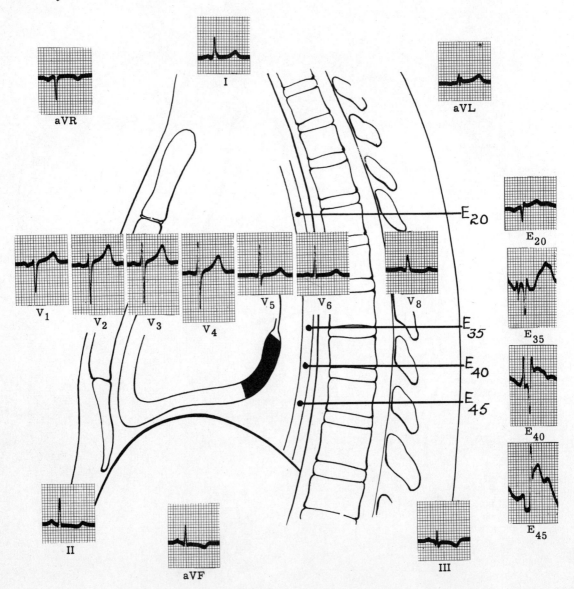

Posterior Wall Infarction Diagnosed by Esophageal Leads. The routine 12-lead electrocardiogram indicates some abnormality of the inferior wall of the left ventricle (inverted T waves in II, III, and aVF), but is not diagnostic of infarction. **Esophageal Leads:** A diphasic P wave is seen at E_{35}, identifying this as the level of the A-V groove. The Qr complex at this level is not necessarily abnormal since this could represent normal cavity potential. At E_{40}, tall upright P waves are seen, indicating a level distal to the A-V groove and therefore indicating that the lead is over the posterior aspect of the left ventricle. In both E_{40} and E_{45} the typical findings of infarction are present: deep Q waves with ST segment elevation. **Clinical Diagnosis:** Myocardial infarction as manifested by typical history and physical findings, including a transitory pericardial friction rub.

Posterior Wall Infarction With Reciprocal Changes:

The reciprocal changes in the precordial leads (as mentioned under inferior wall infarction) may occur and provide a valuable clue to the presence of infarction.

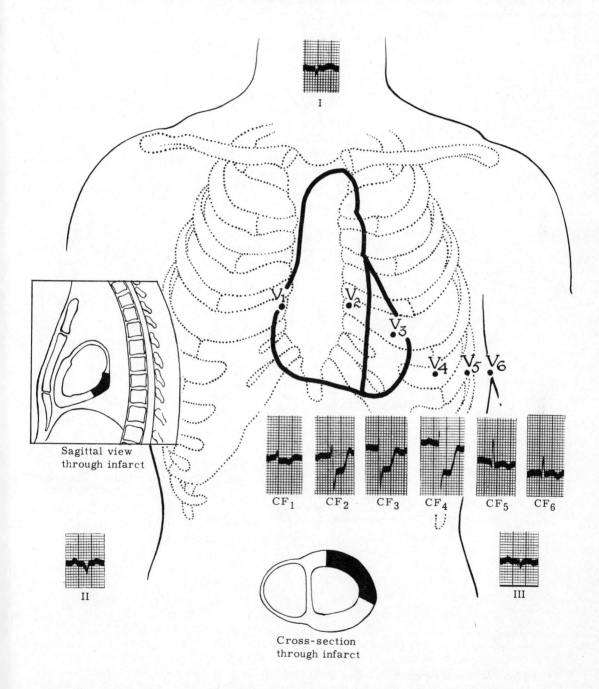

Sagittal view
through infarct

CF₁ CF₂ CF₃ CF₄ CF₅ CF₆

I

II

III

Cross-section
through infarct

Posterior Wall Infarction. This tracing was taken in 1946, which explains the absence of extremity leads and the presence of CF leads. Marked ST depression is seen in CF_{2-4}; the T is inverted in CF_{5-6}; a prominent R is present in CF_1. Since the ST segments are iso-electric in standard leads it can be assumed that the ST segment would be iso-electric in aVF. **Clinical and Autopsy Diagnosis:** Posterior and lateral myocardial infarction.

Inferior and Posterior Lateral Wall Infarction:

The infarct pattern will be seen in leads II, III, aVF, and precordial leads V_{5-8}. A transmural infarct in this area commonly produces changes in right precordial leads (V_{3R}, V_1, V_2) and at times in aVR. Normally the left ventricular potentials are the resultants of activation of the anterior and posterior walls of the left ventricle. If the posterior wall is infarcted, there will be a loss of the normally directed posterior forces and hence an abnormally directed anterior force. This will result in an abnormally tall R wave in the right precordial leads and will simulate the pattern of right ventricular hypertrophy. By vector analysis it can be stated that the initial 0.04 sec. QRS vector is oriented to the right, anteriorly, and superiorly, producing the R waves in V_1 and aVR.

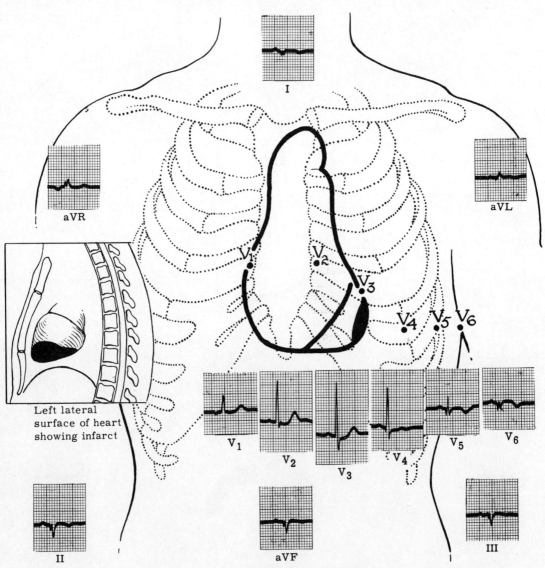

Inferior (and Posterior) Lateral Wall Infarction With Tall R in Right Precordial Leads. Note the infarction pattern in leads I, II, aVF, and V_6 (QS complexes with inverted T waves); tall R waves with ST depression are seen in V_{1-3}; a notched R wave is seen in aVR. The latter findings are a result of inferior and lateral wall infarction and do not indicate right ventricular hypertrophy. **Clinical Diagnosis:** Recent myocardial infarction; no clinical evidence to suggest right ventricular hypertrophy. **Autopsy Diagnosis:** Inferior and lateral wall infarction; normal size right ventricle; occlusion of the left circumflex coronary artery.

SUMMARY OF ELECTROCARDIOGRAPHIC CRITERIA OF
POSTERIOR AND INFERIOR WALL INFARCTION

A. Extremity Leads: Lead aVF is the best lead for determining the presence of inferior wall infarction.
   1. Convex ST segment elevation (early).
   2. The presence of a QS complex or an abnormal Q wave (i.e., a Q wave of 0.04 sec. or more in width and/or 25% or more of the voltage of the R wave in aVF, assuming R = 5 mm. or more). It must be remembered that a QS complex may be a normal finding in aVF in a horizontal heart. In this instance, there must be ST segment and T wave changes in addition to the QS complex in order to interpret the record as that of inferior wall infarction.
   3. T wave inversion occurs later (typically deep and symmetrical inversion).

B. Standard Leads: The pattern similar to aVF is recorded in II and III.

C. Precordial Leads: Usually normal in inferior wall infarction. Early ST segment depression and, later, tall, symmetrical T waves may be seen in leads V_{2-6} as reciprocal changes of the inferior or posterior wall infarction.

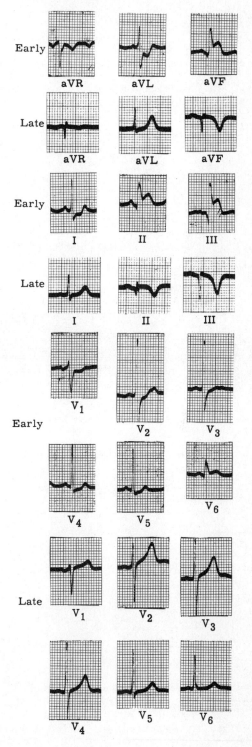

SUBENDOCARDIAL INFARCTION

As stated above, no abnormal Q waves are seen in this type of infarction.* The abnormalities which may be seen in an electrocardiogram are ST segment depression and T wave inversion in leads recorded from the overlying epicardial surface. Reciprocal ST segment elevation and upright T waves will be seen in cavity leads and in epicardial leads recorded from the epicardial surface of the opposite normal myocardium. Thus the pattern in a single electrocardiogram will simulate that seen in myocardial anoxia. However, the latter will be transitory, whereas the former will persist in serial electrocardiograms for weeks or months.

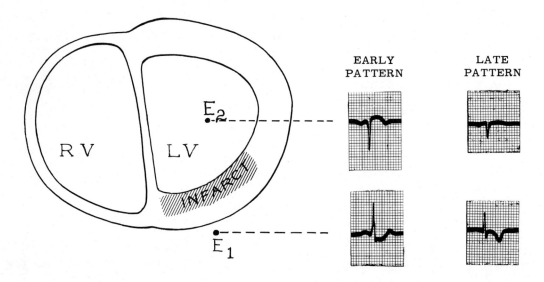

E_1: Left Precordial Lead (e.g., V_{4-6})
E_2: Left Ventricular Cavity Lead (e.g., aVL)

Pattern in Subendocardial Infarction

---

*The concept of an "electrically silent" endocardial layer having a uniform anatomic counterpart throughout the left ventricular wall is subject to revision. These electrically silent endocardial areas are those in which Purkinje fibers penetrate deeply into the myocardium. In those areas of the left ventricle, e.g., the basal portions, where the Purkinje fibers are absent or very scarce, the endocardium will not be electrically silent and will generate an R wave under normal conditions. Thus, endocardial infarction in such an area can produce an abnormal Q wave or QS complex in a surface lead. (See Sodi-Pallares, et al.: Circulation **23**:836, 1961.)

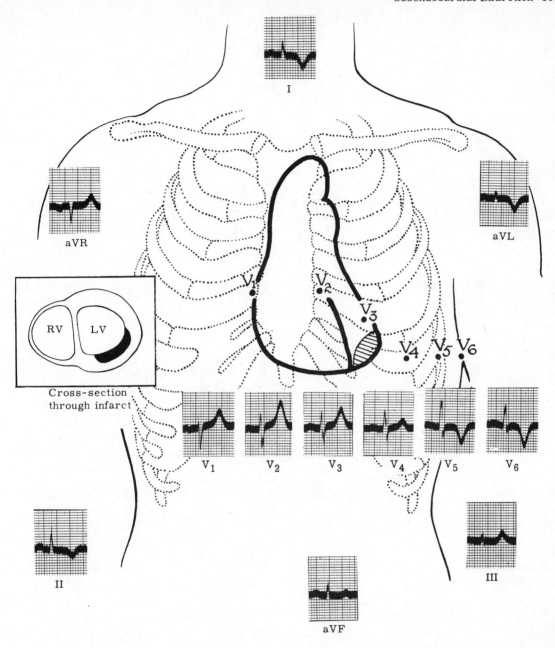

Subendocardial Infarction. Tracing of a 68-year-old man who had suffered a myocardial infarction one month previously. Note the deep, symmetrically inverted T waves in leads I, II, aVL, V_5, and V_6. No abnormal Q waves are seen. Such a pattern in conjunction with the clinical history is consistent with subendocardial infarction involving the anterior and lateral walls of the myocardium. **Autopsy Diagnosis:** Myocardial infarction involving anterior and lateral walls. The area of infarction is not transmural but involves the inner half of the myocardium.

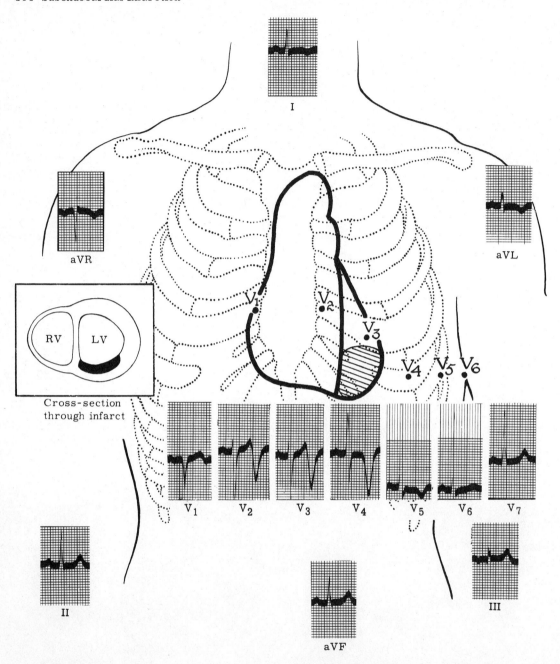

Cross-section through infarct

Subendocardial Infarction. Tracing of a 60-year-old man three weeks after a clinical episode of myocardial infarction. Note the very deep and symmetrically inverted T waves in V_{2-4}, with lesser T wave inversion in V_5, I, and aVL. The above pattern, in conjunction with the clinical history, is consistent with a diagnosis of subendocardial infarction involving the anterior myocardium, with the major area of infarction in the anteroseptal region. **Autopsy Diagnosis:** Anterior wall infarction; the infarction is not transmural but involves the endocardial half of the myocardium. The major area of infarction is anteroseptal.

It must be realized that the preceding classifications are purely arbitrary and that any combination of the above may exist in any one individual.

MULTIPLE INFARCTS

If the electrocardiogram reverts to normal after the initial infarction, a second infarct will produce a pattern as would be expected with initial infarction.

The abnormal Q waves which may persist following the initial infarct (e.g., precordial leads in anterior wall infarction) will not be altered by a second infarct involving the opposite wall (e.g., inferior wall infarction). However, the ST segment elevations which will occur with the second infarct (e.g., in lead aVF in inferior wall infarction) will cause ST segment depression in the area of the initial infarct (e.g., precordial leads in anterior wall infarction). The development of inverted T waves (e.g., in aVF) as a result of the second infarct can cause the previously inverted T waves resulting from the initial infarct (precordial leads) to become upright.

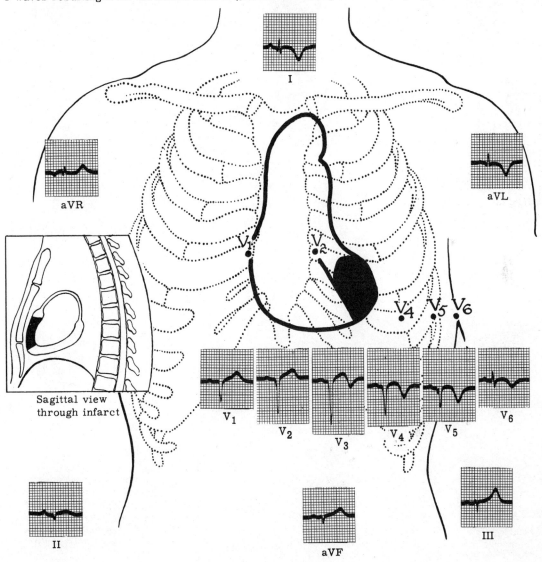

Initial Infarction of Multiple Myocardial Infarctions. There are QS complexes present from V_1 through V_5. The T waves are inverted from V_3 through V_6, I, and aVL. The pattern is indicative of anterior wall infarction. This electrocardiographic pattern was stable for several weeks after the episode of infarction. (See next page.)

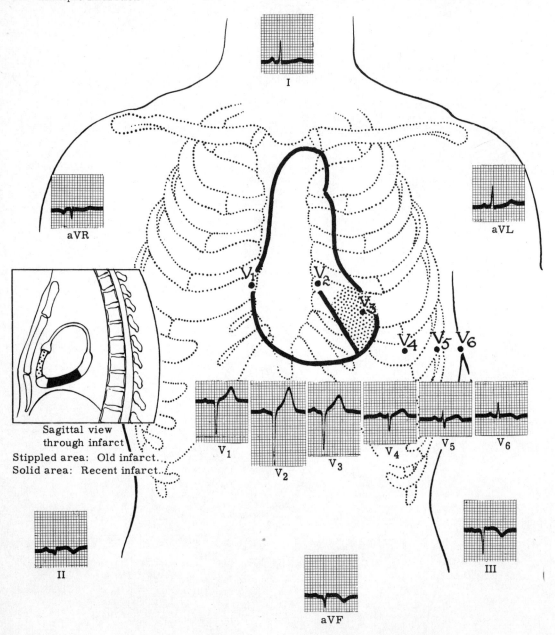

Sagittal view
through infarct
Stippled area: Old infarct.
Solid area: Recent infarct.

Multiple Infarctions. Clinically the patient suffered a second myocardial infarction one month after the tracings on preceding page were taken. A deep Q with inverted T has now appeared in aVF, indicating inferior wall infarction. As a result of this the previously inverted T waves have now become upright in I, aVL, and V_{3-5}.

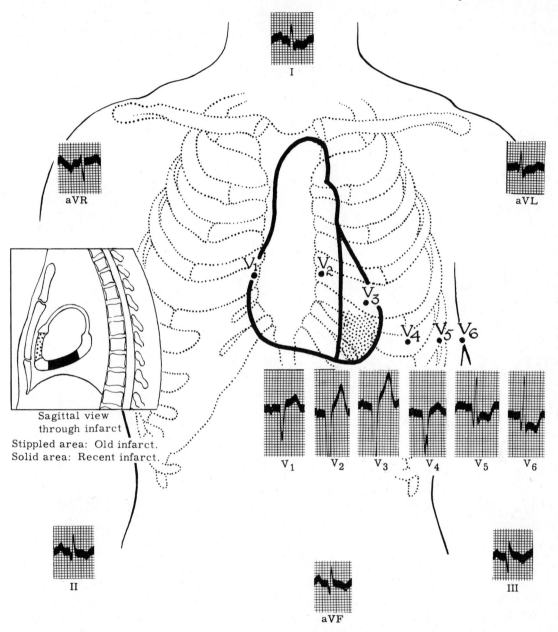

Sagittal view
through infarct
Stippled area: Old infarct.
Solid area: Recent infarct.

Multiple Myocardial Infarctions. The pattern in standard and extremity leads is typical of inferior wall infarction (abnormal Q and T wave inversion in II, III, and aVF). Precordial leads (and I, aVL) indicate anterior wall infarction (QS complexes in V_{2-4}, abnormal Q waves in V_{5-6}, aVL, and I). The ST segment depression in V_{5-6}, I, and aVL suggests reciprocal changes of inferior or posterior wall infarction. **Clinical Diagnosis:** Recent myocardial infarction; old myocardial infarction (by history, ten months previously). **Autopsy Diagnosis:** Old anterior wall infarction; recent inferior and posterior wall infarction; occlusion of left anterior descending and left circumflex arteries.

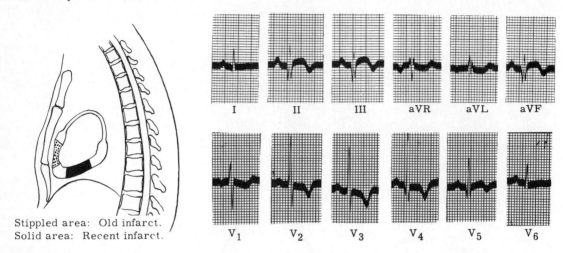

Stippled area: Old infarct.
Solid area: Recent infarct.

Multiple Myocardial Infarctions. The elevated ST segments and inverted T waves in standard and extremity leads (II, III, aVF) are indicative of recent inferior wall infarction. The inverted T waves in V_{2-5} in the precordial leads are indicative of anterior wall infarction; the iso-electric ST segments indicate that this is not as recent as the inferior infarct. **Clinical Diagnosis:** Recent myocardial infarction; old myocardial infarction (by history, one year previously).

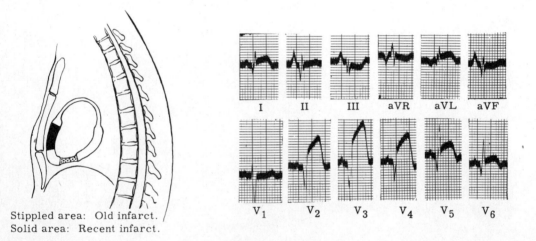

Stippled area: Old infarct.
Solid area: Recent infarct.

Multiple Myocardial Infarctions. The QS complexes and elevated ST segments in the precordial leads and the qr complexes with elevated ST segments in leads I and aVL are indicative of recent anterior wall infarction. Abnormal Q waves in II, III, and aVF is indicative of inferior wall infarction; since the ST segments are iso-electric this is not as recent as the anterior infarct. **Clinical and Autopsy Diagnosis:** Recent anterior wall infarction; old inferior wall infarction; occlusion of left anterior descending and left circumflex arteries.

VENTRICULAR ANEURYSM

An aneurysm of the left ventricular myocardium may result following an episode of myocardial infarction. The most consistent electrocardiographic finding is the persistence of ST segment elevation in the epicardial leads reflecting the area of infarction for a period of months or years. The absence of persistent ST segment elevation does not necessarily indicate the absence of an aneurysm, since this pattern is only seen in approximately 50% of proved cases. Also, the presence of these changes does not necessarily indicate an aneurysm is present.

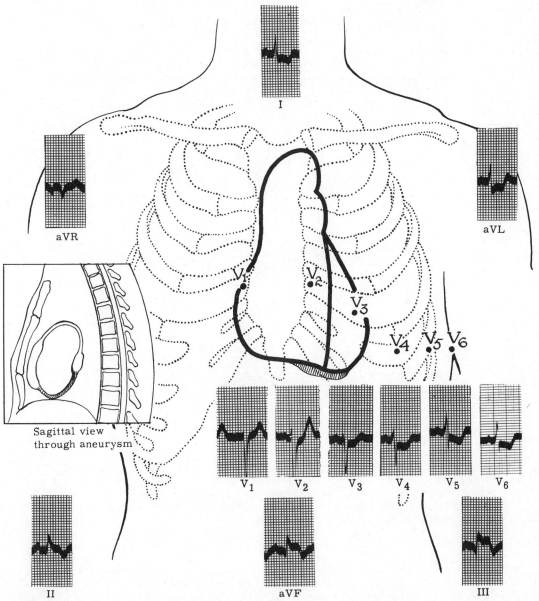

Ventricular Aneurysm. The above tracing is consistent with an early inferior wall infarction as manifested by the ST segment elevation in leads II, III, and aVF and the reciprocal ST segment depression in I, aVL, and V_{2-6}. However, this tracing was taken three months after a clinical episode of myocardial infarction. There was no clinical evidence to suggest more recent infarction. Cardiac fluoroscopy and subsequent autopsy confirmed the diagnosis of ventricular aneurysm involving the inferior and posterior walls of the left ventricle.

DIFFERENTIAL DIAGNOSIS OF MYOCARDIAL INFARCTION

Normal:

   As mentioned above (see pp. 171 and 181), QS complexes with or without inverted T waves may normally be present in aVL or aVF, depending upon heart position. Likewise, QS complexes may normally be seen in V_1 and V_2, especially with clockwise rotation.

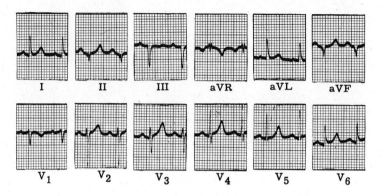

Normal Pattern With QS in aVF. A QS complex with upright T is present in aVF. This could represent the pattern of old inferior wall infarction. However, the heart position is horizontal and therefore a QS may be the normal pattern in aVF.

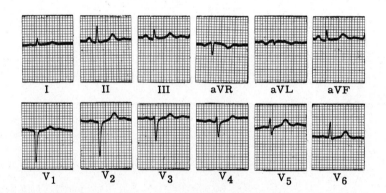

Normal Pattern With QS in V_{1-2}. QS complexes are seen in V_1 and V_2. The R waves progressively increase in height from V_3 to V_6. There are no ST-T abnormalities. Such a pattern can be entirely normal. However, it could represent an old localized anteroseptal infarct. The differential diagnosis will depend upon the clinical picture. Third interspace leads are of value. They were normal in this instance, but if QS complexes were seen in the $3V_{3-4}$ positions it would be indicative of a high anterior wall infarct. **Clinical Diagnosis:** No evidence of heart disease. **Autopsy Diagnosis:** No heart disease; death due to carcinoma.

Left Ventricular Hypertrophy:

   In this condition QS complexes may be seen in V_1 and V_2. On rare occasions QS complexes may extend from V_1 through V_4. Therefore, in the presence of left ventricular hypertrophy, such QS complexes are not necessarily diagnostic of anterior wall infarction.

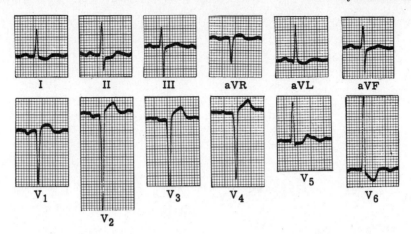

Left Ventricular Hypertrophy. $SV_1 + RV_6 = 47$ mm.; $R = 13$ mm. in aVL; there is ST depression in I, aVL, and V_6. The above criteria are indicative of left ventricular hypertrophy. In addition, QS complexes are present in leads V_{1-4}. This is consistent with anterior wall infarction. **Clinical and Autopsy Diagnosis:** Left ventricular hypertrophy secondary to syphilitic aortitis with aortic insufficiency; no evidence of myocardial infarction.

Right Ventricular Hypertrophy and Dilatation:

In this condition QS complexes may be seen in precordial leads from V_1 (or V_2) through V_5 (or V_6) and therefore simulate anterior wall infarction. However, leads V_3R (or V_1) and aVR will show the pattern of right ventricular hypertrophy.

In association with pulmonary emphysema, a marked left (superior) frontal plane QRS occurs (see p. 292) and may result in prominent Q waves or QS complexes in leads II, III, and aVF, simulating inferior wall infarction.

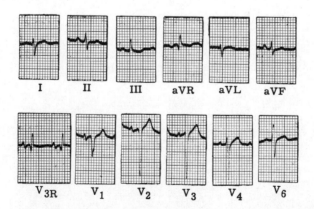

Right Ventricular Hypertrophy. QS complexes with upright T waves are seen in V_{1-3}. This could represent an old anteroseptal infarction. However, there is marked clockwise rotation, as evidenced by a deep S in V_6. Lead V_3R shows the typical pattern of right ventricular hypertrophy. Therefore the QS complexes in V_{1-3} are a reflection of a dilated right ventricle and do not represent infarction. **Clinical and Autopsy Diagnosis:** Right ventricular hypertrophy secondary to chronic pulmonary disease; no evidence of infarction.

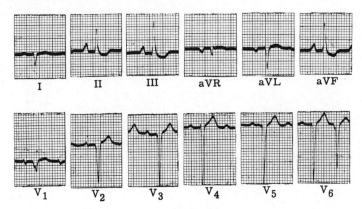

Right Ventricular Hypertrophy. QS complexes are present in leads V_{1-3}. In view of the marked clockwise rotation (rS complexes in leads V_{4-6}) this is not necessarily indicative of infarction, but probably represents leads taken over a greatly dilated right ventricle. The tall P waves in II, III, and aVF, the right axis deviation (+115°) and the ST-T changes in II, III, and aVF are consistent with right atrial and right ventricular hypertrophy. **Clinical and Autopsy Diagnosis:** Right atrial and ventricular hypertrophy and dilatation due to chronic pulmonary disease; no infarction present.

INFARCTION ASSOCIATED WITH BUNDLE BRANCH BLOCK

As a general rule a right bundle branch block does not obscure the pattern of infarction, whereas a left bundle branch block does. The most diagnostic feature of infarction is the abnormal direction of the initial 0.04 sec. QRS vector (i.e., the abnormal Q wave). Since the initial 0.04 sec. QRS vector in uncomplicated right bundle branch is normal, the presence of superimposed infarction can be detected here when it occurs. However, since the initial QRS vector is abnormally directed in left bundle branch block it will obscure the infarction vector and the abnormal Q wave will not appear.

Infarction Associated With Right Bundle Branch Block:
The simultaneous occurrence of a right bundle branch block in association with an infarction pattern indicates infarction of the septum. Anterior wall infarction in association with a right bundle branch block will result in disappearance of the initial r wave (rSR′ of right bundle branch block) in right ventricular epicardial leads, resulting in QR complexes.

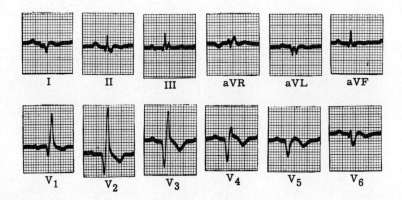

Anterior Wall Infarction in Association With Right Bundle Branch Block. The QRS interval = 0.14 sec.; V.A.T. in V_1 and V_2 = 0.1 sec. The initial r waves of an uncomplicated right bundle branch block normally seen in right precordial leads are not present; deep, wide Q waves indicative of anterior wall infarction are present instead.

Inferior Wall Infarction in Association With Right Bundle Branch Block. Leads aVR, aVL, aVF, and V_1 and V_6 are illustrated. **A:** There is a deep, wide Q with elevated ST segment and inverted T in aVF. This is indicative of recent inferior wall infarction. A 22 mm. R is seen in aVL; this is evidence of left ventricular hypertrophy. The pattern in V_1 is normal. The T is inverted in V_6, probably as a result of partial lateral wall infarction. **B:** Three weeks after A. The QRS interval has increased from 0.08 sec. in (A) to 0.14 sec. in (B). The V.A.T. in V_1 has increased from 0.02 sec. in (A) to 0.11 sec. in (B). Wide R′ waves are seen in aVR and V_1; wide S waves

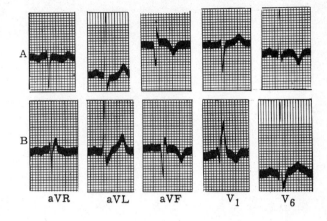

aVR   aVL   aVF V_1 V_6

are seen in aVL and V_6. The pattern of inferior wall infarction in aVF is not altered by the development of the right bundle branch block. This patient recovered. It is reasonable to assume that the right bundle branch block resulted from further infarction involving the interventricular septum.

Posterior Infarction Associated With Right Bundle Branch Block:

A right bundle branch block alters the late forces of ventricular depolarization. Posterior wall infarction alters the initial vector forces in an abnormal anterior direction. This will be evident in the right precordial leads. In addition to the late R′ waves indicative of right bundle branch block, the initial portion of the QRS complex will reveal an abnormally tall R wave (see p. 180). Thus, right precordial leads will reveal a tall slurred R wave or rR′ complex. A similar pattern may be seen in right ventricular hypertrophy associated with a right bundle branch block. There is autopsy evidence that the same pattern can occur in the absence of either posterior wall infarction or right ventricular hypertrophy and is therefore assumed to be the manifestation of a right bundle branch block alone. The reason for this is not known. The ST segments will be depressed in the early stage of infarction and the T waves upright and tall in the late stage of infarction in the same leads.

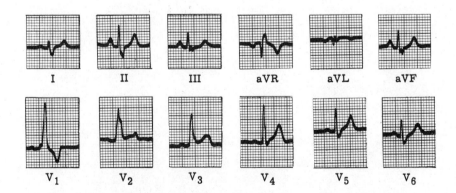

I   II   III   aVR   aVL   aVF

V_1 V_2 V_3 V_4 V_5 V_6

Posterior Infarction plus Right Bundle Branch Block. The QRS interval is 0.12 sec. The wide S waves in leads I, II, III, aVF, V_{5-6} and the late portion of the R waves in V_{1-2-3} are indicative of right bundle branch block. The initial, tall R deflection in V_{1-3} is indicative of associated posterior wall infarction. **Autopsy Diagnosis:** Posterior and septal infarction. It is assumed that the septal infarction produced the right bundle branch block.

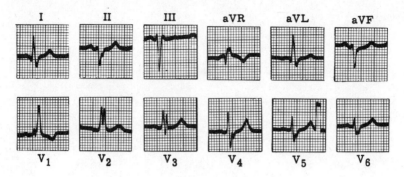

Posterior Infarction plus Right Bundle Branch Block: The QRS interval is 0.13 sec. The wide s waves in I, aVL, and V_{4-6}, the wide r wave in aVR, and the late portion of the R waves in V_{1-2} are indicative of right bundle branch block. The initial R deflections in V_{1-2} indicate abnormal initial anteriorly directed vector forces consistent with posterior wall infarction. In addition the terminal forces are superiorly directed in the frontal plane. **Autopsy Diagnosis:** Posterior and septal infarction. It is likely that the septal infarction produced the right bundle branch block and also the late superior frontal plane axis.

Infarction Associated With Left Bundle Branch Block:

A left bundle branch block may result from myocardial infarction, but one cannot diagnose the latter in the presence of the former. One may be suspicious of infarction if marked ST segment elevation appears in leads which formerly showed the typical left bundle branch pattern. Rarely one may see Q waves in association with a left bundle branch block. This is said to be due to associated infarction of the septum, which allows the initial negativity of the right ventricular cavity to be transmitted into the left cavity and hence into a left ventricular epicardial lead. However, there is little pathologic evidence to support this view; a more likely explanation is the presence of infarction plus a conduction defect in the left ventricle distal to the left bundle (hence not a true left bundle branch block).

Given a left bundle branch electrocardiographic pattern prior to the onset of clinical myocardial infarction, a marked reduction in the voltage of the QRS complexes may offer a clue to the presence of infarction.

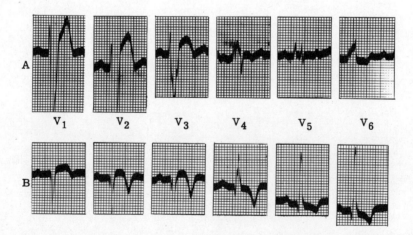

Anterior Wall Infarction in Association With Left Bundle Branch Block. Only the precordial leads are illustrated. A: The patient had suffered an acute myocardial infarction two days previously. A typical left bundle branch block pattern is seen in leads V_{5-6}. Although there is ST segment elevation in leads V_{1-3} and coving of the T in V_{2-3}, it would be hazardous to make an electrocardiographic diagnosis of infarction on this basis in the presence of a left bundle branch block. B: One week after first tracing. The left bundle branch block pattern has disappeared and the pattern of anterior wall infarction has become evident.

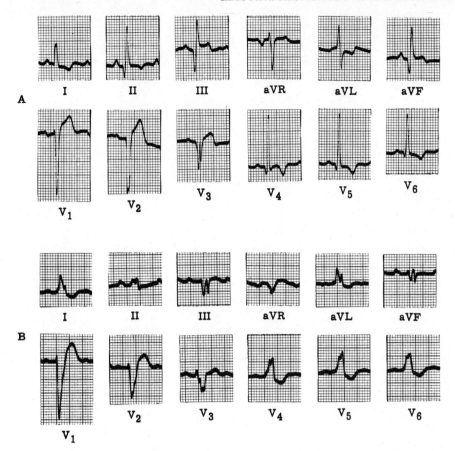

Infarction Associated with Left Bundle Branch Block. A: The deep, wide Q waves with ST-T changes in II, III, and aVF are indicative of inferior wall infarction. The QS complexes in V_{2-3} and abnormal q waves with T inversion in V_{4-6} are indicative of anterior wall infarction. $SV_1 + RV_5 = 40$ mm. and is consistent with left ventricular hypertrophy. Clinically, the patient had suffered two episodes of myocardial infarction. **B:** Following a third clinical episode of myocardial infarction, the electrocardiogram now demonstrates a left bundle branch block and the previous signs of infarction and hypertrophy are gone. **Autopsy Diagnosis:** Left ventricular hypertrophy, old infarction involving anterior and inferior portions of the left ventricle; recent septal infarction. The latter probably explains the left bundle branch block.

Inferior Wall Infarction in Association With Left Bundle Branch Block.
A. The patient had suffered an acute myocardial infarction one day previously. The electrocardiographic pattern is that of a left bundle branch block.

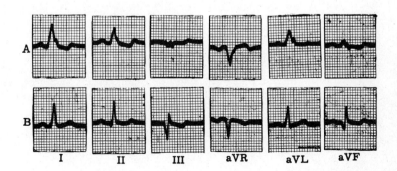

B. Seven days after (A) there was no clinical evidence of further coronary insufficiency or infarction. The left bundle branch pattern has disappeared, uncovering a definite pattern of inferior wall infarction as evidenced by the deep, wide Q in aVF (also II and III).
It is likely that the left bundle branch block in (A) was due to temporary coronary insufficiency in the region of the left bundle branch.

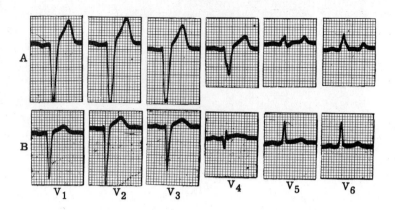

V_1 V_2 V_3 V_4 V_5 V_6

EFFECT OF FURTHER CORONARY INSUFFICIENCY ON THE INFARCT PATTERN

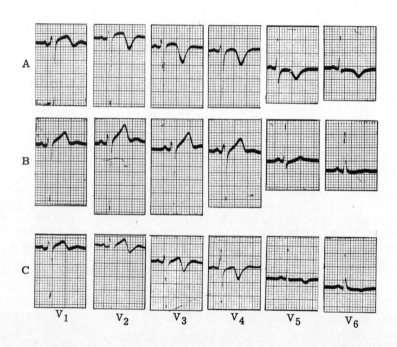

V_1 V_2 V_3 V_4 V_5 V_6

Coronary Insufficiency Superimposed Upon Infarction. (Only the precordial leads are illustrated.)
A: Represents the stable electrocardiographic pattern of a clinical myocardial infarct two months old. B: One day after initial tracing. The T waves are now upright (except in V_6) in precordial leads. The pattern looks more normal, but the inverted T waves of established infarction could not suddenly become upright in one day. This therefore indicates further coronary insufficiency (the patient was having chest pain at the time this record was taken). C: One day after (B). The T waves are again inverted in precordial leads, similar to (A).

PERI-INFARCTION BLOCK: (See p. 294.)

Chapter 12

NORMAL CARDIAC RHYTHM
AND THE ATRIAL ARRHYTHMIAS

PHYSIOLOGY OF CARDIAC RHYTHM

In order to better understand disturbances of cardiac rhythm, a brief review of some of the physiologic properties of the heart is indicated. Some of these concepts have been discussed in Chapter 2.

<u>Rhythmicity</u>:

Normally the sinus node forms stimuli at a faster rate than any other neuromuscular tissue of the heart. Thus the sinus node is the principal pacemaker of the heart and controls the cardiac rate. When stimulus formation in the sinus node is depressed or ceases, secondary pacemakers in the A-V node, the bundle branches, or the ventricles can take over. Stimulus formation is slower in the A-V node than in the sinus node and still slower in the bundle branches and ventricles.

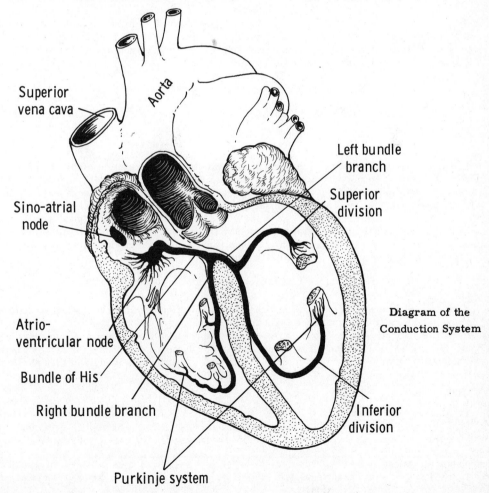

Superior vena cava

Aorta

Left bundle branch

Superior division

Sino-atrial node

Atrio-ventricular node

Bundle of His

Right bundle branch

Inferior division

Purkinje system

Diagram of the Conduction System

Conduction:

Ordinarily an electrical stimulus spreads in all directions from its point of origin. When the spread of a stimulus is hindered in all directions but one, this is known as "unidirectional block." Normally, unidirectional block exists in the A-V node, resulting in **forward conduction** to the bundle of His. The reverse is known as **retrograde conduction**.

Refractory Period:

When heart muscle is stimulated it cannot respond to a second stimulus until a certain time elapses. This is known as the refractory period. The duration of this period in the ventricles approximates the Q-T interval. The refractory period consists of an **absolute refractory period**, during which no stimulus can initiate a response, followed by a **partial or relative refractory period**, during which a response can be elicited by a stronger than average stimulus.

A period of "supernormal recovery" has also been described during which the heart can respond to a stimulus which would be too weak to cause a response at any other period in the cardiac cycle. In the ventricles, the supernormal period corresponds to the terminal portion of the T wave.

EFFECT OF THE AUTONOMIC NERVOUS SYSTEM ON CARDIAC RHYTHM

Although stimulus formation is automatic, it can be modified by the autonomic nervous system. The sinus and A-V nodes are predominantly under vagal influence and, to a lesser degree, under the influence of the sympathetic nervous system. The ventricles are exclusively under sympathetic control. The sympathetic system has a stimulating effect on the heart rate; the parasympathetic system (vagus) has a depressant effect. Vagal stimulation increases conductivity in the atrial muscle but delays conduction in the A-V node. Since the latter effect is greater, the net effect is a slowing of the ventricular rate.

EFFECT OF DIGITALIS, QUINIDINE, AND PROCAINAMIDE ON CARDIAC RHYTHM

Digitalis:

Digitalis has a dual effect on cardiac rhythm, one direct and the other indirect. Its direct effect is to slow conductivity through the atrial myocardium and to delay conduction through the A-V node. Its indirect effect is strong vagal stimulation, which increases conductivity through the atrial myocardium and delays conduction through the A-V node. The net effect of this dual action on the A-V node is to slow the ventricular rate. The effect of digitalis on abnormal atrial rates is unique. At ectopic atrial rates of 160 to 200, digitalis can abolish the ectopic rhythm. At atrial rates of 300 or more, digitalis usually increases the atrial rate. Both of these latter effects are thought to be due to vagal stimulation. *

Quinidine:

Quinidine likewise has a dual action. Its direct effect is to slow conduction through the atrium and the A-V node and to suppress myocardial irritability. Its indirect effect is that of weak vagal depression, which results in a delayed conduction through the atrium and increased conduction through the A-V node. The direct and indirect actions on the A-V node balance one another; the net effect is to slow conduction through the atrium, thus first slowing and then abolishing an ectopic atrial rhythm.

Procainamide (Pronestyl®):

The effect of procainamide is similar to that of quinidine. However, procainamide is much more effective against the ventricular ectopic arrhythmias than those originating in the atria.

---

*Experimental work by Scherf indicates that this vagal effect does not always depend upon the ectopic atrial rate but that vagal stimulation may either **slow** or **increase** the atrial rate regardless of the initial ectopic atrial rate.

SUMMARY OF EFFECTS OF DIGITALIS AND QUINIDINE

	Quinidine	Digitalis
Vagal effect	Decreased	Increased
Absolute refractory period	No effect (or shortened)	Shortened
Conduction in atria	Delayed	1. Delayed (direct effect) 2. Accelerated (indirect effect)
Effect on A-V node	1. Direct: delayed conduction 2. Indirect: accelerated conduction Net effect: slightly accelerated conduction	1. Direct: delayed conduction 2. Indirect: delayed conduction Net effect: markedly delayed conduction
Net effect on atrial rate*	Decreased	1. "Slow" rates (160 to 200): decreased 2. "Fast" rates (300+): accelerated
Net effect on ventricular rate*	May be accelerated due to slight effect on A-V node	Decreased due to marked effect on A-V node

*In the presence of atrial tachycardia, flutter, or fibrillation.

NORMAL AND ABNORMAL CARDIAC RHYTHMS

Diagram of Cardiac Conduction:
    The following type of diagram will be used to illustrate the electrocardiographic tracings of normal and abnormal conduction.

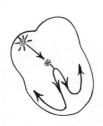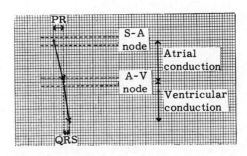

Diagram of Cardiac Conduction. (The normal delay in the A-V node is not illustrated.)

SINUS RHYTHMS

Regular Sinus Rhythm:
This is the normal rhythm of the heart.   The average rate is 60 to 100 beats per minute.

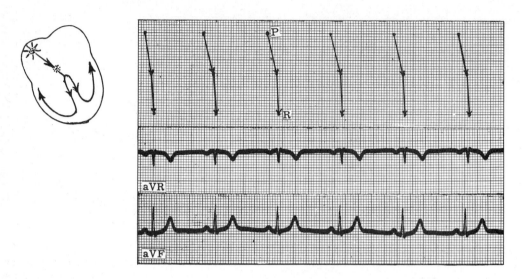

Regular Sinus Rhythm. R-R = 0.96 sec.   Rate = 63.   The P is normally inverted in aVR and normally upright in aVF.

Sinus Tachycardia:
A regular sinus rhythm with a rate in excess of 100. Sinus tachycardia does not usually exceed 160 beats per minute in the adult.

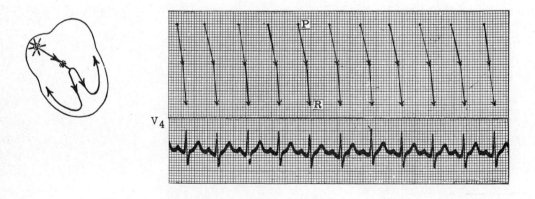

Sinus Tachycardia. R-R = 0.48 sec. Rate = 125

Sinus Bradycardia:
A regular sinus rhythm with a rate under 60 per minute.

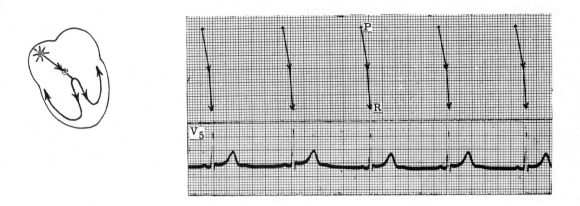

Sinus Bradycardia. R-R = 1. 20 sec. Rate = 50

Sinus Arrhythmia:
The impulse arises normally in the S-A node. The arrhythmia is manifested by alternating periods of slower and more rapid heart rates. The variations are usually related to respiration, the rate increasing with inspiration and decreasing with expiration. This condition is more common in children than adults and is frequently associated with sinus bradycardia.

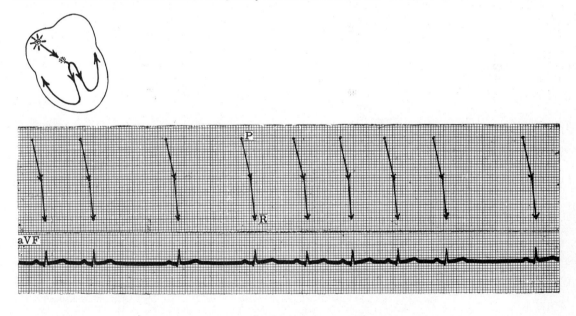

Sinus Arrhythmia. Slowing of the Rate During Expiration

Clinical Significance:
Sinus tachycardia, sinus bradycardia, and sinus arrhythmia do not in themselves indicate any organic heart disease.

Sinus Arrest (Atrial Standstill):

This denotes a pause in the cardiac rhythm due to a momentary failure of the sinus node to initiate an impulse. This results in a prolonged diastolic pause between two complexes. The pause is not necessarily an exact multiple of the normal P-P interval. Usually only a single beat is dropped at a time. If the sinus node remains inactive for a longer period of time, atrial stand-still results. This may result in the A-V node or a ventricle becoming the pacemaker and in-itiating nodal or ventricular ectopic beats until the sinus node resumes its function.

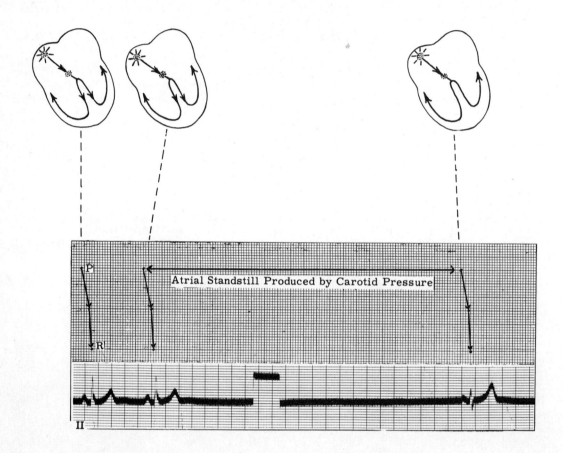

Atrial Standstill (Lead II). The patient was a 25-year-old "vagotonic" individual. The rhythm at the start of the record is regular sinus with a rate of 63. Following right carotid sinus pres-sure complete asystole is produced for 4.6 sec. The first beat following asystole is sinus con-ducted but shows aberrant intraventricular conduction. (See p. 265.)

Clinical Significance:

Sinus arrest and atrial standstill are the result of increased vagal tone. They can occur in normal "vagotonic" individuals, can be produced by carotid sinus stimulation, digitalis or quini-dine, or organic heart disease involving the S-A node (inflammatory involvement from rheumatic fever or infarction of the node).

ABNORMAL ATRIAL RHYTHMS

ATRIAL PREMATURE BEATS

An atrial premature beat (or premature contraction) results from a secondary stimulus arising in an ectopic focus anywhere in either atrium. An atrial excitation (P′) takes place prematurely. Usually it will initiate a ventricular complex with a normal or basic* QRS configuration. Since the normal spread of excitation is from the upper end to the lower end of the atrium, the P wave is normally inverted in aVR and high esophageal leads and upright in aVF and low esophageal leads. An atrial ectopic stimulus arising in the upper end of the atrium will result in P′ waves having this same normal direction. An impulse arising in the lower end of the atrium will stimulate the atrium in a foot-to-head direction, producing upright P′ waves in aVR and high esophageal leads, and inverted P′ waves in aVF and low esophageal leads. The P′-R interval may be shorter or longer than the basic P-R interval. In most instances there is not a full compensatory pause (see p. 240) in association with this arrhythmia. That is, the R-R interval between the normal beats preceding and following the premature beat is not double the normal R-R interval.

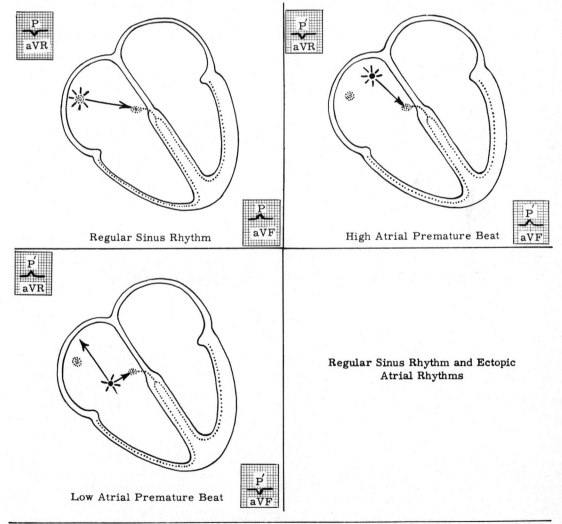

Regular Sinus Rhythm

High Atrial Premature Beat

Low Atrial Premature Beat

Regular Sinus Rhythm and Ectopic Atrial Rhythms

*The term "basic" is used to describe the configuration of the QRS complex associated with the regular sinus-conducted beats. Thus in a bundle branch block, the basic QRS complex will be wide and slurred and an atrial premature beat will likewise produce a QRS complex of the bundle branch type.

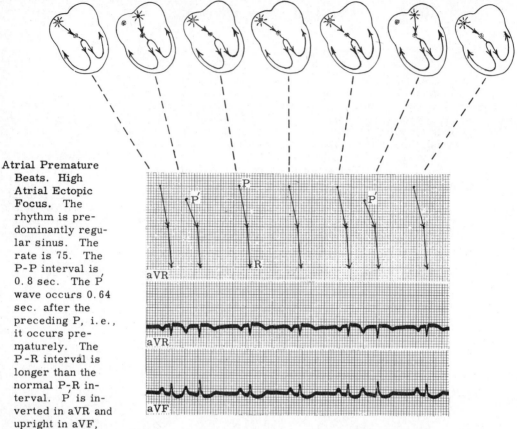

Atrial Premature Beats. High Atrial Ectopic Focus. The rhythm is predominantly regular sinus. The rate is 75. The P-P interval is 0.8 sec. The P' wave occurs 0.64 sec. after the preceding P, i.e., it occurs prematurely. The P'-R interval is longer than the normal P-R interval. P' is inverted in aVR and upright in aVF, indicating a high atrial ectopic focus. The normal configuration of the QRS complex of the premature beat indicates that conduction through the A-V node and ventricles is normal.

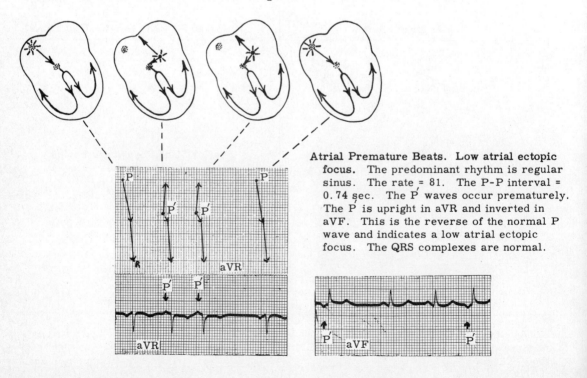

Atrial Premature Beats. Low atrial ectopic focus. The predominant rhythm is regular sinus. The rate = 81. The P-P interval = 0.74 sec. The P' waves occur prematurely. The P' is upright in aVR and inverted in aVF. This is the reverse of the normal P wave and indicates a low atrial ectopic focus. The QRS complexes are normal.

Blocked Atrial Premature Contractions:

If the P' wave occurs very soon after a normal beat, the ventricle will still be refractory and will not respond. This is known as a blocked atrial premature beat.

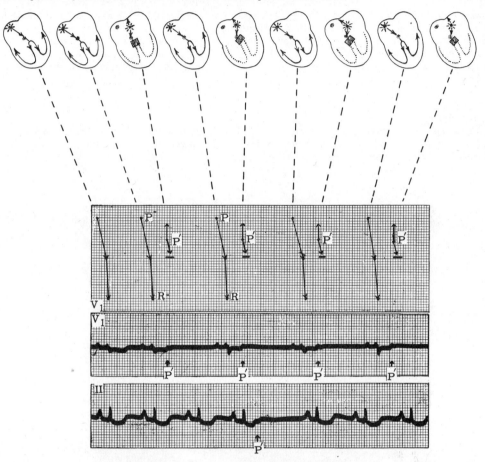

Blocked Atrial Premature Contractions: V_1. The first two beats are sinus conducted. The P-P interval = 0.68 sec. An atrial complex (P') follows the second QRS complex. The P-P' interval = 0.36 sec. This atrial complex is occurring prematurely. Since it follows so closely after the QRS, the ventricle is still refractory and does not respond. A full compensatory pause does not follow. The cycle is repeated for the next three sinus conducted beats, producing an atrial bigeminal rhythm, i.e., one regular sinus conducted beat followed by one blocked atrial premature beat. **II:** One blocked premature atrial contraction is seen.

Premature atrial foci arising in the middle of the atrium will produce flat or diphasic P' waves in aVR and aVF.

Aberrant intraventricular conduction may be associated with atrial premature beats. This will be discussed on p. 265.

Clinical Significance:

Atrial premature beats usually occur in normal individuals. At times they may occur secondary to stimulation from emotional disturbances, tobacco, or tea or coffee. Digitalis uncommonly produces this arrhythmia. Almost any form of organic heart disease may be responsible, and in such instances this arrhythmia may be the precursor of paroxysmal atrial tachycardia and atrial fibrillation. As a general rule, a diagnosis of organic heart disease must not be made solely on the electrocardiographic finding of atrial premature contractions.

WANDERING PACEMAKER

In this disturbance of cardiac rhythm some of the impulses originate in the S-A node, whereas others originate from various foci in the atrium and even in the A-V node. As a result there will be a variation in rhythm, a changing configuration of the P′ wave and a changing P′-R interval. Normally inverted P or P′ waves in aVR and upright P or P′ waves in aVF will result from impulses arising in the S-A node and the upper portion of the atrium; upright P′ waves in aVR and inverted P′ waves in aVF will result from impulses arising in the lower portion of the atrium or A-V node.

Clinical Significance:

This arrhythmia may occur in normal individuals. It can result from increased vagal tone. Digitalis may be the etiologic factor. Various forms of organic heart disease, notably acute rheumatic fever, can also produce this arrhythmia.

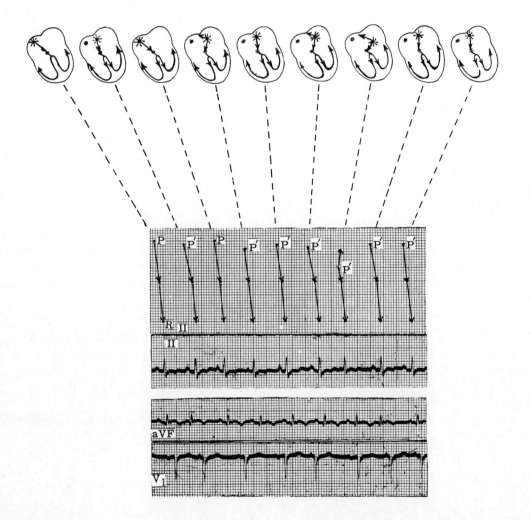

Wandering Pacemaker. Each QRS complex is preceded by an atrial wave. However, the configuration of the P wave frequently changes in height and direction and the P-R interval varies. This indicates that the pacemaker is shifting from the sinus node to varying portions of the atrium.

PAROXYSMAL ATRIAL TACHYCARDIA

Paroxysmal atrial tachycardia is a regular rhythm with a rate of 160 to 220. On occasion this rhythm may exist with a rate of 100 or lower or may exceed 300.

Etiology and Incidence:

Paroxysmal atrial tachycardia most commonly occurs in normal individuals who show no clinical evidence of heart disease. It may occur in relation to emotional trauma. Rheumatic mitral valvular disease, thyrotoxicosis, and coronary artery disease are less common etiologic factors.

Mechanism:

This arrhythmia results from an ectopic focus located in either atrium which regularly discharges stimuli at the above-mentioned rates. The ventricle responds to each atrial stimulus, producing a perfectly regular ventricular rhythm. There are rare exceptions to the typical regularity of atrial tachycardia. These are (1) multiple atrial foci instead of a single focus, producing an atrial tachycardia of the wandering pacemaker type, and (2) introduction of premature beats from other foci interrupting the regularity of the rhythm.

Electrocardiographic Pattern:

Paroxysmal atrial tachycardia merely consists of a continuous run of atrial premature beats. With the rare exceptions of the above-mentioned conditions, each P' wave will be followed by a ventricular complex. As is true also of atrial premature beats (see p. 203), the direction of the P' waves in leads aVR, aVF, and esophageal leads will indicate the site of origin (high or low) of the atrial ectopic focus.

The QRS complexes and T waves are of normal (or basic) configuration. However, with prolonged tachycardia the ST segment may become depressed and the T waves inverted in left ventricular epicardial leads as a result of anoxia.

In this arrhythmia the impulse spreads through atrial muscle more slowly than a normal sinus beat or an atrial premature beat. Thus the P'-R interval is often prolonged. The P' wave may therefore be buried in the preceding ventricular (QRS) complex, simulating an A-V nodal tachycardia (see p. 234).

Ventricular aberration can occur with paroxysmal atrial tachycardia (see p. 249).

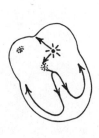
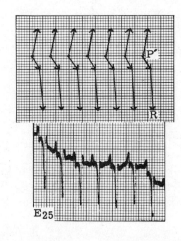
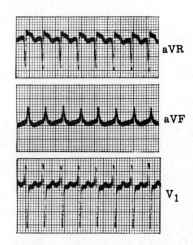

Paroxysmal Atrial Tachycardia. The ventricular rhythm is regular at a rate of 215. The QRS complexes are normal. No definite evidence of atrial activity can be seen in leads aVR, aVF, and V₁. Lead E₂₅ shows an upright P' preceding each QRS complex, indicating a low atrial ectopic focus.

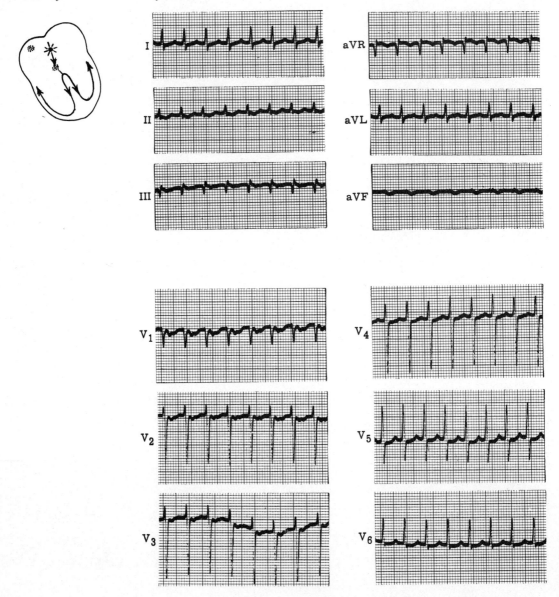

Paroxysmal Atrial Tachycardia. A regular ventricular rhythm is seen with a ventricular rate of 188. The QRS complexes are not widened. P´ waves are evident in V_1 and V_2. The minor ST depressions seen in precordial leads could be the result of prominent T_a waves or could represent myocardial anoxia secondary to the tachycardia.

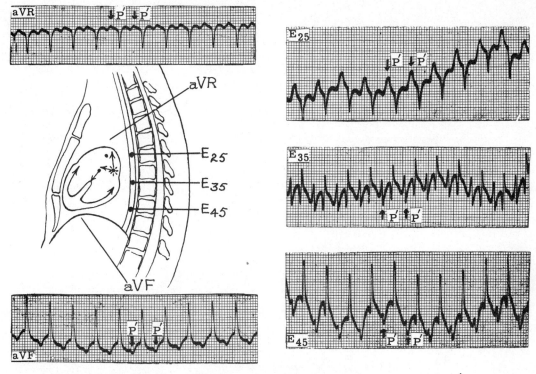

Paroxysmal Atrial Tachycardia. The atrial and ventricular rates are 170. The P′ waves (indicated by arrows) are upright in aVR, inverted in aVF and E₄₅, diphasic in E₃₅, and upright in E₂₅, indicating an ectopic focus low in the atrium (or A-V node).

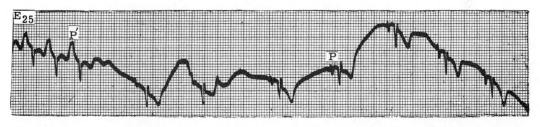

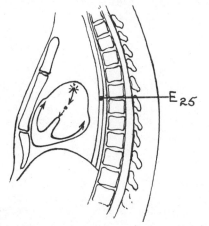

E₂₅: Reversion to Regular Sinus Rhythm With Quinidine. Note the change from the large upright P′ waves of the atrial tachycardia to the smaller diphasic P waves of the regular sinus rhythm. The wavy baseline illustrates one of the technical difficulties encountered in taking esophageal leads.

Differential Diagnosis:

A. Sinus Tachycardia: A paroxysmal atrial tachycardia arising from an ectopic focus high in the atrium and therefore producing normally directed P' waves may be indistinguishable from a sinus tachycardia at rates of approximately 140 to 160 in one single electrocardiogram. A constant R-R interval will favor a diagnosis of paroxysmal atrial tachycardia. The response to carotid sinus pressure may solve this problem. In paroxysmal atrial tachycardia this maneuver may abruptly terminate the attack. In sinus tachycardia there may be some gradual and slight sinus slowing. If there is no response to carotid sinus pressure, one must then compare the pattern of the P (or P') waves of the tachycardia to the pattern present during slower regular sinus rhythm. If there is a difference in configuration of the atrial complexes in the two tracings, a diagnosis of paroxysmal atrial tachycardia is justified. The above refers to an electrocardiographic differential diagnosis and does not include the points of clinical difference between these two rhythms.

B. Nodal and Ventricular Tachycardia: These will be discussed under their respective headings.

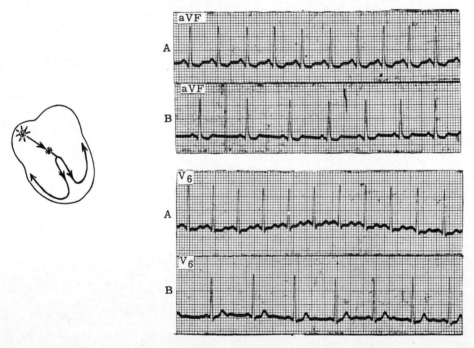

Sinus Tachycardia. Response to Carotid Sinus Pressure. The upper strips of aVF and V_6 show a tachycardia with a rate of 150. This is more likely a sinus tachycardia, but a relatively slow ectopic atrial tachycardia cannot be excluded. The lower strips of aVF and V_6 show the response to carotid pressure. There is slowing of the heart rate with gradual increase as the pressure is stopped. This definitely indicates that the upper strips represent sinus tachycardia.

Clinical Significance:

The tachycardia may last for a few seconds, minutes, hours, or days. Persistence of this arrhythmia in an individual with a diseased myocardium can precipitate congestive heart failure and coronary insufficiency. Even in a normal individual the persistence of the tachycardia for days can produce heart failure. It is therefore urgent that this arrhythmia be diagnosed and treated promptly.

Prognosis:

The prognosis of paroxysmal atrial tachycardia depends on the status of the heart irrespective of the tachycardia. If properly treated and if there is no known underlying cause, this arrhythmia will in no way reduce the patient's life expectancy. Such patients are prone to have recurrences unless controlled by digitalis and/or quinidine in maintenance doses. These patients must be assured that their paroxysms are not indicative of heart disease and that the prognosis is excellent.

ATRIAL FLUTTER

Atrial flutter is manifested by a regular atrial rate, usually 220 to 350 (the author has observed one case with an atrial rate of 430), with varying degrees of A-V block, usually 2:1 or 4:1. The ventricular rhythm is most often regular, being one-half or one-fourth the atrial rate. Occasionally, as a result of a constantly changing A-V block, the ventricular rhythm is irregular.

Etiology and Incidence:

Atrial flutter may occur in normal individuals. However, there is usually underlying organic heart disease, notably coronary artery disease, rheumatic mitral valvular disease, or associated hyperthyroidism. It commonly occurs during the course of quinidine therapy for atrial fibrillation. It is seen much less commonly in association with trauma to the heart, metastatic malignancy involving the heart, and the various myocarditides.

Mechanism:

Since the work of Sir Thomas Lewis it had been accepted that atrial flutter results from a "circus" movement in the atrium. The work of Scherf and Prinzmetal has shown that atrial flutter results from a single ectopic atrial focus. Thus, except for the difference in A-V conduction, atrial tachycardia and atrial flutter differ only in frequency of atrial rates. Sir Thomas Lewis' still-valid observations of the influence of the atrial rate upon A-V conduction testify further to the identity of the basic mechanism of the two conditions. With atrial rates of 160 to 220 (atrial tachycardia), vagal stimulation produces asystole followed by reversion to regular sinus rhythm; with rates of 220 to 300, varying degrees of A-V block result without a change in the atrial rate; with rates of 300 or more atrial fibrillation results*. This explains the reversion of paroxysmal atrial tachycardia to regular sinus rhythm with carotid sinus pressure (vagal influence)†; the abrupt but temporary slowing of the ventricular rhythm in atrial flutter with carotid sinus pressure (vagal influence); and the conversion of atrial flutter to atrial fibrillation with digitalis (vagal influence).

This "unitarian" concept is by no means universally accepted. Three different schools of thought are defended by (1) the "circus" movement advocates, (2) the adherents of the unitarian concept, and (3) those who believe that both mechanisms operate under differing conditions. For clinical purposes the question is academic, however.

Electrocardiographic Pattern:

With atrial rates of less than 200 the P′ waves of atrial flutter will be identical with those of atrial tachycardia. As the atrial rate increases, a more prominent T_a wave will appear. The direction of the T_a wave is opposite to that of the P′. As the atrial rate continues to increase (over 300), the amplitude of the T_a wave will be equal to that of the P′ wave, producing a "saw-toothed" appearance. The direction of the P′ wave will indicate the site of origin of the ectopic atrial focus. The QRS complexes are of normal (or basic) configuration if no other cardiac abnormalities exist.

Atrial Tachycardia-Flutter. Note the increasing prominence of the T_a wave with increasing atrial rates. (Reproduced, with permission, from Prinzmetal, et al., The Auricular Arrhythmias. Charles C Thomas, 1952.)

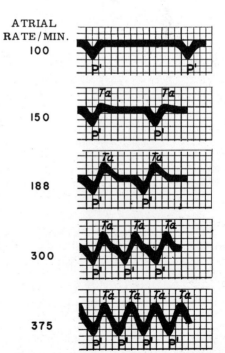

ATRIAL RATE/MIN.
100
150
188
300
375

---

*See p. 198, note. †In very rare instances, a 1:1 paroxysmal atrial tachycardia has been changed by carotid sinus pressure into a 2:1 atrial "flutter." Scherf has reported one such case and the author has observed another.

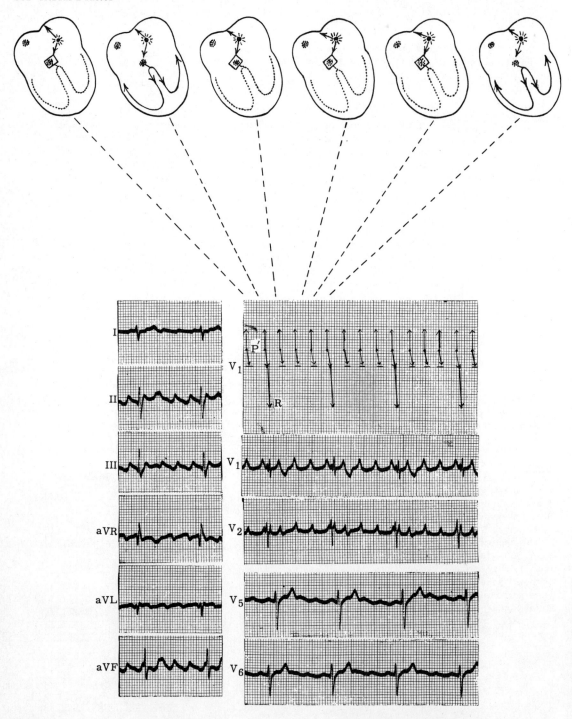

Atrial Flutter. The atria are beating regularly at a rate of 240. The P′ waves have a "saw-toothed" appearance in II, III, and aVF. The ventricles are beating regularly at a rate of 60. Every fourth atrial stimulus penetrates the A-V node and results in ventricular stimulation. Thus this is a 4:1 atrial flutter. In addition, the pattern is that of an incomplete right bundle branch block (rsR in V₁; QRS = 0.08 sec.). **Clinical Diagnosis:** Mitral stenosis.

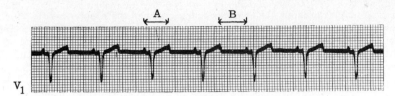

Atrial Flutter with Inconstant Atrial Rate. A 2:1 atrial flutter is present. The ventricular rhythm is regular at a rate of 75. The P′-P′ interval in which a QRS complex intervenes (A) is 0.38 sec. The P′-P′ interval with no intervening QRS complex (B) is 0.41 sec. This difference in rate is thought to result from a reflex mechanism induced by the ventricular contraction.

Differential Diagnosis of Atrial Flutter:
A. Paroxysmal Atrial Tachycardia: Basically there is no difference between atrial tachycardia and atrial flutter. Therefore both of these rhythms can be defined as atrial tachycardia with a certain degree of A-V block, i.e., 1:1, 2:1, 4:1, etc. At times such a rhythm with a 2:1 block may be mistaken for an atrial tachycardia with 1:1 conduction or even regular sinus rhythm because one of the P′ waves is buried in the QRS complex. In such an instance, carotid sinus pressure will be helpful in making the differentiation by increasing the degree of A-V block.

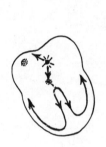
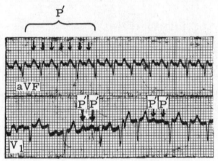

Atrial Flutter (Paroxysmal Atrial Tachycardia with 2:1 A-V Block). Lead aVF: The ventricular rhythm is regular; the rate = 215. At first glance only one atrial contraction is seen for each QRS complex. However, upon closer inspection another P′ wave may be present immediately following the QRS complex. **Lead V₁:** With carotid sinus pressure the degree of A-V block is temporarily increased and an atrial rate of 430 is present. This proves that the pattern in aVF is an atrial flutter (or tachycardia) with 2:1 A-V block.

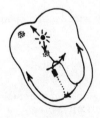
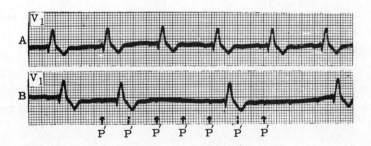

Atrial Flutter Simulating Regular Sinus Rhythm. **A.** The ventricular rate is 72; the pattern is that of a right bundle branch block. Only one atrial wave is seen preceding each QRS complex, which suggests regular sinus rhythm. Other leads offered no further information. **B.** Taken during carotid sinus pressure. This produces further A-V block and clearly demonstrates a flutter with an atrial rate of 144. This proves that the rhythm in (A) is a 2:1 atrial flutter.

B. Atrial Fibrillation: With rapid atrial rates many leads of the electrocardiogram will not clearly show the regularly recurring P′ waves. If the ventricular response is irregular this will simulate atrial fibrillation. Lead V_1, which most commonly best records the atrial impulses, will usually show the regular P′ waves even though no other lead of the 12-lead electrocardiogram will. Carotid sinus pressure, by increasing the degree of A-V block, is also of aid.

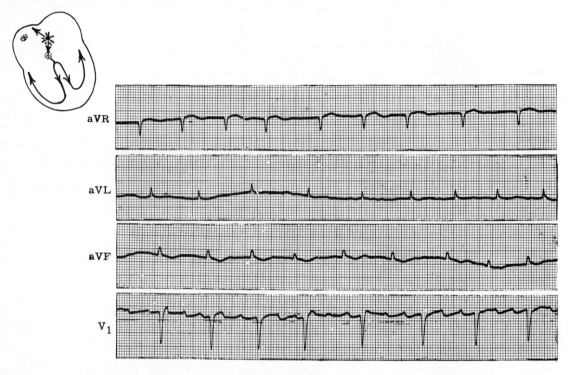

Atrial Flutter Simulating Atrial Fibrillation. Leads aVR, aVL, and aVF reveal an irregular ventricular rhythm with no evidence of regular atrial activity. Other leads, except V_1, showed a similar pattern. This would be termed atrial fibrillation. Lead V_1 shows a regular atrial rhythm at a rate of 210. The ventricular rhythm is irregular. This is an atrial flutter with irregular ventricular response.

Clinical Significance:
    Atrial flutter may be paroxysmal or chronic. The urgency of therapy will depend upon the ventricular rate, as in paroxysmal atrial tachycardia.

Prognosis:
    The prognosis of atrial flutter will depend on the nature of the underlying heart disease. If no heart disease is present the prognosis is the same as that of paroxysmal atrial tachycardia.

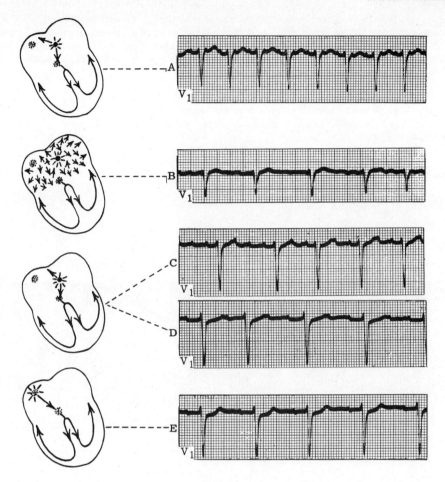

Atrial Flutter; Response to Digitalis and Quinidine.

A. Before Therapy: Atrial flutter with 2:1 A-V block. The atrial rate is 272; the ventricular rate is 136.

B. After Digitalization: The rhythm is now atrial fibrillation; the ventricular rate has been slowed to 80.

C. During Initial Quinidine Therapy: Quinidine has changed the atrial fibrillation to atrial flutter. The atrial rate is 272 (as in A), but due to the blocking action of digitalis on the A-V node there is 3:1 and 4:1 A-V block, resulting in a ventricular rate of 85.

D. During Continued Quinidine Therapy: Atrial flutter persists, but the atrial rate has been reduced to 200. There is 2:1 and 3:1 A-V block resulting in a ventricular rate of 75.

E. Further Quinidine Therapy: The rhythm has reverted to regular sinus.

ATRIAL FIBRILLATION

Atrial fibrillation is a totally irregular atrial rhythm manifested by an irregular ventricular rhythm occurring at rates of less than 50 to more than 200.

Etiology and Incidence:
    Atrial fibrillation is most commonly seen in association with coronary artery disease, rheumatic mitral valvular disease, and hyperthyroidism. It also may occur in perfectly normal persons, either in paroxysmal or chronic, persistent form. Less common etiologic factors include those listed under atrial flutter. (See p. 211.)

<u>Mechanism:</u>

The human atrium can respond regularly to a stimulus only up to a certain rate. This is usually in the range of 350 to 400 per minute. At faster rates than this the atrium can no longer respond completely to each stimulus. A chaotic disturbance with asynchronous contractions of the atria results.

The ventricular rhythm is totally irregular because the majority of the atrial impulses reaching the A-V node are too weak to result in its stimulation. Only the "strongest" atrial stimuli activate the A-V node, and since this does not occur in any regular sequence, the ventricular response is irregular.

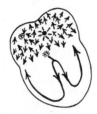

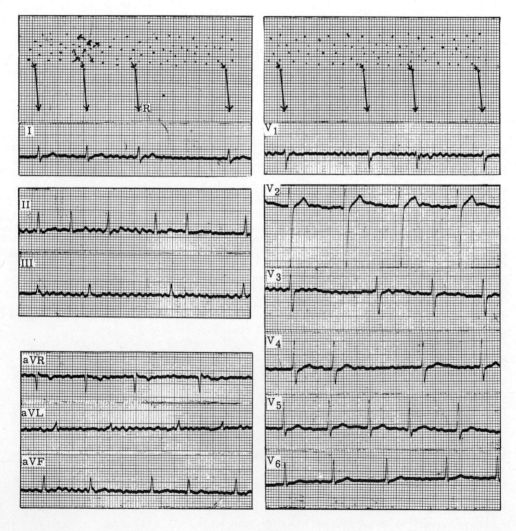

Atrial Fibrillation. Atrial activity is manifested by rapid, small, irregular waves. The ventricular rhythm is completely irregular.

Electrocardiographic Pattern:

The atrial impulses are recorded as small waves which are totally irregular and vary in size and shape from beat to beat. These are called F waves. They are usually most prominent in V_1 in the routine electrocardiogram. The ventricular rhythm is irregular. The QRS complexes and T waves are usually of normal or basic configuration (see p. 203, note). With rapid sustained atrial fibrillation, ST segment and T wave changes can occur as the result of secondary myocardial anoxia.

Differential Diagnosis:

A. Atrial Flutter: This has already been discussed (see p. 214). At times the rhythm may alternate between flutter and fibrillation in a single tracing. There are borderline cases in which a precise differentiation cannot be made. In such instances the terms "flutter-fibrillation," "coarse fibrillation," or "impure flutter" may be used. However, it is better to reserve the term "flutter" for those records with perfectly regular atrial contractions, and fibrillation for all those that are irregular. The presence of coarse fibrillatory waves favors an etiological diagnosis of rheumatic mitral valve disease or thyrotoxicosis. Fine fibrillatory waves are more commonly associated with arteriosclerotic or hypertensive cardiovascular disease.

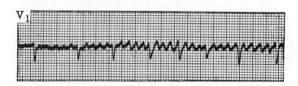

Atrial Flutter-fibrillation. On the right-hand portion of the strip, regularly recurring atrial complexes are seen which simulate flutter waves. These occur at a rate of 500 per minute. This is too rapid for true flutter. The atrial complexes on the left-hand portion of the strip are typical of atrial fibrillation. It is simplest to call the above atrial fibrillation. It could also be called "flutter-fibrillation," "coarse fibrillation," or "impure flutter."

B. Atrial Tachycardia: A rapid atrial fibrillation with a ventricular rhythm of 200 may simulate an atrial tachycardia. However, on careful measurement of many R-R intervals the former rhythm will show variation, whereas the latter will be perfectly regular. Carotid sinus pressure may terminate a tachycardia but will only produce some ventricular slowing in atrial fibrillation.

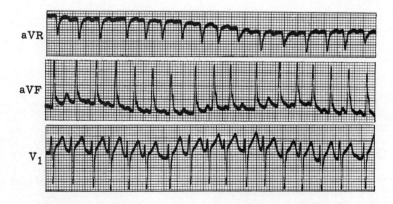

Rapid Atrial Fibrillation Simulating Tachycardia. A rapid ventricular rhythm is present at a rate of 200. At first glance this has the appearance of paroxysmal atrial tachycardia. However, upon more careful inspection, it is seen that the ventricular rhythm is not regular, indicating a rapid atrial fibrillation.

Clinical Significance:

Atrial fibrillation is a much less efficient cardiac mechanism than regular sinus rhythm because it reduces cardiac output. It also leads to the formation of atrial thrombi, with the danger of pulmonary and systemic arterial embolism. Even in the normal person, atrial fibrillation persisting for years can lead to cardiac dilatation and hypertrophy. For these reasons, an attempt to revert this arrhythmia to regular sinus rhythm is indicated in most cases.

Prognosis:

The prognosis of atrial fibrillation depends on the nature of any underlying disease. If the ventricular rate can be kept in a normal range, the prognosis from the atrial fibrillation is by no means poor. However, one can never be certain of this, since such a patient may dislodge a mural thrombus from either atrium and develop serious or even fatal pulmonary or systemic embolism.

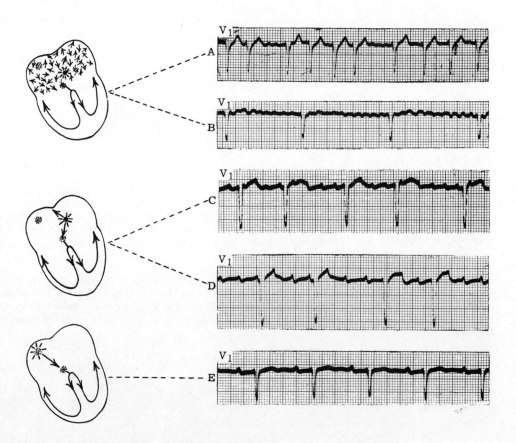

Atrial Fibrillation. Treatment with digitalis and quinidine.
A. Before Therapy: Atrial fibrillation; ventricular rate = 120.
B. After Digitalization: Atrial fibrillation; ventricular rate = 50.
C. During Initial Quinidine Therapy: Atrial flutter; atrial rate = 300; there is a varying A-V block (3:1 to 5:1), resulting in a ventricular rate of 75.
D. During Continued Quinidine Therapy: Atrial flutter persists, but the atrial rate has been reduced to 210; there is a varying A-V block, resulting in a ventricular rate of 65.
E. Further Quinidine Therapy: Regular sinus rhythm; rate = 68.

SUMMARY OF THE ATRIAL ARRHYTHMIAS

An ectopic focus in the atrium is responsible for the development of atrial premature contractions, atrial tachycardia, atrial flutter (which can also be called atrial tachycardia with A-V block), and atrial fibrillation. The rate at which this ectopic atrial focus discharges will determine the type of the atrial arrhythmia.* This concept is not universally accepted, however; a "circus" movement may play a role in the mechanism of the atrial arrhythmias.

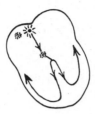

Ectopic Focus in the Atrium (Upper End)

Rate of Discharge of Atrial Ectopic Focus	Arrhythmia
Occasional discharge at a rate slower than the basic sinus rhythm. Atrial premature contractions.	
About 160 to about 220. Atrial tachycardia (with 1:1 conduction).	
About 220 to about 350 Atrial flutter (i.e., atrial tachycardia with A-V block).	
Over 350 Atrial fibrillation.	

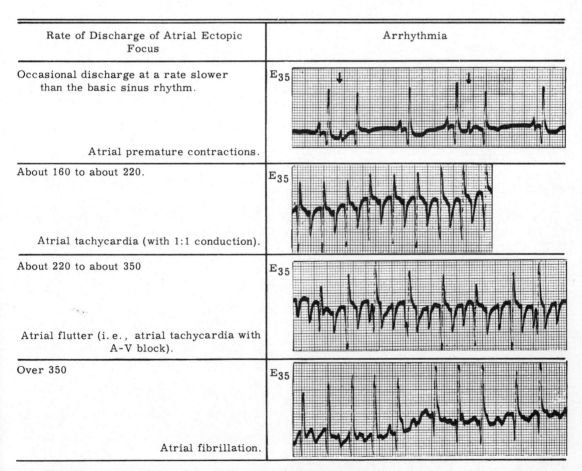

The above are portions of a continuous lead E_{35} electrocardiogram of one patient. The above rhythms were all manifest within a single five minute period.

*This is the unitarian theory of the atrial arrhymias as proposed by Scherf and Prinzmetal.

Chapter 13

DISTURBANCES OF
ATRIOVENTRICULAR CONDUCTION

ATRIOVENTRICULAR BLOCK

Atrioventricular block is a disturbance in conduction between the normal sinus impulse and the eventual ventricular response. It may be complete or incomplete.

Classification:

A. Incomplete:
    1. First degree.
    2. Second degree.
        a. Periodic A-V block.
        b. Constant A-V block.
        c. Wenckebach A-V block.

B. Complete (third degree).

Etiology and Incidence:

First degree A-V block may occur in the absence of any evidence of organic heart disease. Practically every known acute infectious disease may cause this abnormality. It is quite common in acute rheumatic fever. Digitalis and quinidine may produce a first degree A-V block. Coronary artery disease and certain congenital heart lesions may be etiologic factors.

Second and third degree A-V blocks are usually on an organic basis. Digitalis toxicity, infectious diseases (especially diphtheria), coronary artery disease, and myocardial infarction resulting from occlusion of the right coronary artery (the major blood supply to the A-V node) are common causes of the abnormal rhythm.

Mechanism:

Atrioventricular block results from either functional or pathologic defect in the A-V node or bundle of His with resulting delay in the conduction of the impulse. Functional block can occur as the result of increased vagal stimulation. The A-V block produced by digitalis toxicity is in part due to vagal stimulation.

The degree of delay in A-V conduction will determine the type of A-V block: (1) If all atrial impulses are conducted to the ventricles but the conductivity is delayed (i.e., PR >0.20 sec.), a first degree A-V block results. (2) If some of the atrial impulses are conducted to the ventricles and others are not, second degree A-V block results. (3) If all atrial impulses are blocked at the A-V node, a second cardiac pacemaker, either in the A-V node or in the ventricle, stimulates the ventricles; complete (third degree) A-V block is the result.

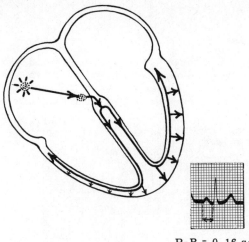

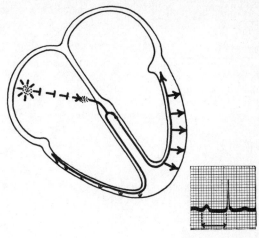

P-R = 0. 16 sec.   P-R = 0. 38 sec.

Normal A-V Conduction. No abnormal delay in spread of impulse from the S-A
node through the A-V node and bundle of
His. This produces a normal P-R
interval.

First Degree A-V Block. Delay in conduction
through the A-V node or bundle of His (or
through atria). This produces a lengthening
of the P-R interval.

Differential Diagnosis:
   The diagnosis of first degree A-V block is rarely made clinically. Second degree A-V block
may clinically be mistaken for any other arrhythmia with an irregular ventricular rhythm. A
complete A-V block with a ventricular rate of ±50 may be mistaken for a sinus bradycardia.
Therefore, an electrocardiogram is essential for the correct diagnosis.

Clinical Significance and Prognosis:
   The clinical significance and the prognosis of A-V block depend on the etiology. That due to
vagal stimulation is of no clinical significance in itself. Heart block due to digitalis toxicity, if
properly treated, does not alter the prognosis of the individual patient. The sudden change from
a regular sinus rhythm to a complete heart block is one cause for the clinical entity known as the
Stokes-Adams syndrome.

   Heart block occurring in association with many acute infectious diseases (except rheumatic
fever) is of little clinical significance in itself. The finding of a first or second degree A-V block
in acute rheumatic fever is an indication of rheumatic myocarditis. The A-V block usually dis-
appears as the disease becomes inactive, but occasionally this disturbance in conduction persists
long after all other signs of rheumatic activity have disappeared. Heart block in diphtheria indicates a severe myocarditis. However, with recovery from the disease, there is no evidence of
resulting chronic myocarditis.

   The significance and prognosis of heart block in association with coronary artery disease will
depend upon the severity of the latter disease. Many individuals are able to tolerate a complete
heart block for years with few or no symptoms.

   The Stokes-Adams syndrome associated with complete A-V block carries a serious prognosis.
Death may occur due to ventricular standstill or ventricular fibrillation.

ELECTROCARDIOGRAPHIC PATTERNS

First Degree Block:

In this condition there is a disturbance in conduction between the S-A and the A-V nodes or a delay in conduction through the A-V node. This results in prolongation of the P-R interval above the upper limit of normal (0.2 sec.). With slow heart rates the interval may be prolonged to 0.6 sec. Rare instances of P-R intervals of 0.7 to 0.8 sec. have been reported. The rhythm remains regular. No dropped beats occur.

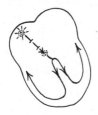

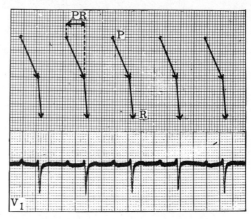

First Degree A-V Block.
The P-R interval is
prolonged to 0.28 sec.

Second Degree Periodic Block:

Periodically the ventricle fails to respond to the atrial stimulation. This may occur at any interval. For example, only five ventricular complexes may follow six atrial complexes, the sixth P wave not being followed by a QRS complex. The seventh to eleventh subsequent atrial contractions will again initiate ventricular responses, but the twelfth will not. The above example would be termed a 6:5 A-V block. The P-P interval is constant throughout. This rhythm is not uncommonly associated with first degree A-V block.

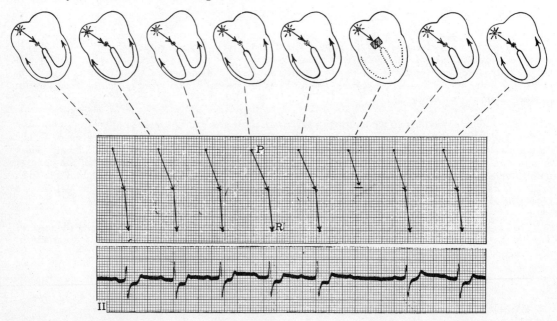

Periodic Second Degree A-V Block. After five sinus-conducted beats, the sixth atrial impulse fails to produce ventricular stimulation. The seventh atrial impulse again initiates ventricular response. The cycle is then repeated. This can be called a 6:5 A-V block. Since there is some progressive lengthening of the P-R interval, it could also be called a Wenckebach block. The ST segment depression is probably the result of digitalis (see p. 275).

Second Degree Constant Block:

With more severe A-V block the ventricles respond even less frequently. A ventricular complex will follow every second, third, or fourth atrial beat, resulting in 2:1, 3:1, or 4:1 A-V block. The atrial rate (P-P interval) is constant. The ventricular response may be a continuing change from 1:1 conduction to 2:1 or 4:1 A-V block.

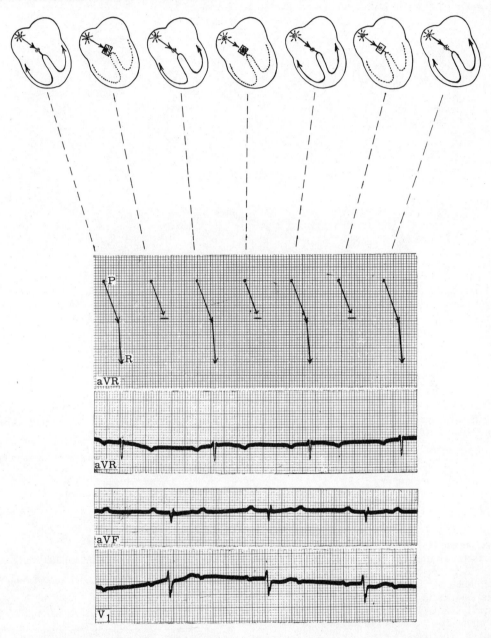

2:1 A-V Block. The atrial rhythm is regular at a rate of 82. Every second atrial beat produces ventricular stimulation.

Second Degree Wenckebach Type of Block:

    A single ventricular beat is dropped in a cyclic fashion. With the first atrial impulse of the cycle there is usually a normal P-R interval. With each succeeding beat the P-R interval becomes progressively longer, until after several (usually three to six) beats an atrial contraction fails to initiate a ventricular response. A long diastolic pause results, and the cycle is then resumed. The number of beats in each cycle is not necessarily constant.

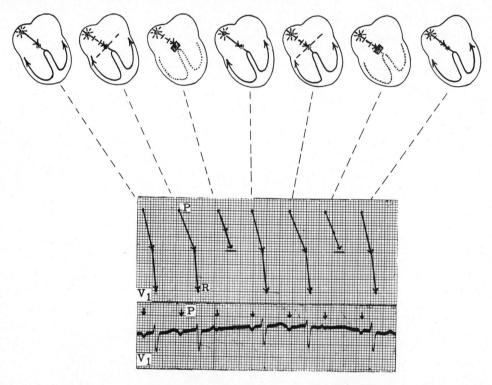

Second Degree A-V Block of Wenckebach Type. The atrial rhythm is regular. (The P waves are identified by arrows.) Every third atrial beat fails to produce a ventricular response. The first P-R = 0.16 sec., the second = 0.28 sec.

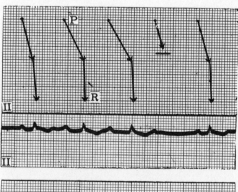

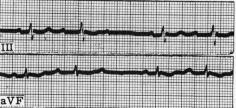

Second Degree A-V Block of Wenckebach Type. The atrial rhythm is regular. In lead II, the first PR interval = 0.18 sec., the second = 0.28, and the third = 0.36 sec. The fourth atrial beat fails to activate the ventricle. In leads III and aVF, the cycle consists of only two sinus-conducted beats followed by the dropped ventricular beat.

Complete (Third Degree) Block:

In this condition the atria and ventricles beat entirely independently of one another. The atrial rhythm is usually regular, and the atrial rate is that of average regular sinus rhythm. However, the atrial rhythm may at times be an atrial tachycardia or atrial fibrillation. The ventricular rhythm is usually quite regular but of much slower rate (20 to 60). The ventricle may respond to a pacemaker in the A-V node, producing QRS complexes which appear normal; or may respond to a pacemaker in either ventricle, producing QRS complexes which have the appearance of ventricular premature beats. The latter is termed idioventricular rhythm.

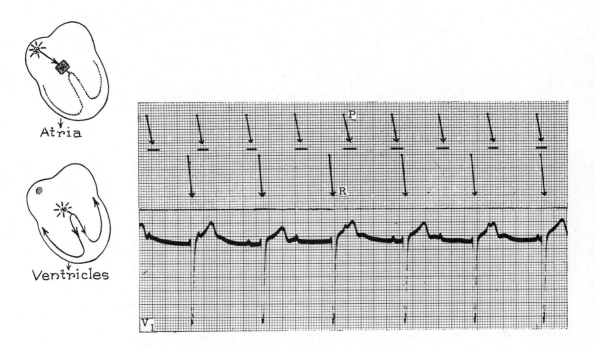

Atria

Ventricles

Diagram of Complete Heart Block. The atria are activated by impulses arising normally in the S-A node. In this example the atrial rate = 72. The atrial impulses do not activate the ventricles. A second cardiac pacemaker is located near the A-V node and stimulates the ventricles. The ventricular rate = 54. The atrial and ventricular rhythms are independent of each other.

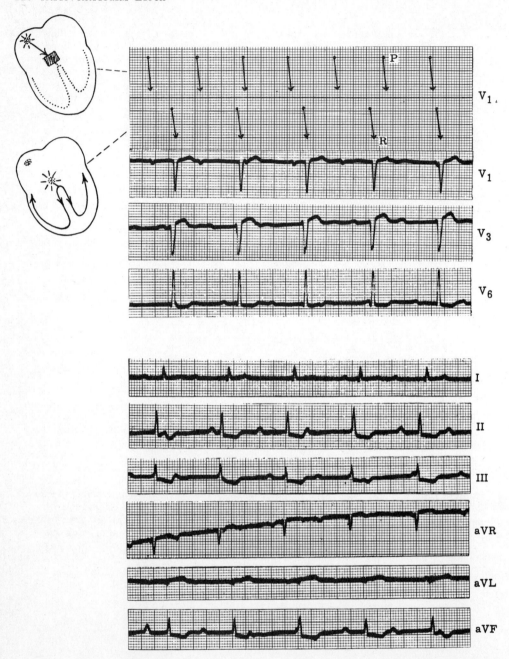

Complete A-V Block. The atrial rhythm is regular at a rate of 82. The ventricular rhythm is regular at a rate of 60. There is no relationship between the two rhythms, the atria responding to the sinus node and the ventricles responding to a second independent pacemaker. Since the QRS complexes are of normal duration, this latter pacemaker is in or close to the A-V node. The apparent widening of some of the QRS complexes (fifth QRS in lead III and third QRS in lead aVF) is the result of fortuitous superimposition of the P wave and the QRS complex.

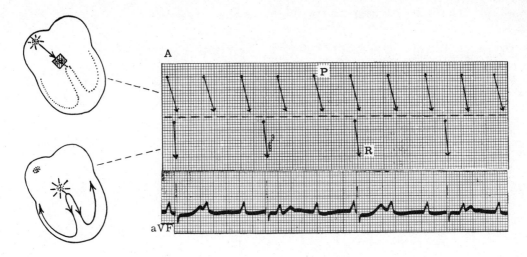

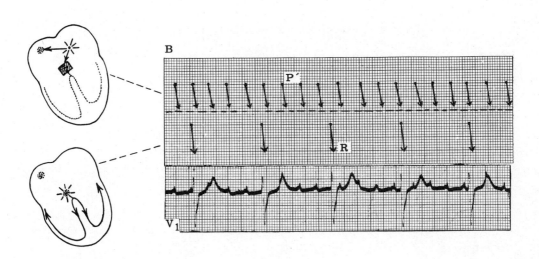

Complete A-V Block. **A:** A regular sinus atrial rhythm at a rate of 107 exists with an independent ventricular rhythm at a rate of 43. **B:** The atrial rate is now rapid at a rate of 230. This indicates atrial tachycardia (or flutter). The ventricular rhythm is regular at a rate of 55. This is still a complete heart block and not a 4:1 flutter since there is no constant relationship between the QRS complex and the preceding atrial wave. (Note that the atrial rhythm is not perfectly regular. This is a rare exception to the general rule that the atrial rhythm of atrial tachycardia is regular. It is believed that the ventricular contractions "reflexly" alter the P-P interval (see p. 212).

ATRIOVENTRICULAR NODAL RHYTHMS

Nodal Premature Beats:

In this condition an ectopic focus arises in the A-V node. The impulse then spreads upward into the atrium and downward into the ventricle. This produces an upright P′ in aVR and high esophageal leads and an inverted P′ in aVF and low esophageal leads. The QRS-T complexes are of normal (or basic) configuration.

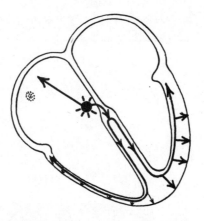

Cardiac Impulse Arising in A-V Node

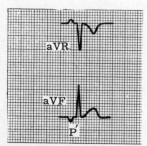

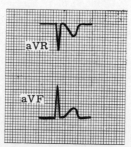

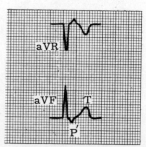

High A-V nodal focus. Note upright P′ in aVR and inverted P′ in aVF preceding the QRS complex.

Mid A-V nodal focus. P′ buried in QRS complex.

Low A-V nodal focus. Note upright P′ in aVR and inverted P′ in aVF following the QRS complex.

High A-V Nodal Premature Beats:

The ectopic focus is believed to arise in the upper portion of the node. The atrium is activated in a retrograde fashion prior to activation of the ventricle. This produces a normal or short P'-R interval. Such a beat is indistinguishable from an atrial ectopic beat arising from a low atrial focus and therefore is best referred to as a supraventricular premature beat.

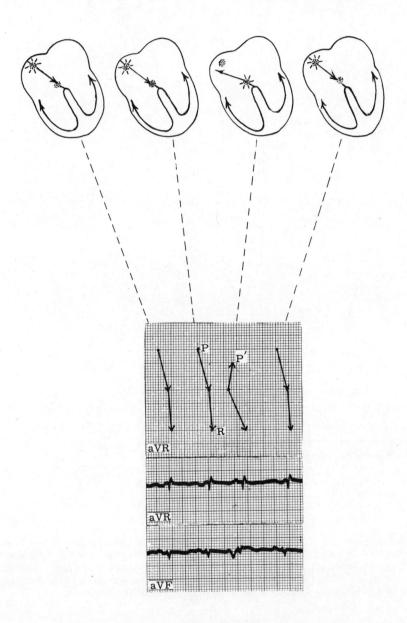

High A-V Nodal Premature Beats. The first, second, and fourth beats are sinus-conducted; the P-R interval = 0.14 sec. The third beat has an upright P' in aVR and an inverted P' in aVF, indicating retrograde atrial conduction. The P'-R interval = 0.08 sec. The QRS-T complexes are normal. It is postulated that the impulse arises in the upper portion of the A-V node and produces retrograde atrial stimulation prior to ventricular stimulation. An identical pattern could result from an ectopic focus low in the atrium. A more inclusive term would be "supraventricular premature beats."

Mid A-V Nodal Premature Beats:
The P wave is buried in the QRS complex and may not be visible.

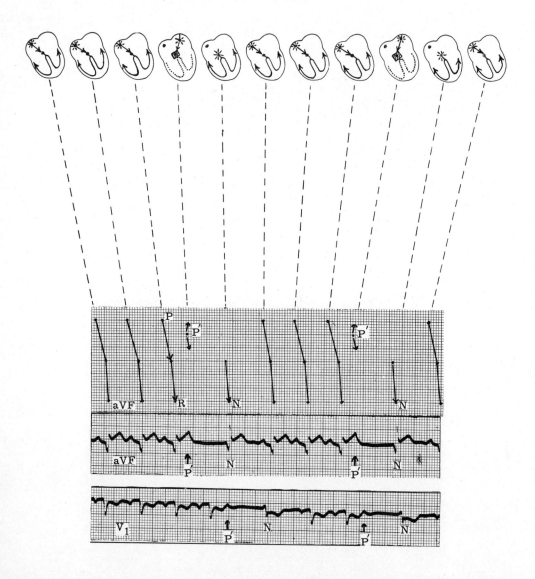

Mid A-V Nodal Beats. Blocked premature atrial contractions (P′) are indicated by the arrows in aVF and V₁. Each is followed by a ventricular complex (N) which is similar to those of the regular sinus beats. However, no evidence of atrial activity can be seen preceding or following the ventricular complex. These beats are therefore termed mid-nodal A-V beats. In addition lead aVF reveals a deep, wide Q wave indicative of inferior wall infarction.

<u>Low A-V Nodal Premature Beats:</u>

The P' wave follows the QRS complex. The atria are stimulated in a retrograde fashion but are activated after ventricular excitation.

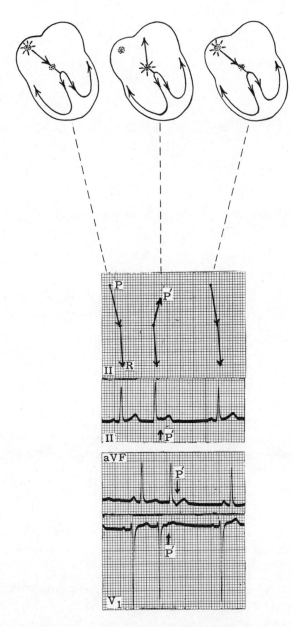

Low A-V Nodal Premature Beats. One premature beat is seen in each lead. The QRS complex is normal and is not preceded by an atrial wave, indicating that it is arising from an ectopic stimulus in the A-V node. Each such QRS complex is followed by a P' wave (indicated by arrow). This is inverted in aVF, indicating retrograde atrial conduction.

<u>Clinical Significance:</u>

Nodal premature beats have the same clinical significance as atrial premature beats.

Reciprocal Beats:

The P' wave may follow the QRS complex by a fairly long interval. If the ventricle is no longer refractory, the atrial stimulation resulting from the A-V nodal stimulus may in turn re-activate the ventricle and produce another QRS-T complex of normal (or basic) configuration. This is known as a reciprocal beat.

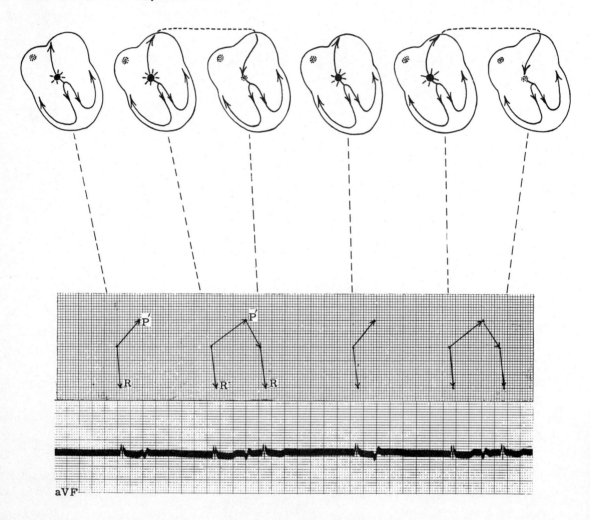

A-V Nodal Rhythm With Reciprocal Beats. The first two ventricular complexes are not preceded by atrial activity. Both are followed by P' waves produced by retrograde atrial conduction. The second atrial beat follows the ventricular beat by a sufficiently long period of time to allow the ventricle to respond again to this retrograde atrial impulse. The cycle is then repeated.

A-V Nodal Rhythm:

The A-V node acts as the cardiac pacemaker. Each complete complex has the same appearance as a nodal premature beat. The rhythm is regular, and the rate may vary from 40 to 80. Similar to the types of nodal premature beats, an A-V nodal rhythm may arise from a high, middle, or low nodal focus. That arising from a high nodal focus has been termed "coronary sinus" rhythm.

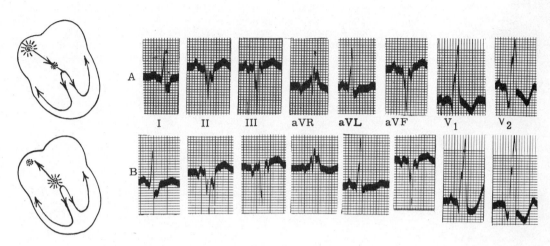

A-V Nodal Rhythm (Coronary sinus rhythm). A: The rhythm is regular sinus, as evidenced by the upright P waves in II, III, and aVF and the inverted P in aVR. In addition, the pattern is that of a right bundle branch block (wide, notched R in V_{1-2}; QRS = 0.15 sec.) with anterior wall infarction (deep, wide Q in V_{1-2}). B: The P' waves are now inverted in II, III, and aVF and upright in aVR. This is indicative of a high A-V nodal rhythm.

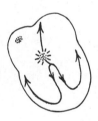

A-V Nodal Rhythm. A regular ventricular rhythm is present at a rate of 70. No atrial activity precedes the QRS complexes. An atrial wave intermingled with the T wave is seen following each QRS complex. The P is upright and the T is inverted in aVR; the P and T are inverted in aVF, indicating retrograde atrial conduction.

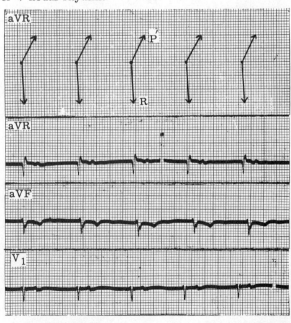

Clinical Significance:

Nodal rhythm may be transient or permanent. Transient nodal rhythm may be seen in normal people. It may be produced by carotid sinus pressure or may result from digitalis or quinidine administration. Transient or permanent nodal rhythm results from a variety of organic heart diseases, e.g., rheumatic fever, other acute infectious myocarditides, and coronary artery disease.

ATRIOVENTRICULAR NODAL TACHYCARDIA

In A-V nodal tachycardia the A-V node acts as the primary cardiac pacemaker. The rate can vary from 120 to 200. The ventricular rhythm is regular. The $\overset{\prime}{P}$ waves may precede, be buried in, or follow the QRS complexes, depending upon the site of origin in the A-V node. The electrocardiographic pattern of each entire complex is identical with that of a nodal premature beat. With a rapid rate it is impossible to tell whether any given $\overset{\prime}{P}$ wave is related to the preceding QRS complex or to the following complex. Actually one cannot differentiate the electrocardiographic pattern produced by nodal tachycardia from that produced by an atrial tachycardia arising in a low atrial ectopic focus. Therefore, the more inclusive term, supraventricular tachycardia, is applicable.

<u>Clinical Significance:</u>
The same as for atrial tachycardia (see p. 210).

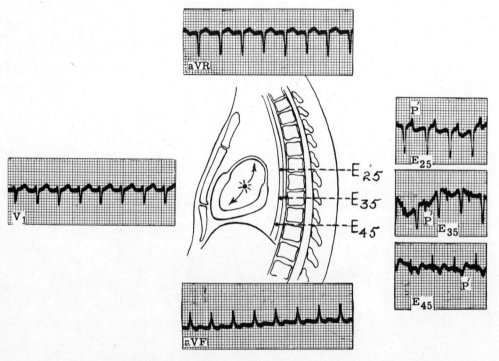

Leads aVR, aVF, and V_1 reveal a tachycardia with a ventricular rate of 182. No atrial activity can be identified. In esophageal leads the atrial waves are readily visible. At E_{45} the $\overset{\prime}{P}$ is inverted, and at E_{25} the $\overset{\prime}{P}$ is upright. This is the reverse of the normal direction, indicating an ectopic focus in the A-V node or lower portion of the atrium.

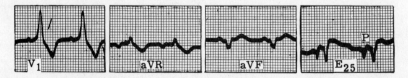

After conversion with intravenous digitalis. The P wave is now normally inverted at E_{25}. The basic pattern is that of a Wolff-Parkinson-White syndrome. (See p. 261.)

Supraventricular (A-V Nodal or Low Atrial) Paroxysmal Tachycardia

Chapter 14

THE VENTRICULAR ARRHYTHMIAS

INTRAVENTRICULAR CONDUCTION DEFECT

In this condition the QRS interval is prolonged over 0.1 sec. No other electrocardiographic abnormalities need be present.

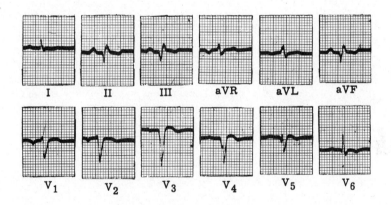

I	II	III	aVR	aVL	aVF
V_1	V_2	V_3	V_4	V_5	V_6

Intraventricular Conduction Defect. The electrocardiogram shows evidence of anterior (QS complexes in V_{3-4}; inverted T waves V_{3-6}) and inferior wall (deep Q waves with inverted T waves in II, III, and aVF) infarction. In addition the QRS interval is widened to 0.1 to 0.12 sec. The pattern is not that of either a right or left bundle branch block. It is therefore classified as an intraventricular conduction defect.

Focal Intraventricular Block:

Occasionally an intraventricular conduction defect will be seen only in a few leads and the remainder of the leads will have normal QRS intervals. This results from localized disease of the ventricular myocardium, usually infarction.

Since this is usually evident in precordial leads and not in frontal plane leads which cannot be explained on the basis of vector concept (i.e., the QRS interval at any given time is a constant and hence cannot vary from lead to lead), it must be due to the proximity effect of the precordial electrodes.

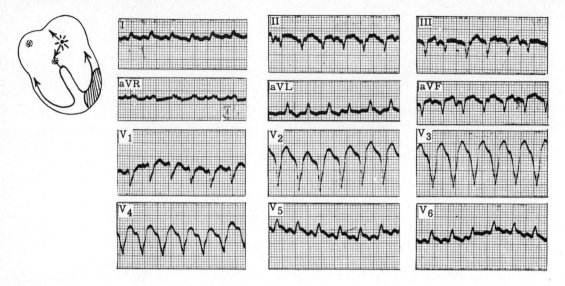

Focal Intraventricular Block. The QRS interval in leads I, II, III, aVR, aVL, aVF, V_5, and V_6 is 0.08 sec. In leads V_{1-4} the QRS interval is widened to 0.14 sec. This indicates a localized or focal intraventricular conduction defect in the anteroseptal region of the myocardium (zone of infarction). (See p. 249 for other details of this electrocardiogram.)

Clinical Significance:

An intraventricular conduction defect may result from the administration of digitalis or quinidine. It may result from a variety of organic diseases, most commonly coronary artery disease with local myocardial destruction, the infectious myocarditides, and certain forms of congenital heart disease.

VENTRICULAR PREMATURE BEATS

Ventricular premature beats (or contractions) are those which arise from an ectopic focus in any portion of the ventricular myocardium.

Etiology and Incidence:

Ventricular premature beats are commonly seen in association with any form of organic heart disease, especially coronary artery disease and any of the myocarditides. They are often the result of drug intoxication, digitalis being the commonest offender and quinidine a less common cause. They may occur in normal individuals, but much less commonly than supraventricular premature beats.

Mechanism:

Ventricular premature beats result from an irritable focus in any portion of the ventricular myocardium. The impulse arising from this ectopic focus will activate the ventricles. Since this impulse usually does not activate the atria, the regular sinoatrial rhythm is not disturbed. The regular sinus impulse following the premature beat will usually not activate the ventricle since the latter is still refractory from the premature contraction. The ventricle will respond to the next normal sinus impulse. Therefore the interval between the two sinus beats preceding and following the premature beat will be exactly twice the regular sinus rate. This is known as a compensatory pause (see p. 240, top).

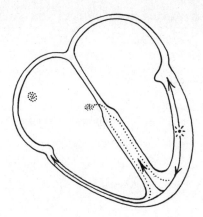

Ectopic Focus in Ventricle Producing Ventricular Premature Beat

Differential Diagnosis:

    Clinically, ventricular premature beats may be mistaken for atrial premature beats. The presence of numerous ventricular premature beats may lead to a mistaken clinical diagnosis of atrial fibrillation. Electrocardiographically there is little difficulty in diagnosis. Accelerated conduction beats may be mistaken for ventricular premature contractions (see p. 265, top).

Clinical Significance:

    Digitalis is a common cause of ventricular premature contractions and characteristically produces ventricular bigeminy. On the other hand, one may see frequent ventricular premature beats (or even bigeminy) in a patient with congestive heart failure who has not received digitalis. These may then disappear following digitalization. One can see how important an accurate history is in such a circumstance, since the ventricular premature beats as a manifestation of heart failure could indicate a need for digitalis or could indicate digitalis intoxication.

    Ventricular ectopic beats occurring in association with acute myocardial infarction require immediate therapy since they may be the precursors of such serious or even fatal arrhythmias as ventricular tachycardia or ventricular fibrillation.

Prognosis:

    The nature of the underlying heart disease rather than the presence of the ventricular premature beats per se will determine the prognosis. The presence of numerous and multifocal ventricular premature beats in the presence of serious heart disease (e. g., acute myocardial infarction) worsens the prognosis. In the absence of organic heart disease, ventricular premature beats have no significance and do not affect prognosis.

ELECTROCARDIOGRAPHIC PATTERNS

The QRS complex is prolonged over 0.1 sec. and has a bizarre appearance, being notched and slurred. The ST segment and the T wave are usually displaced in the direction opposite to the main deflection of the QRS complex.

Ventricular premature beats arising from a single ectopic focus have the same configuration in any one lead. Those arising from different ectopic foci show differing patterns in any one lead.

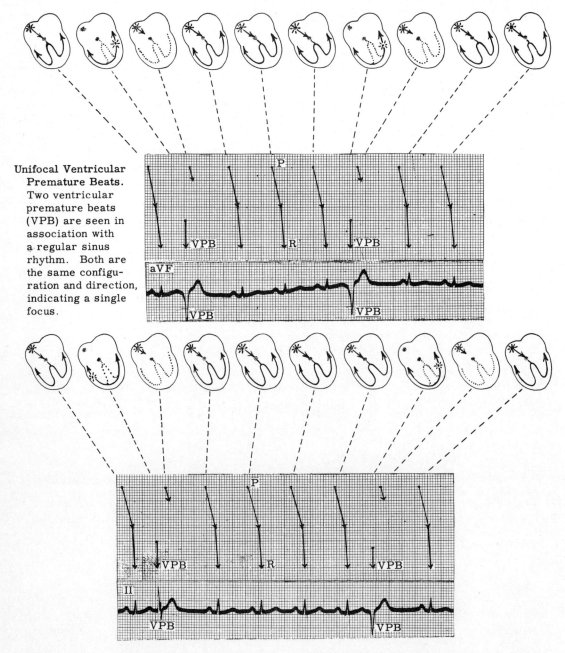

Unifocal Ventricular Premature Beats. Two ventricular premature beats (VPB) are seen in association with a regular sinus rhythm. Both are the same configuration and direction, indicating a single focus.

Multifocal Ventricular Premature Beats. Two ventricular premature beats (VPB) are seen in association with a regular sinus rhythm. The major deflection of the first is upright; that of the second is downward. This indicates two different ventricular foci.

Depending upon when the ventricular premature beat occurs, the independent normal atrial beats may precede, be hidden in, or follow the QRS. A retrograde Ṕ may follow the QRS. The occurrence of a normal P wave preceding the QRS complex of the premature ventricular beat is purely fortuitous. It may be impossible to distinguish such a beat from an accelerated conduction beat (see p. 264).

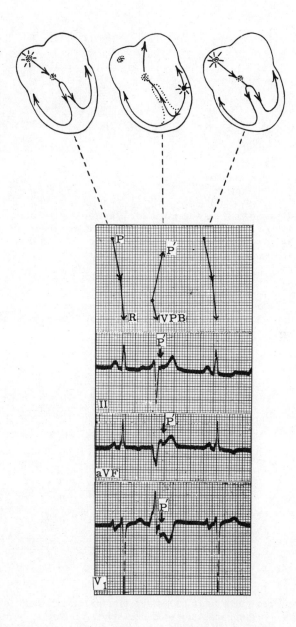

Ventricular Premature Contractions. In the illustrated leads a wide slurred QRS complex is seen between two regular sinus beats. These are not preceded by an atrial complex and hence are premature ventricular contractions. Ṕ waves are seen following each of these. The direction of the Ṕ wave (inverted in II and aVF) is opposite that of the normal P, indicating a reverse direction of atrial stimulation. These are retrograde atrial contractions resulting from the premature ventricular beat.

Since the normal sinus rhythm is usually not disturbed, a full compensatory pause follows the ventricular premature beat.

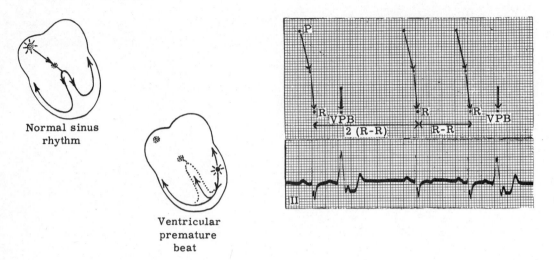

Normal sinus
rhythm

Ventricular
premature
beat

Ventricular Premature Beats; Compensatory Pause. Ventricular premature beats are seen following the first and third sinus beats. The R-R interval for the sinus rhythm (measured between the second and third sinus beats) = 0.8 sec. The R-R interval between the first and third sinus beats = 1.6 sec. Hence, a full compensatory pause exists.

If the sinus rhythm is slow, a ventricular premature beat can occur between two normal sinus beats without altering the R-R interval. This is known as an **interpolated beat.**

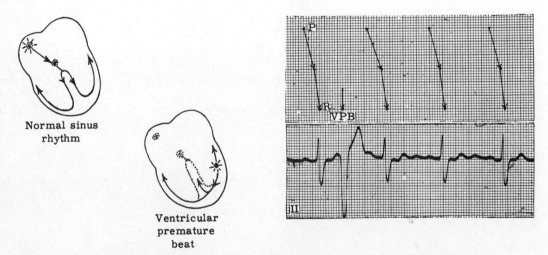

Normal sinus
rhythm

Ventricular
premature
beat

Interpolated Ventricular Premature Beat. A ventricular premature beat is seen between the first and second sinus beats. A compensatory pause does not follow the premature contraction. The slight variation in the R-R interval is due to sinus arrhythmia. The QRS interval of the sinus beats = 0.15 sec., indicating an intraventricular conduction defect.

Ventricular premature beats may occur in association with any other arrhythmia.

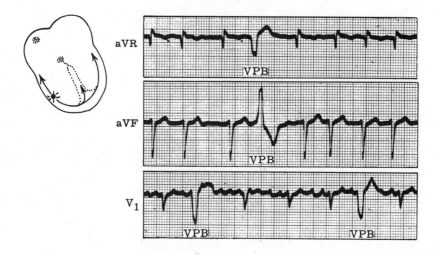

Ventricular Premature Contractions in Association With Atrial Fibrillation

Ventricular Premature Contractions During the Refractory Period:

Since the Q-T interval approximates the refractory period of the heart cycle, a ventricular premature contraction usually occurs after the T wave of the preceding beat (see p. 198). However, on occasion a ventricular ectopic beat may begin during the inscription of the preceding T wave, i.e., during the relative refractory period. This indicates a strong ectopic stimulus and clinically is more serious.

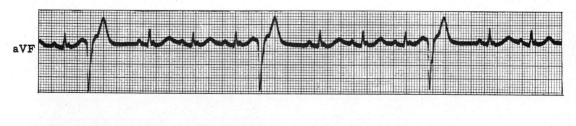

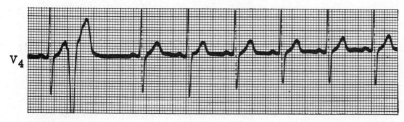

Ventricular Premature Contractions During the Refractory Period. Above are two electrocardiographic strips from two patients. Ventricular ectopic beats are seen occurring before completion of the T wave of the preceding beat.

Differentiation of Site of Ectopic Beat:

One can distinguish between ventricular premature beats arising in either the left or right ventricle. If the major QRS deflection is upright in right precordial leads (V_1) and downward in left precordial leads (V_{5-6}), the ectopic focus is in the left ventricle. The reverse is true for right ventricular premature beats.

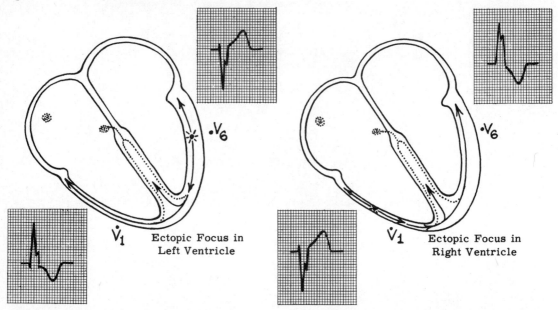

| Ectopic Focus in Left Ventricle | Ectopic Focus in Right Ventricle |

The main spread of the impulse is away from the electrode at V_6, resulting in a downward QRS deflection; it is towards the electrode at V_1 resulting in an upright QRS deflection.

The main spread of the impulse is away from the electrode at V_1 resulting in a downward QRS deflection; it is toward the electrode at V_6 resulting in an upright QRS deflection.

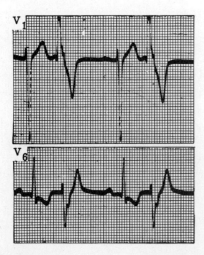

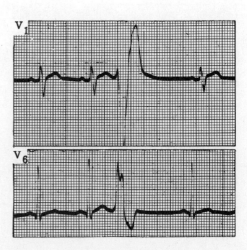

Ventricular Premature Beats of Left Ventricular Origin. The main deflection of the ventricular premature beats is upright in V_1 and downward in V_6, indicating an ectopic focus in the left ventricle.

Ventricular Premature Beats of Right Ventricular Origin. The main deflection of the ventricular premature beats is downward in V_1 and upright in V_6, indicating an ectopic focus in the right ventricle.

Ventricular Bigeminy:

The rhythm alternates between a regular sinus beat (or any basic arrhythmia) and a ventricular premature beat. There is usually a constant interval between the sinus beat and the ventricular premature beat, i.e., fixed coupling, indicating that by some means the sinus beat controls the discharge of the ventricular ectopic focus.

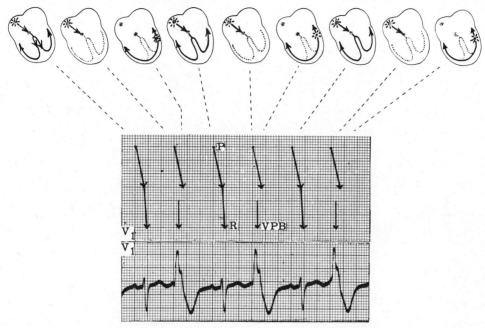

Ventricular Bigeminy. The rhythm is a regular sinus beat followed by a ventricular premature beat, a pause, and then repetition of this sequence. The time interval between the sinus beat and the ventricular premature beat is perfectly constant (fixed coupling). The P waves of the sinus rhythm fortuitously precede the first two ectopic beats. The P wave is buried (fused) in the QRS complex of the third ectopic beat (fusion beat).

Post-Extrasystolic T Wave Change:

Occasionally the T wave of the basic complex following a premature ventricular contraction will have a different configuration than the basic T wave of the other sinus-conducted beats. For example, the basic T wave will be upright and the T wave of the complex following the premature beat will be inverted. It is believed by some that this is indicative of organic heart disease.

Change in the T Wave Following a Ventricular Premature Beat.
The T waves of the complex preceding the premature beat are upright. Those following are diphasic to inverted. The strips illustrated are from two different patients. Both were clinically diagnosed as idiopathic (Fiedler's) myocarditis.

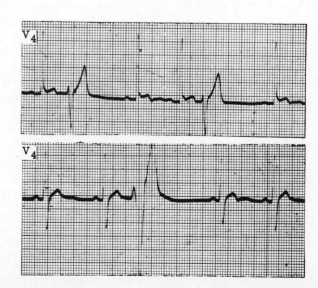

In the presence of myocardial infarction, a ventricular premature beat may show some of the typical features of an infarct pattern. As mentioned above (see p. 194) one cannot usually diagnose an infarct in the presence of a left bundle branch block. However, a ventricular premature beat in such a circumstance may show the infarct pattern.

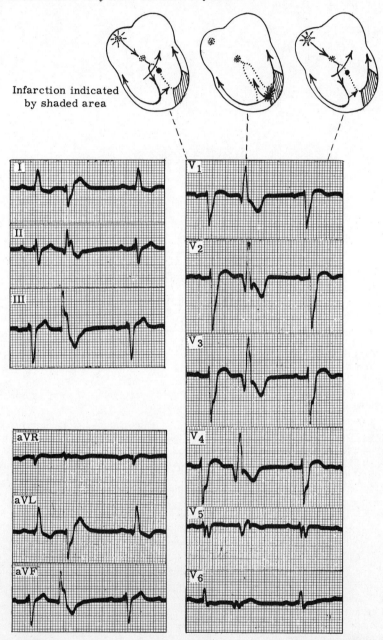

Infarction indicated
by shaded area

Ventricular Premature Contractions as an Indication of Myocardial Infarction. The first and third complexes in each lead are sinus conducted beats. The pattern is indicative of a left bundle branch block. An electrocardiographic diagnosis of infarction cannot be made in the presence of this pattern. The second complex in each lead is a premature ventricular contraction. The major QRS deflection is upright in V_1 and downward in V_6, indicating a left ventricular focus. Deep Q waves are part of the complex of these beats and are characteristic of an infarct pattern. Although an electrocardiographic diagnosis of infarction based on the appearance of premature ventricular contractions is not conclusive, it is strongly suggestive. **Clinical Diagnosis:** Arteriosclerotic heart disease; history of myocardial infarction one year previously.

VENTRICULAR TACHYCARDIA

Ventricular tachycardia is a rapid heart action, with a rate usually varying from 140 to 220 beats per minute. The rhythm is usually slightly irregular.

Etiology and Incidence:

Ventricular tachycardia is most commonly associated with recent myocardial infarction. It may occur in association with hypertensive and arteriosclerotic heart disease. Digitalis toxicity or quinidine toxicity may induce ventricular tachycardia. It is rarely seen in individuals with no clinical evidence of organic heart disease. In the latter instance it has been reported to occur in association with the Wolff-Parkinson-White syndrome (see p. 258).

Mechanism:

Ventricular tachycardia results from a rapidly discharging focus (usually single) in the ventricular myocardium.

Clinical Significance:

Ventricular tachycardia is practically always indicative of serious organic heart disease or serious drug (digitalis or quinidine) intoxication.

Prognosis:

Ventricular tachycardia is a very serious arrhythmia. Unless successfully terminated, the mortality will be very high. Prognosis depends also upon the nature of the underlying heart disease.

ELECTROCARDIOGRAPHIC PATTERNS

The rhythm is a rapid succession of ventricular premature beats, each complex having the exact appearance of a ventricular premature beat. With a rapid rate it may be impossible to separate the QRS complexes from the ST segments and T waves, and the tracing has the appearance of a series of wide, large undulations. The ventricular rhythm is usually slightly irregular.

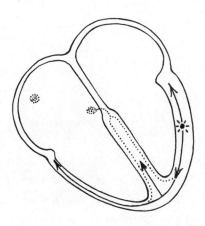

Ventricular Tachycardia and Ventricular Premature Contractions. The first three strips are indicative of ventricular tachycardia with a ventricular rate of 240. The lower strip was taken following conversion to regular sinus rhythm. One ventricular premature beat is seen. This has a QRS configuration similar to that of the tachycardia. This suggests that both are arising from the same ectopic focus located in the left ventricle.

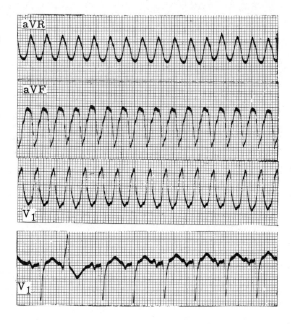

The normal sinus rhythm usually continues independently of the ventricular tachycardia. The P waves may not be seen with any regularity in the standard 12-lead electrocardiogram, but esophageal leads will clearly record the sinus beats. Retrograde P' waves may occur just as in an isolated ventricular premature beat or a low nodal premature beat.

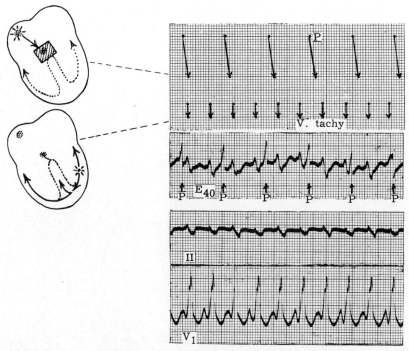

Ventricular Tachycardia. Leads II and V_1 reveal a tachycardia with a ventricular rate of 173. There is suggestive evidence of atrial activity, but one could not be positive of this. The QRS complexes are wide and slurred. Esophageal lead E_{40} clearly identifies the atrial contractions (indicated by arrows). They occur regularly at a rate of 95. This, therefore, is a ventricular tachycardia. The ventricles respond to an ectopic left ventricular focus discharging at a rate of 173. The atria respond to the normal sinus pacemaker at a rate of 95.

Ventricular tachycardia may occur independently in the presence of any atrial arrhythmia. However, it is usually impossible to diagnose the atrial arrhythmia at this time without the use of esophageal leads.

Bidirectional ventricular tachycardia is the term applied to a form of ventricular tachycardia in which the QRS complexes in any one lead alternate in opposite directions; i.e., the QRS complex of one ventricular beat is upright and that of the following is downward.

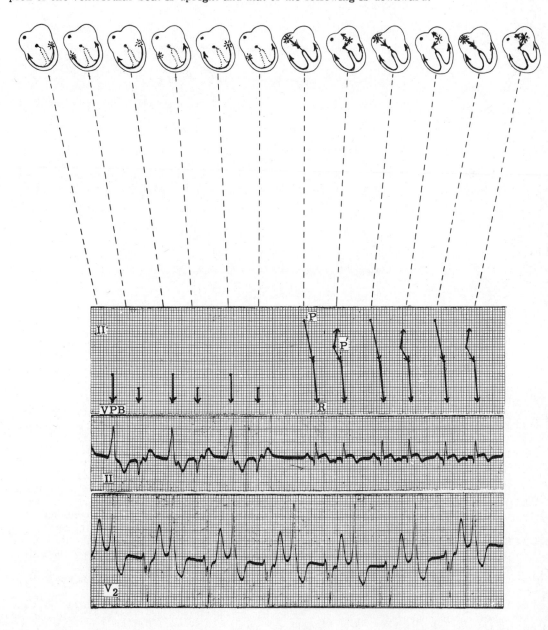

Bidirectional Ventricular Tachycardia. The first portion of II and all of V_2 show a series of ventricular premature contractions occurring in a bidirectional fashion. The ventricular rate is 128. The bidirectional ventricular tachycardia did not result from digitalis in this case. The second half of the lead II strip reveals a regular sinus rhythm alternating with atrial premature contractions. The Q and inverted T in II is evidence of inferior wall infarction.

Differential Diagnosis:
A. Atrial Fibrillation (or Supraventricular Tachycardia) With Bundle Branch Block: Such a pattern may be indistinguishable from a ventricular tachycardia. If the ectopic focus is arising in the upper portion of the atrium and the P′ waves are clearly recorded (as in esophageal leads), the P′ waves will indicate a normal direction of atrial stimulation (inverted in aVR and high esophageal leads; upright in aVF and low esophageal leads) and therefore identify the rhythm as atrial in origin.

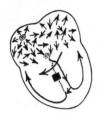 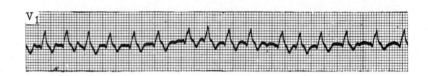

A: An irregular rhythm is seen with a ventricular rate of 170. The QRS complexes are wide and notched. This could represent a ventricular tachycardia, but the degree of irregularity would be unusual.

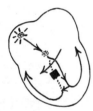 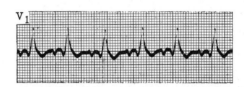

B: The rhythm is now regular sinus. The QRS complexes remain wide and are similar to those seen in (A). (The wide Q and absent initial r indicate the presence of anterior wall infarction in association with right bundle branch block.)

Rapid Atrial Fibrillation With a Right Bundle Branch Block Simulating Ventricular Tachycardia

However, if the supraventricular tachycardia is the result of an ectopic focus in the lower portion of the atrium (or A-V node), the P′ waves will indicate the reverse direction of atrial stimulation and are indistinguishable from retrograde P′ waves resulting from ventricular tachycardia. One will therefore have to rely on other criteria for the differential diagnosis.
1. Supraventricular tachycardia is practically always perfectly regular, i.e., the R-R interval is constant. Ventricular tachycardia is usually slightly irregular, i.e., the R-R interval is not absolutely constant.
2. Carotid stimulation may terminate an episode of supraventricular tachycardia but will have no effect on a ventricular tachycardia.
3. Differentiation may be impossible until the tachycardia stops and the subsequent QRS complexes can be observed.

PAROXYSMAL VENTRICULAR VS. SUPRAVENTRICULAR TACHYCARDIA

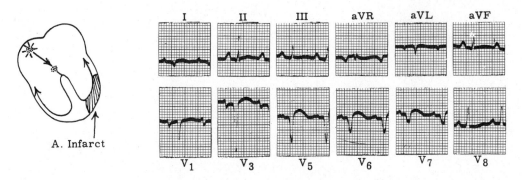

A. Infarct

The pattern is that of extensive anterior wall infarction (QS complexes in
I, aVL, and V_{1-7}, with ST segment elevation in V_{3-7}).

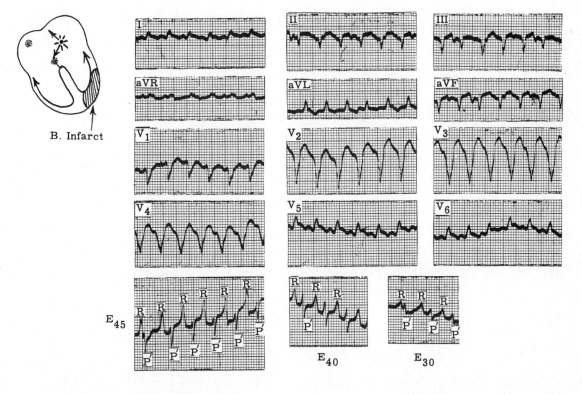

B. Infarct

One day after the tracing at top of page was taken: a tachycardia is now present. The ventricular rhythm is perfectly regular at a rate of 187. The QRS complexes are now inverted in II, III, and aVF. The QRS complexes are wide in V_{3-5} and are typical of ventricular tachycardia. However, the QRS complexes are not widened in other leads. This therefore suggests focal intraventricular block. Suggestive atrial activity is seen in some of the leads. **Esophageal Leads:** Definite atrial activity is now seen. The atrial rate is exactly the same as the ventricular rate. The P waves are inverted at E_{45} and upright at E_{30}, indicating retrograde atrial conduction. The above record could be called a ventricular tachycardia with 1:1 retrograde atrial conduction. However, since the QRS complexes are not widened in all leads, this tracing more probably represents supraventricular conduction with the pacemaker in the lower portion of the atria (explaining the reverse direction of the P' wave), aberrant intraventricular conduction (explaining the change in II, III, and aVF), and focal intraventricular block (explaining the localized widening of the QRS complexes in V_{2-4}). Following treatment with intramuscular quinidine, the pattern reverted to that seen above.

B. Supraventricular Tachycardia With Accelerated Conduction: Such a pattern will simulate that of supraventricular tachycardia with bundle branch block. (See p. 266.)

VENTRICULAR FIBRILLATION

Ventricular fibrillation is a rapid, irregular cardiac rhythm. The diagnosis must be made electrocardiographically since the peripheral pulses are not palpable and the heart beat is usually inaudible.

Etiology and Incidence:
The same conditions which give rise to ventricular tachycardia can result in ventricular fibrillation. The most common cause is acute myocardial infarction and is an explanation for many of the sudden deaths in this disease. It can occur as the terminal manifestation of any organic heart disease. Digitalis or quinidine toxicity can produce this rhythm. It occurs during surgical procedures performed under general anesthesia, in which case hypoxia is the common precipitating factor. Electric shock may produce ventricular fibrillation. Hypothermia, either naturally occurring or induced as an adjunct for surgery (unless a by-pass circulation is used), commonly produces ventricular fibrillation when the body temperature falls below 28° C.

Mechanism:
Ventricular fibrillation results from a rapid discharge of impulses from single or multiple foci in the ventricles. The ventricles are unable to respond completely and effectively to each stimulus.

Electrocardiographic Pattern:
Since the ventricular contractions are erratic, the electrocardiogram shows bizarre ventricular patterns of varying size and configuration. The rate is rapid and irregular. The atria may continue to respond to sinus node stimulation, but P waves are not visible without the aid of esophageal leads.

Differential Diagnosis:
Since there is no palpable or auscultatory evidence of cardiac action, ventricular fibrillation cannot be clinically differentiated from ventricular standstill. It is essential to differentiate these two conditions electrocardiographically, since the drugs (epinephrine and ephedrine) which are useful in treatment of ventricular standstill are contraindicated in ventricular fibrillation.

Clinical Significance:
Ventricular fibrillation is the most serious arrhythmia which occurs. Since it is often preceded by ventricular premature beats and ventricular tachycardia, the latter rhythms in the presence of serious organic heart disease (e. g., acute myocardial infarction) must be treated promptly. However, since ventricular fibrillation may occur without warning in an individual with an acute myocardial infarct, many authorities advise the routine use of quinidine (0. 4 Gm. four times daily) to attempt to prevent this arrhythmia.

Ventricular fibrillation may occur in transient paroxysms and be the cause of the Stokes-Adams syndrome.

Prognosis:
The prognosis is exceedingly poor in the presence of ventricular fibrillation. Since recovery is rare if this arrhythmia has continued for five minutes, immediate electrocardiographic diagnosis and prompt therapy is necessary for recovery.

The prognosis is better when this arrhythmia occurs during surgery even though the anesthetist cannot differentiate this rhythm from ventricular standstill without an electrocardiogram. In either event prompt exposure of the heart will allow for immediate diagnosis and treatment.

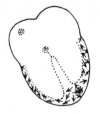

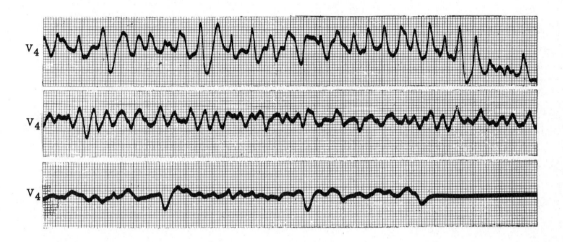

Ventricular Fibrillation. Portions of a continuous strip of lead V_4 taken on a patient dying of a myocardial infarct. The ventricular complexes are rapid, irregular, and bizarre. This is typical of ventricular fibrillation. The tracing terminates with asystole.

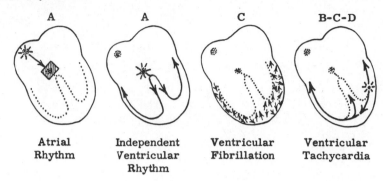

A	A	C	B-C-D
Atrial Rhythm	Independent Ventricular Rhythm	Ventricular Fibrillation	Ventricular Tachycardia

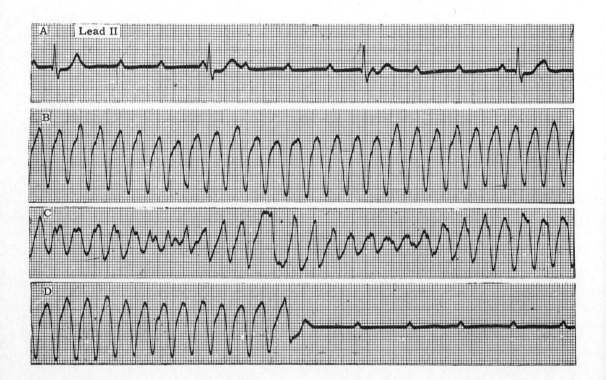

Stokes-Adams Syndrome. Complete heart block with ventricular tachycardia, ventricular fibrillation, and ventricular asystole.

A. Complete Heart Block: The atrial rate is 92, the ventricular rate 25.

B. Ventricular Tachycardia: The ventricular rate is 200. The QRS complexes are wide, undulating waves.

C. Ventricular Fibrillation Interspersed With Ventricular Tachycardia: The QRS complexes are more bizarre during the period of ventricular fibrillation and vary in size and configuration from beat to beat.

D. Ventricular Tachycardia Terminating in Ventricular Asystole: Atrial activity is now seen. The patient died shortly thereafter. This tracing illustrates the arrhythmias associated with the Stokes-Adams syndrome.

Chapter 15

THE PARARRHYTHMIAS

A pararrhythmia is an abnormal rhythm in which two pacemakers discharge independently of each other; each at differing times can activate the ventricles. One center is usually in the S-A node. By definition, a pararrhythmia does not disturb the conduction of the normal sinus impulse. Complete A-V block, a common example of two independent rhythms, is therefore not a pararrhythmia since it "blocks" conduction of the sinus impulse through the A-V node.

Such a mechanism, consisting of two independent rhythms activating the heart at different times, could not exist unless the more rapid rhythm were somehow prevented from assuming complete control of the heart. The protective mechanism which prevents this from happening is known as a "protective block" or "entrance block."

There are two types of pararrhythmias: (1) parasystole and (2) A-V dissociation with interference.

PARASYSTOLE

A parasystolic rhythm is a pararrhythmia in which one pacemaker is in the S-A node and the second is in an ectopic site.

Incidence and Significance:
    Parasystole is an uncommon form of arrhythmia. It is most commonly seen in association with organic heart disease of varying etiology.

Mechanism and Electrocardiographic Patterns:
    The most common type of parasystole is one in which the slower ectopic center (more often in the ventricle than the atrium) competes with the more rapid S-A center for control of the heart. The ventricles will be activated by one or the other pacemaker, depending upon the refractoriness of the A-V node and ventricles at any particular moment. The slower ectopic center will produce an electrocardiographic complex having the appearance of an ectopic beat. The electrocardiographic criteria of parasystole are (1) that there is no constant time relationship between the sinus beat and the ectopic beat (in contrast to fixed coupling; see p. 243); and (2) that the time interval between ectopic beats (i. e., parasystolic contractions) will be constant or will be an exact multiple of a common denominator. The least common denominator will represent the actual rate of discharge of the ectopic focus.

A less common form of parasystole is one in which the rate of impulse formation of the ectopic focus is more rapid than that of the normal S-A pacemaker. In an attempt to explain why the more rapid ectopic pacemaker does not assume complete control of the heart and produce an entirely ectopic rhythm or ectopic tachycardia, it has been postulated that some of the impulses originating in the ectopic center are blocked and that this allows the normal S-A center to activate the heart at that given moment. This is known as "exit block."

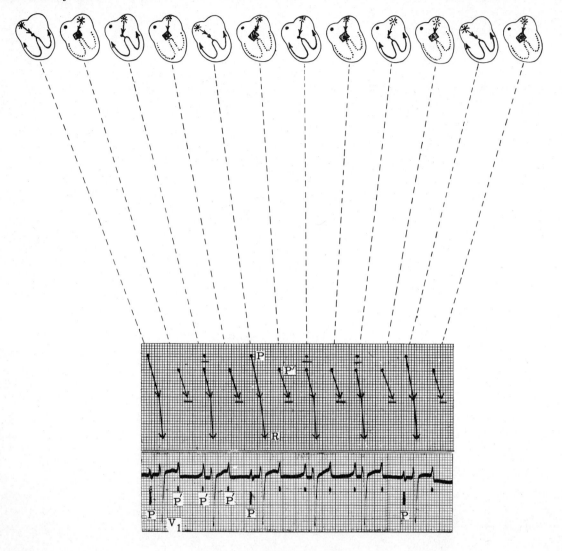

Atrial Parasystole. Two types of atrial complexes are seen. The normal P waves occur at intervals of 1.56 sec. and 2.34 sec. These are both multiples of 0.78 sec., indicating a normal sinus rhythm at a rate of 77 per min. Each P wave is not visible at the 0.78 sec. interval because the ectopic atrial (parasystolic) pacemaker is discharging more rapidly. This latter focus produces the P′ waves. These occur at a rate of 150 per minute. The ventricle only responds to every second P′ wave (atrial flutter with 2:1 A-V block). The P and P′ waves are both competing for the ventricular response; since the rate of the P′ waves is more rapid, it dominates the ventricular response. This is an uncommon example of parasystole because (1) the ectopic focus is in the atrium and (2) the atrial ectopic focus rate is more rapid than the S-A pacemaker rate.

Ventricular Parasystole:

Beats 1, 3, 4, 6, and 8 (see below) are regular sinus, normal complexes. The rate of the sinus rhythm as determined by the R-R interval between two successive sinus beats (3 and 4) is 67. Beats 2, 5, and 7 are ventricular ectopic in origin. The intervals between a ventricular ectopic beat and the preceding sinus beat are as follows: 1 and 2 = 0.85 sec., 4 and 5 = 0.69 sec., and 6 and 7 = 0.74 sec. Therefore, this is not fixed coupling. The intervals between the ventricular ectopic beats are as follows: 2 and 5 = 2.56 sec., and 5 and 7 = 1.92 sec. These are both multiples of 0.64 sec., indicating a ventricular parasystolic rate of 94 per minute.

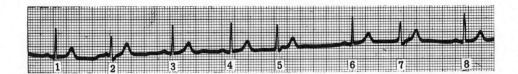

Ventricular Parasystole

A-V DISSOCIATION WITH INTERFERENCE

A-V dissociation with interference is probably the most difficult arrhythmia for the non-specialist to understand. This is largely due to confusion arising from differing definitions and terminology. Basically, A-V dissociation with interference consists of an A-V nodal rhythm whose normal ventricular rhythm is disturbed ("interfered with") by occasional atrial conducted beats.

Incidence and Significance:

This uncommon arrhythmia most often occurs as a result of coronary artery disease, rheumatic carditis, other myocarditides, and digitalis or quinidine poisoning.

Mechanism and Electrocardiographic Patterns:

Two pacemakers exist, one in the A-V node and the other in the atrium, usually in the S-A node. The A-V nodal pacemaker is more rapid than the S-A (or ectopic atrial) pacemaker, and, on occasion (again depending upon refractoriness), the higher atrial center is able to activate the heart and thereby interfere with the more dominant A-V nodal rhythm. "Interference dissociation" and "incomplete A-V dissociation" are synonyms for this arrhythmia. As is true of parasystoles also, a protective mechanism must be present to protect the slower atrial pacemaker. When such a mechanism does not exist, "interference" cannot occur and complete A-V dissociation results. The only difference between complete A-V dissociation and complete heart block is the respective rates of the two pacemakers. In complete heart block the atrial rate is more rapid than the A-V nodal (or idioventricular) rate. In complete A-V dissociation the atrial rate is slower than the A-V nodal rate.

Electrocardiographic Pattern:

The basic rhythm is A-V nodal. An independent slower atrial rhythm is present. On occasions the ventricle responds to the atrial stimulus, thereby interfering with the regularity of the A-V nodal rhythm.

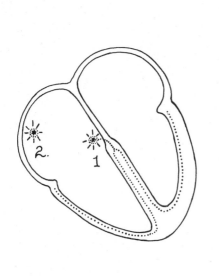 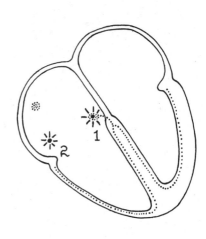

1. Pacemaker in A-V node. 2. Second pacemaker in S-A node interfering with (1).

1. Pacemaker in A-V node. 2. Second pacemaker in lower end of atrium interfering with (1).

A-V Dissociation With Interference

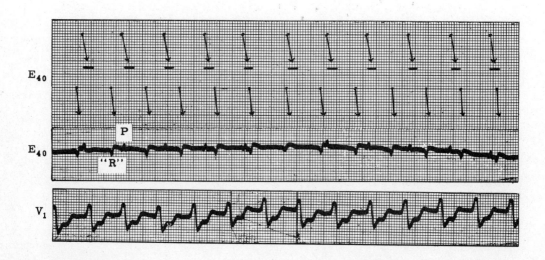

Complete A-V Dissociation. The ventricular rhythm is regular at a rate of 113. An independent atrial rhythm is present at a rate of 94. There is no relationship between the two rhythms. Since the ventricular rhythm is regular and of A-V nodal origin, it is evident that no atrial impulse has activated the ventricle and hence there is no interference. The arrhythmia can readily be diagnosed in E_{40} but could not be resolved by V_1 alone.

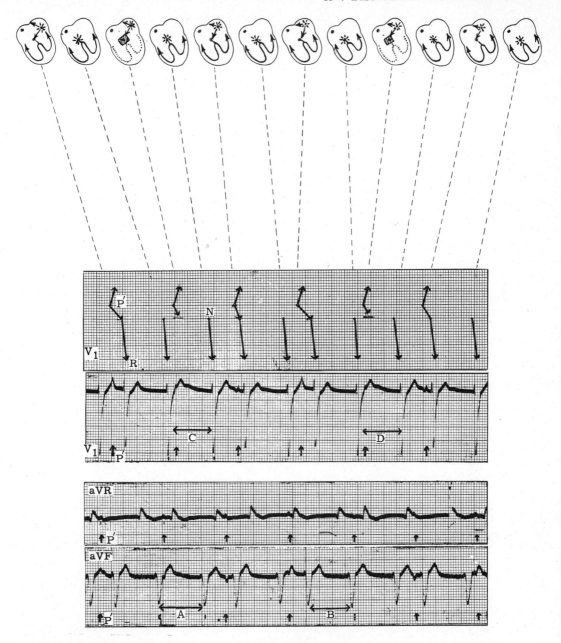

A-V Dissociation With Interference (Interference Dissociation, Incomplete A-V Dissociation).
Two rhythms are evident on study of this record.
1. A regular atrial rhythm (indicated by arrows) is present at a rate of 60. The P′ waves are
   upright in aVR and inverted in aVF, indicating an ectopic focus low in the atrium. These
   atrial stimuli initiate some of the ventricular complexes seen. P′-R varies from 0.1-0.28 sec.
2. In addition, QRS complexes are seen which are of the same configuration as those resulting
   from the above atrial stimuli. They are not preceded by P′ waves and therefore are of A-V
   nodal (N) origin. The A-V nodal rate can be determined when two nodal beats are seen in
   sequence. These are marked at A, C, and D. The R-R interval is 0.7 sec., resulting in a
   basic A-V nodal rhythm of 85. B has the same R-R interval, but this is fortuitous since the
   first ventricular beat results from the atrial stimulus. In this illustration there is an A-V
   nodal rhythm at a basic rate of 85. However, the ectopic atrial focus interferes with this
   rhythm by also stimulating the ventricles. This produces an irregular ventricular rhythm.
Clinical Diagnosis: Arteriosclerotic heart disease.

Chapter 16

ACCELERATED CONDUCTION

Accelerated conduction is the electrocardiographic term used to identify the following electrocardiographic patterns:
1. Wolff-Parkinson-White (W-P-W) syndrome.
2. Isolated accelerated conduction beats.
3. Aberrant intraventricular conduction in association with the atrial arrhythmias.

<u>Etiology and Incidence:</u>
The Wolff-Parkinson-White syndrome usually occurs in individuals with no evidence of organic heart disease. It may occur secondary to organic disease which involves the A-V node, notably myocardial infarction and acute rheumatic fever. Similarly, isolated accelerated conduction beats may be seen in normal individuals. Isolated or transient runs of accelerated conduction may be seen during cardiac catheterization or surgical manipulation of the heart.

<u>Mechanism:</u>
The atrial impulse originates in the S-A node; hence this is a normal sinus mechanism. The most acceptable explanation for it is the presence of an accessory pathway of specialized conduction tissue which bypasses the A-V node. This pathway arises from intercommunicating fibers from the three atrial internodal tracts (see p. 40). It normally takes about 0.09 sec. for a stimulus to pass from the S-A node to the A-V node. The remaining time elapsing prior to ventricular activation - i.e., the remainder of the duration of the P-R interval - results from a normal delay of the impulse in the A-V node. In accelerated conduction the accessory pathway, which bypasses the A-V node, communicates with a branch of the I-V conduction system, resulting in premature activation of a portion of the ventricular myocardium. This is followed by activation of the remaining ventricular myocardium via normal A-V conduction (in addition to the accessory pathway) or by spread of the activation wave from the original site of activation, by way of the accessory tract, into the remainder of the I-V conduction system.

<u>Clinical Significance:</u>
The electrocardiographic pattern of accelerated conduction has no clinical significance itself. However, individuals who have this pattern are prone to have paroxysmal attacks of an atrial arrhythmia. This is usually paroxysmal atrial tachycardia (i.e., 1:1 conduction) and, less commonly, atrial flutter (i.e., atrial tachycardia with A-V block) or atrial fibrillation. (See p. 234.) Paroxysmal ventricular tachycardia has been described as a rare occurrence in association with the W-P-W syndrome, but in the author's opinion this has not been documented.

<u>Prognosis:</u>
Accelerated conduction in the normal individual does not alter the normal life expectancy. Its presence in association with organic heart disease does not alter the prognosis of the underlying disease process.

ELECTROCARDIOGRAPHIC PATTERNS

Due to the accelerated conduction that results from the accessory pathway bypassing the A-V node with early activation of a portion of the ventricle, the P-R interval is shortened. This is usually under 0.1 sec., but may be any length shorter than that of a normally conducted sinus beat in the same individual. As a result of early stimulation of one portion of the ventricle and later stimulation of the remainder, the QRS complexes are wide and slurred. Typically the initial portion of the R wave has a slurred appearance (the delta wave). Frequently the ST segments and the T waves are opposite to the major deflection of the QRS complex. Thus the ventricular complex resembles that of bundle branch block.

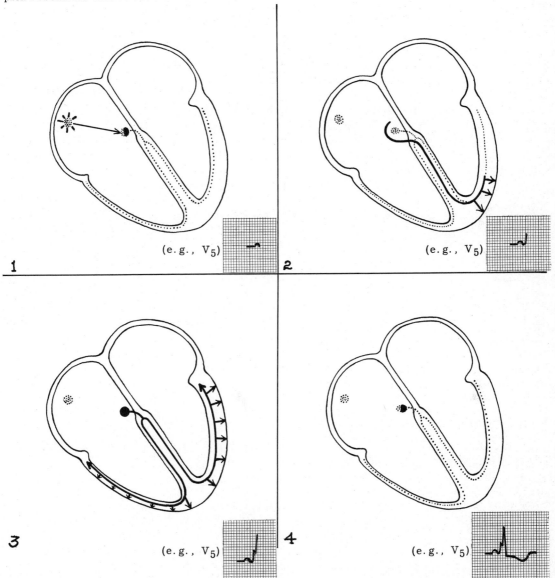

Diagram of Accelerated Conduction.
1. The impulse arises normally in the S-A node and traverses a normal pathway to the A-V node.
2. Intercommunicating fibers from the internodal atrial tracts bypass the A-V node and activate a branch of the I-V conducting system, which results in premature activation of a portion of the ventricular myocardium.
3. The A-V node, which has been activated in a normal fashion and has delayed transmission of the impulse, now activates the I-V conducting system in a normal manner, completing ventricular depolarization.
4. Depolarization and repolarization are complete.

The usual accelerated conduction beat has a normal P-J interval. That is, the interval from the beginning of the P wave to the end of the QRS complex is the same in any one individual for an accelerated conduction beat and a normally conducted sinus beat. Thus the common pattern is a short P-R interval, a wide and slurred QRS complex, and a normal P-J interval.

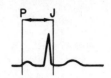

Normal sinus beat.

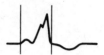

Usual accelerated conduction beat; short P-R interval, wide and slurred QRS complex, normal P-J interval.

Variations of the above pattern may occur. These are:

A. Short P-R interval with wide QRS and shortened P-J interval; it is postulated that the premature ventricular stimulation excited the remainder of the ventricular myocardium before the latter could be activated through a normal pathway. This shortens the P-J interval. However, one cannot know whether this P-J interval is short or normal unless normally conducted sinus beats are seen in the same tracing or in serial tracings.

Accelerated conduction beat with short P-R interval, wide and slurred QRS complex, but short P-J interval.

B. Short P-R interval with normal QRS-T complexes and a short P-J interval; it is believed that the fibers that bypass the A-V node enter and activate the bundle of His prematurely, and ventricular activation occurs in a normal fashion. This (except for the short P-R interval) is indistinguishable from a normally conducted sinus rhythm. If the P-R interval is ±0.12 sec. it cannot be so distinguished unless normally conducted sinus beats are seen with longer P-R intervals.

Accelerated conduction beat with short P-R interval, but normal QRS-T complex and short P-J interval.

Variations in the Electrocardiographic Pattern of Accelerated Conduction

Wolff-Parkinson-White Syndrome:

The entire electrocardiogram may show the pattern of accelerated conduction. This is the classical example of the Wolff-Parkinson-White syndrome. Although the term W-P-W syndrome is commonly used to denote the electrocardiographic pattern, the original description requires the additional presence of associated paroxysmal supraventricular tachycardia.

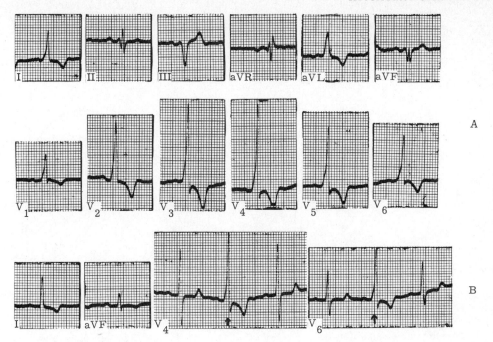

Accelerated Conduction.

A. Sinus rhythm; P-R = 0.14 sec.; QRS = 0.14 sec. The major slurring of the QRS occurs in the initial portion of the R wave and is evident in I, aVL, and all precordial leads (delta wave). The ST segment and T waves are directed opposite to the major QRS deflection in each lead. The one unusual feature of this record, which otherwise is typical of accelerated conduction, is the relatively long P-R interval (0.14 sec.).

B. Two days after A. Spontaneous reversion to normal I-V conduction except for the isolated beats, which are marked with arrows. The P-R interval during normal I-V conduction = 0.2 sec. The P-R interval during accelerated conduction = 0.14 sec. Although the latter is relatively long for this syndrome, it is appreciably shorter than the P-R interval of normally **conducted beats.**

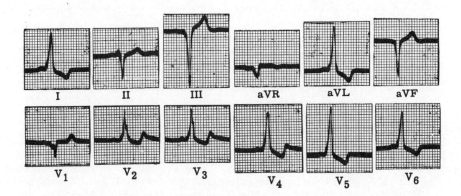

Accelerated Conduction: Wolff-Parkinson-White Syndrome. Typical electrocardiographic pattern. P-R interval = 0.1 sec.; QRS = 0.12 sec. The initial portion of the R is slurred in leads I, aVL and V_{2-6}. There is ST depression and T wave inversion in the latter leads. The QS complexes in leads III and aVF do not indicate inferior wall infarction. Because of the abnormal I-V conduction, one cannot diagnose infarction. **Clinical Diagnosis:** A 26-year-old white male with no clinical evidence of organic heart disease. He did have occasional episodes of paroxysmal supraventricular tachycardia (see p. 234).

Accelerated Conduction With Normal QRS Complexes:

It is theorized that all of the atrial impulses bypass the A-V node, producing a short P-R interval, and enter the I-V conducting system distal to the A-V node. This results in normal ventricular repolarization and depolarization, producing normal QRS complexes and normal T waves.

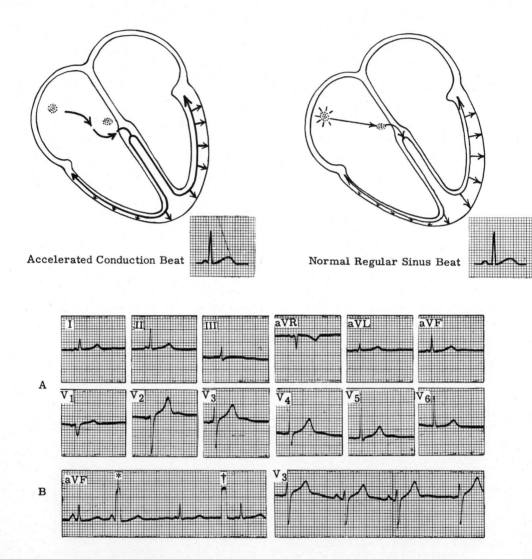

Accelerated Conduction Beat

Normal Regular Sinus Beat

Accelerated Conduction With Normal QRS Complexes.
A. **Standard Leads**: No axis deviation; the P waves are upright in all leads; P-R = 0.09 to 0.10 sec.; QRS = 0.06 sec. **Extremity Leads**: Semi-vertical heart; the P is inverted in aVR and upright in aVF. This excludes the possibility of a nodal rhythm. **Precordial Leads**: Normal. The above pattern could represent a normal regular sinus rhythm with an unusually short P-R interval. However, the latter finding strongly suggests accelerated conduction.
B. **Leads aVF and V_3**: Complexes are seen with larger P waves and a P-R interval of 0.14 sec. These are therefore the normal beats, and the other beats do represent accelerated conduction with normal QRS complexes. The P-J interval of the accelerated conduction beat = 0.16 sec. The P-J of the normally conducted beat = 0.2 sec.

---

*Standardization of the machine has distorted the second QRS complex.
†Standardization of machine.

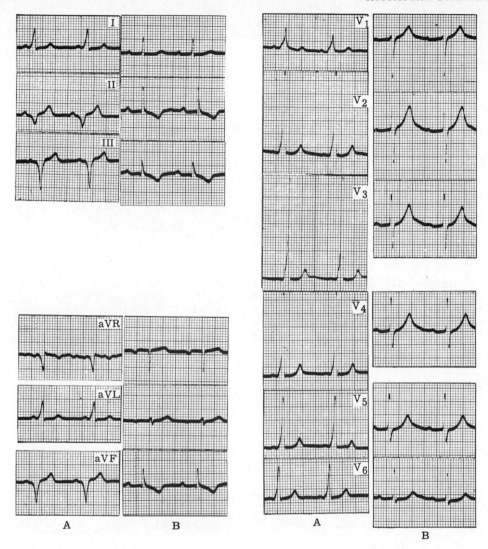

Accelerated Conduction: Wolff-Parkinson-White Syndrome.
  A. The typical characteristics of accelerated conduction are present: P-R = 0.1 sec.; QRS =
     0.12 sec.; there is slurring of the initial upstroke of the R wave in I, aVL, and all precordial
     leads. Because of the abnormal I-V conduction, the QS complex in II, III, and aVF does not
     prove inferior wall infarction. From this electrocardiographic pattern alone, the diagnosis
     of organic heart disease cannot be made.
  B. Following conversion with quinidine. The P-R interval is now 0.24 sec., the QRS interval is
     0.06 sec., and the QRS complexes are now normal in appearance. The T waves are inverted
     in II, III, and aVF. This indicates some abnormality involving the inferior wall of the left
     ventricle. This could be the result of inferior wall infarction but is by no means diagnostic
     of it.
Clinical Diagnosis: Arteriosclerotic heart disease; history of previous myocardial infarction.

Individual accelerated conduction beats may be seen. These may occur as isolated complexes or may occur in a regular recurring sequence.

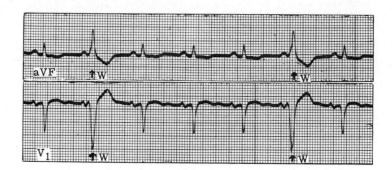

Isolated Acceleration Conduction Beats. The basic rhythm is regular sinus, with a P-R interval of 0.17 sec. At the arrows there are QRS complexes (W) which have the appearance of premature ventricular contractions. However, each is preceded by a P wave. These P waves do not occur prematurely because the P-P interval is constant. The P-R interval for these beats is 0.1 sec. Hence these are accelerated conduction beats.

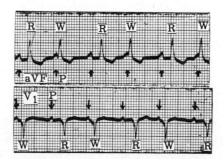

Alternating Accelerated Conduction Beats. The P waves are indicated by arrows. The P-P interval is constant throughout. The regular sinus beats (R) have a P-R of 0.18 sec. Each alternate beat has a very short P-R interval (0.06 to 0.08 sec.). The QRS complexes (W) following the short P-R interval are quite similar to those of the normal sinus beats. The P-J interval is shorter with the W beats. This record is that of alternating accelerated conduction, with the latter showing normal QRS complexes and a short P-J.

Aberrant intraventricular conduction may be seen in association with any of the atrial arrhythmias. In this instance the QRS complexes are wide and slurred during the period of the arrhythmia, but are normal in the absence of the arrhythmia. It is postulated that accelerated conduction due to bypassing of the A-V node explains this pattern. An alternative explanation is that it is caused by normal A-V excitation with bundle branch block-type activation of the ventricles in association with ectopic atrial discharge.

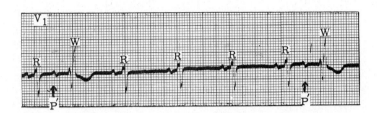

Premature Atrial Contractions With Aberrant Intraventricular Conduction. The predominant rhythm is regular sinus (R). The P-R interval is 0.16 sec., and the P-P interval is 0.82 sec. P waves (arrows) occur prematurely. The resulting QRS complexes (W) are wide and of different configuration. This represents premature atrial contractions with aberrant (or accelerated) conduction. The P'-R interval is longer (0.24 sec.) than the P-R interval of the sinus-conducted beats.

Differential Diagnosis:

A. Isolated Accelerated Conduction Beats vs. Atrial Premature Contractions With Aberrant Intraventricular Conduction: Both complexes will show P waves with wide, slurred QRS complexes. The P-R interval will be shorter with the former than the latter. However, since accelerated conduction is believed to be a sinus conducted rhythm, the P waves will be normal and the P-P interval will be constant in the former. In the latter, the P' wave may have a different configuration than the normal P, and the P-P interval will not be constant, since the atrial contraction is occurring prematurely.

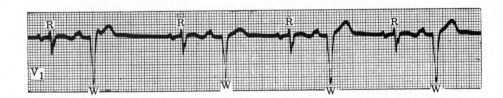

Atrial Bigeminy With Aberrant Intraventricular Conduction. Each regular sinus-conducted beat (R) is followed by a beat with a wide, bizarre QRS complex (W). This simulates a ventricular premature contraction. However, each such complex is preceded by an atrial complex which occurs prematurely and is of a different configuration than the normal P wave. This rhythm is therefore an atrial bigeminy with aberrant (or accelerated) conduction.

B. Supraventricular Tachycardia With Aberrant Intraventricular Conduction vs. Supraventricular Tachycardia With Bundle Branch Block vs. Ventricular Tachycardia: The points of differential diagnosis will be the same as given on p. 248. It may be impossible to arrive at the correct diagnosis until the arrhythmia ceases.

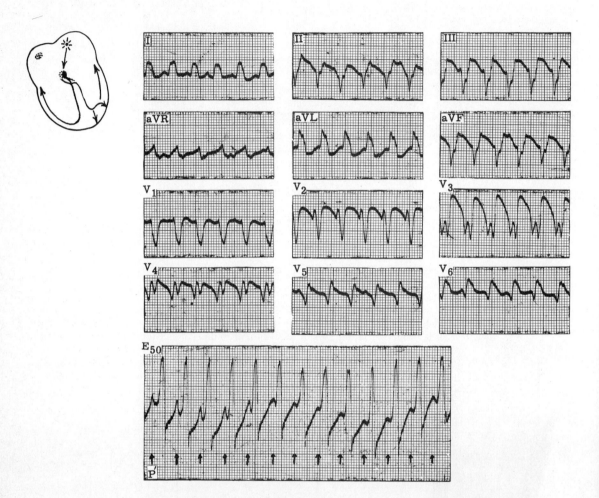

Paroxysmal Atrial Tachycardia With Accelerated Conduction. The patient had suffered a recent myocardial infarction. The electrocardiogram prior to the onset of the tachycardia revealed a regular sinus rhythm, normal QRS interval, and a typical infarction pattern involving both the anterior and inferior walls. This electrocardiogram reveals a tachycardia with a regular ventricular rhythm at a rate of 171. The QRS complexes are now wide and bizarre. Although there is some evidence of atrial activity, this cannot be identified in any regular fashion. From a study of the routine 12 leads this could be called ventricular tachycardia. The esophageal lead, E_{50}, shows definite atrial activity at the same rate of 171. The atrial waves (arrows) are upright and therefore indicate a focus high in the atrium. A P' wave precedes each QRS complex. The P'-R interval varies from 0.04 to 0.10 sec. This therefore represents a paroxysmal atrial tachycardia with accelerated conduction (explaining the short P'-R interval and the wide QRS complexes). The variable (but always short) P'-R interval is consistent with accelerated conduction.

Chapter 17

MISCELLANEOUS ABNORMAL
ELECTROCARDIOGRAPHIC PATTERNS

The electrocardiogram is frequently interpreted as abnormal because of ST segment and T wave changes. Because these often do not permit an etiologic diagnosis, they are referred to as "nonspecific" changes. Proper evaluation will depend upon the clinical evaluation of the patient and serial electrocardiographic studies.

PERICARDITIS

The earliest electrocardiographic evidence of pericarditis is ST segment elevation in those leads reflecting the epicardial surface of the involved area (due to epicardial currents of injury) Typically the ST segment elevation assumes a concave curvature in contrast to the usual convex curvature seen in myocardial infarction. Since pericarditis is usually a diffuse disease, these changes will be seen in all leads reflecting epicardial potential. A cavity lead (such as aVR) will show ST segment depression. These early segment changes can exactly simulate the normal variant described on p. 86. Clinical evaluation and serial electrocardiograms will be necessary to differentiate these two conditions. Occasionally the disease process will be localized and therefore seen only in those leads reflecting the involved area.

After a period of days the ST segments become iso-electric and the T waves begin to invert. The T wave inversion may appear while the ST segment is still elevated.

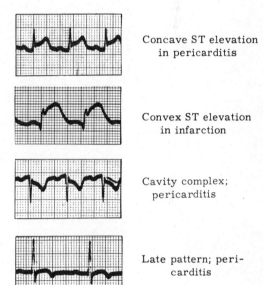

Concave ST elevation in pericarditis

Convex ST elevation in infarction

Cavity complex; pericarditis

Late pattern; pericarditis

Electrocardiographic Patterns in Pericarditis and Infarction

In "benign" pericarditis the electrocardiogram returns to normal within a period of weeks. In more chronic pericarditides (e.g., tuberculosis), the T wave abnormalities may persist for many months.

In a mild case of "benign" pericarditis T wave inversion may never appear. The early ST segment elevations will be seen, and these will then return to the iso-electric line with normally upright T waves persisting. Conversely, T wave inversion may be seen without ST segment elevation ever being evident.

Abnormal Q waves or QS complexes are not seen in pericarditis.

In pericarditis with effusion, the QRS complexes are of low voltage.

Uremic pericarditis rarely produces a typical electrocardiographic pattern of pericarditis.

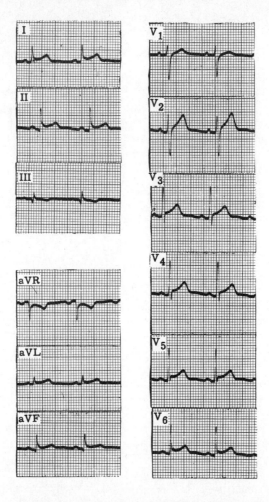

Acute Pericarditis. ST segment elevation with concave upward curvature is seen in leads I, II, aVL, aVF, and V_{2-6}. Reciprocal ST segment depression is seen in cavity lead aVR. **Clinical Diagnosis:** Acute "benign" pericarditis.

Acute Pericarditis. There is ST segment elevation with a concave upward curvature in
leads I, II, III, aVF, and V$_{2-6}$. There is reciprocal ST depression in aVR (cavity potential). The P-R inverval is short, 0.1 sec.,
and the P is upright in II, III, and aVF. This
could be regular sinus rhythm or accelerated
conduction. **Clinical and Autopsy Diagnosis:**
Carcinoma of the esophagus, with rupture;
secondary mediastinitis and pericarditis.

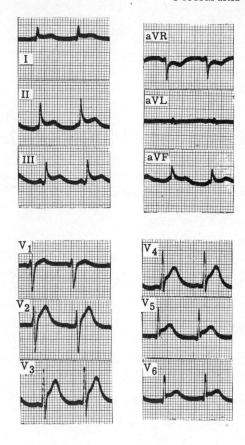

Rarely one may see deep, symmetrically inverted T waves simulating those of infarction.

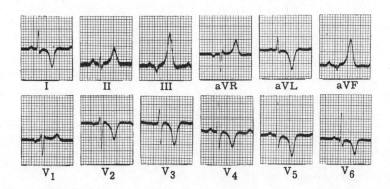

Pericarditis (Late Pattern). Deep, symmetrically inverted T waves in I, aVL, and V$_{2-6}$.
  Clinical Diagnosis: Acute rheumatic fever in a 25-year-old white male; persistent pericardial
friction rub.

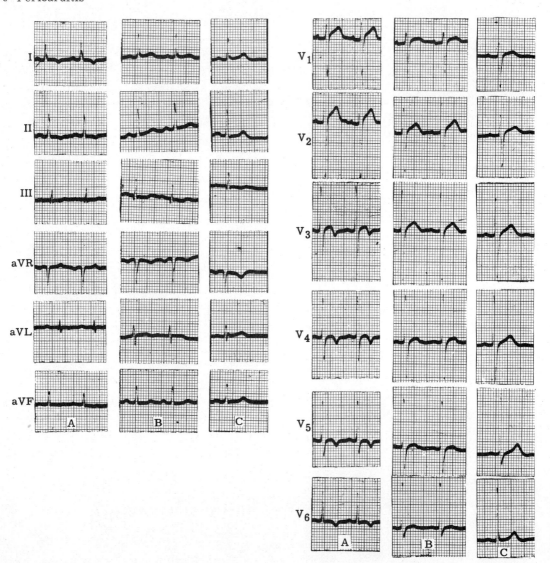

Acute Pericarditis Associated With Serum Sickness.
A. The T waves are inverted in leads I, II, aVL, aVF, and V$_{3-6}$. This pattern is consistent with pericarditis, but one could not diagnose this from the electrocardiogram. Clinically the patient had a severe serum sickness secondary to tetanus antitoxin and had a pericardial friction rub at the time this tracing was taken.
B. Taken 20 hours after (A). Cortisone had been given. The T waves have now become upright but are still of low voltage.
C. Taken 48 hours after (B). Cortisone continued. The electrocardiogram is now normal.
(M. J. Goldman and F. Lau: New England J. Med. **250**:278, 1954.)

MYOCARDITIS

Almost every known acute infectious disease can involve the myocardium and thereby produce electrocardiographic abnormalities. The electrocardiogram below is an example. These may be:

1. Prolongation of the P-R interval.
2. Lengthening of the Q-T$_C$ interval.
3. Various arrhythmias.
4. ST segment depression and/or T wave inversion in left ventricular epicardial leads.

Similar nonspecific changes are seen in chronic myocarditides, beri-beri, amyloidosis, etc.

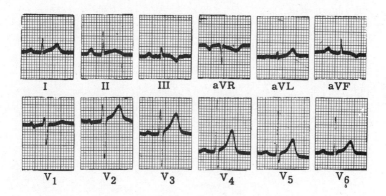

Acute Rheumatic Fever. The abnormalities are a prolonged P-R interval of 0.24 sec. and an inverted T in aVF. The electrocardiogram returned to normal when the rheumatic process became clinically inactive.

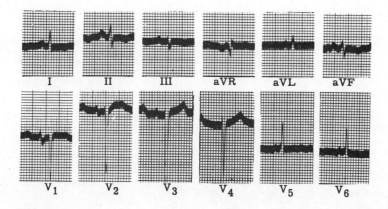

Chronic Beri-beri Heart Disease. The abnormalities are: inverted T waves in I, II, III, and aVF and flat T waves in V_{5-6}. **Autopsy Diagnosis:** Cardiac hypertrophy, endocardial fibrosis, and myocardial changes consistent with beri-beri.

HYPERTHYROIDISM

This disease is typically characterized by tachycardia. One may also see ST segment elevation with T wave inversion in left ventricular epicardial leads. The mechanism producing this
electrocardiographic change is unknown.

Hyperthyroidism.
  A. Taken prior to therapy for hyper-
     thyroidism. Rate = 110. The T
     waves are inverted in I, II, III,
     aVF, and V_6; flat in aVL, and
     diphasic in V_{2-5}. These changes
     are nonspecific. $R_{V5} + S_{V1}$ = 40
     mm. Ordinarily this would be
     suggestive of left ventricular
     hypertrophy, but these voltage
     criteria are invalid in the pres-
     ence of hyperthyroidism.
  B. Taken when patient was euthyroid.
     The electrocardiogram is now
     within normal limits.

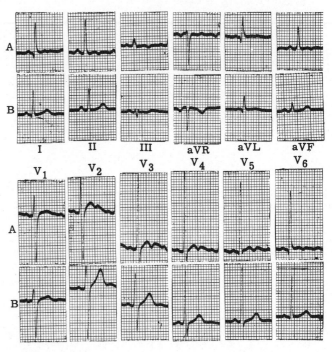

MYXEDEMA

Bradycardia, prolongation of the P-R interval, low voltage of the QRS complexes, and
flattened T waves are the common electrocardiographic findings in myxedema.

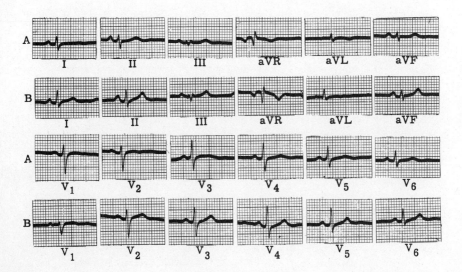

Myxedema.
  A. The QRS complexes are of low voltage and the T waves are of low amplitude in all leads.
  B. Three Weeks After Thyroid Therapy: The T waves are now of normal amplitude, and there is
     a slight increase in the QRS voltage.

TRAUMATIC HEART DISEASE

This can result from penetrating or nonpenetrating injuries to the heart. The electrocardiographic abnormalities may be:
1. Arrhythmias of various types.
2. A pattern consistent with pericarditis.
3. Nonspecific ST segment and T wave changes.
4. An infarct pattern resulting from extensive myocardial trauma or actual traumatic coronary occlusion.

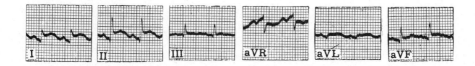

Cardiac Trauma. The above individual sustained a gunshot wound of the chest. The bullet traumatized the epicardial half of the myocardium at the apex of the heart (as visualized at surgery). Precordial leads could not be taken because of the chest injury. Marked concave ST segment elevation is seen in leads I, II, aVL, and aVF; reciprocal ST depression is present in aVR. Such a pattern is consistent with either early myocardial infarction or pericarditis, but in this instance was due to trauma.

NEUROMUSCULAR DISEASES

Such diseases as myotonia atrophica, Friedreich's ataxia, and progressive muscular dystrophy may produce electrocardiographic abnormalities such as:
1. Prolongation of the P-R interval.
2. Arrhythmias of various types.
3. Nonspecific ST segment and T wave changes.

Myotonia Atrophica. The patient was a 46-year-old male. The electrocardiogram reveals an atrial flutter with 2:1 A-V block in standard and extremity leads and a changing block in V_1.

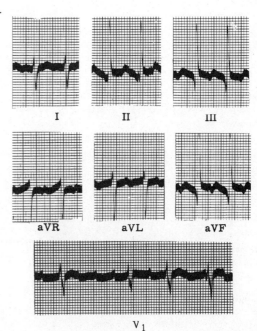

MALIGNANCY INVOLVING THE HEART

Primary cardiac malignancy is a rare condition. However, metastatic involvement of the heart is not uncommon and is frequently not diagnosed during life.

An arrhythmia may be a manifestation of cardiac malignancy. The sudden appearance of atrial tachycardia or atrial fibrillation in a patient with known extracardiac malignancy should arouse suspicion of pericardial or atrial metastatic disease.

Diffuse malignant involvement of the pericardium can produce a pattern of pericarditis.

Extensive but localized involvement can produce a pattern indistinguishable from myocardial infarction.

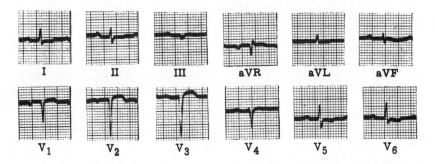

Tumor of the Heart. Complexes are of low voltage in frontal plane leads. QS complexes are present in V_1 and V_2; there are minute r waves in V_{3-4}; there is slight ST elevation of V_{2-3}; the T waves are inverted in V_{5-6}. The above findings are typical of anterior wall infarction, but in this case were the result of metastatic bronchogenic carcinoma to the anterior wall of the left ventricle. The electrocardiogram records the electrically "dead or silent" area and of course cannot differentiate between death of heart muscle due to infarction and replacement and death of heart muscle due to tumor.

REFRIGERATION

With the increasing use of refrigeration in surgery it is essential to be aware of the changes which will occur electrocardiographically. Bradycardia and prolongation of the QT interval are to be expected at temperatures of 30°C; the latter is not due to hypocalcemia. Various atrial arrhythmias and heart block are not uncommon. Fatal arrhythmias, cardiac arrest, or ventricular fibrillation may occur during the induction period of refrigeration or at temperatures far below 30°C. It is therefore essential to have constant electrocardiographic guidance when this procedure is used.

Effect of Refrigeration. A: Before refrigeration. B-D: During refrigeration. All illustrations are lead II. A: QTc = 0.41 sec. B: A-V nodal rhythm; rate = 45. C: QTc = 0.52 sec. D: Ventricular fibrillation.

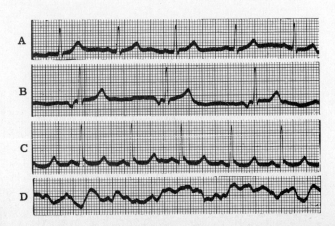

EFFECTS OF DRUGS ON THE ELECTROCARDIOGRAM

DIGITALIS

This is by far the most commonly used drug which produces electrocardiographic abnormalities.

Digitalis Effect:

Digitalis commonly produces ST segment depression in ventricular epicardial leads. Characteristically, the ST segment assumes a rounded, concave ("scooped") configuration or an oblique line descending from the ST junction. Due to the ST segment depression the T wave may be "dragged" downward, giving the appearance of T wave inversion. In addition there is a shortening of the Q-T interval resulting from a shortening of electrical systole. It must be emphasized that the above findings will be seen in most individuals who are adequately digitalized. This represents digitalis effect but not digitalis toxicity.

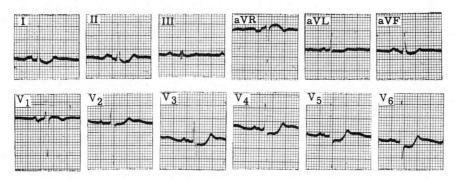

Digitalis Effect. Note the typical rounded ST segment depression in I, II, aVF, and V_{2-6}. There is reciprocal ST elevation in aVR. These changes are characteristic of digitalis effect, but do not indicate digitalis toxicity. Note also the notched P waves, the typical "P mitrale." This patient has mitral stenosis.

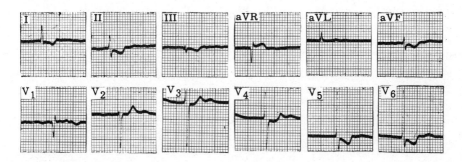

Digitalis Effect. Note the ST segment depression. This produces an oblique downward configuration of the first portion of the ST in leads I, II, III, aVF, V_5, and V_6. There is a rounded ST segment depression in V_3 and V_4. As a result the T waves are "dragged" downward. There is reciprocal ST elevation in aVR. The above changes are indicative of digitalis effect, but do not indicate digitalis toxicity. The rhythm is atrial fibrillation.

Digitalis Toxicity:
   Any arrhythmia may result from overdigitalization. The most common arrhythmias are sinus bradycardia, first degree A-V block, isolated ventricular premature beats arising from single or multiple foci, and ventricular bigeminy.

Digitalis Toxicity, Ventricular Bigeminy.
Regular sinus rhythm alternating with ventricular premature contractions (left ventricular origin). ST segment depression and T wave inversion in the sinus-conducted beats are seen in V_6. The latter could also be the result of digitalis.

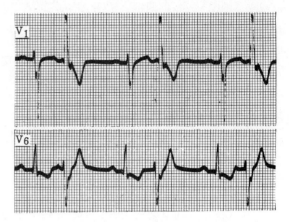

   Associated with the injudicious dosages of purified digitalis preparations and the frequent administration of potent diuretic agents which can cause hypokalemia, digitalis toxicity as manifested by serious arrhythmias is unfortunately being observed more frequently. In addition to the arrhythmias mentioned above, paroxysmal atrial tachycardia, usually with block and an atrial rate of 200 or less, is quite common. Less common are atrial flutter (atrial rate over 250) and atrial fibrillation. It is important to realize that the appearance of these three rhythms in a patient who has been in regular sinus rhythm and has received adequate doses of digitalis (and especially if diuretics have also been given) is more an indication of digitalis toxicity than an indication for further digitalis therapy.

   Less common arrhythmias resulting from digitalis intoxication are second and third degree A-V block, A-V nodal rhythm, A-V dissociation, ventricular tachycardia, and ventricular fibrillation.

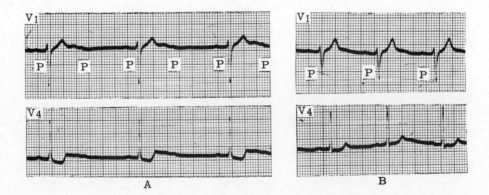

Digitalis Toxicity. Second Degree 2:1 A-V Block.
A. The atrial rhythm is regular at a rate of 86. The ventricle responds to every second atrial beat, resulting in a ventricular rate of 43. There is ST segment depression in V_4. This rhythm has resulted from digitalis intoxication.
B. Digitalis Discontinued: The rhythm is now regular sinus. There is much less ST segment depression in V_4.

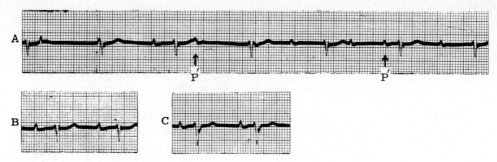

Digitalis Toxicity. Complete Heart Block. The patient had been in regular sinus rhythm. He then received increasing doses of digitalis.

A. Complete Heart Block: The atrial rate is 66 and the ventricular rate is 52. The QRS complexes are of normal configuration, indicating that the second pacemaker is in the A-V node. In addition there are blocked atrial premature contractions (indicated by the arrows).

B. Four Days After (A) (Digitalis Discontinued): First degree heart block; P-R = 0.3 sec.

C. One Week After (B): P-R has been reduced to 0.24 sec.

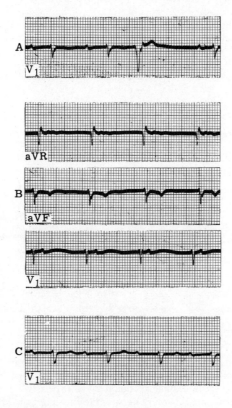

Digitalis Toxicity. A-V Nodal Rhythm.

A. First degree A-V block (P-R = 0.32 sec.). One ventricular premature beat is seen. The P-R interval of the first sinus beat after the ectopic beat is shorter, 0.24 sec.

B. Increasing doses of digitalis have been given. The rhythm is now A-V nodal. P′ waves are seen. These are upright in aVR and inverted in aVF, indicating a reverse spread through the atrium. This results from retrograde atrial stimulation secondary to the A-V nodal rhythm.

C. Six days after (B). Digitalis withheld. The rhythm is again regular sinus (P-R = 0.32 sec.).

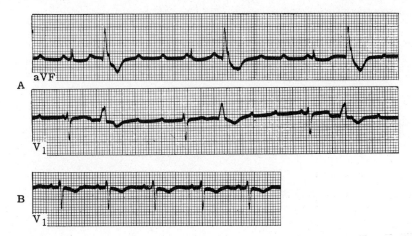

Digitalis Toxicity. Atrial Tachycardia, Complete Heart Block, and Ventricular Bigeminy. The patient had been in regular sinus rhythm and received large doses of digitalis.

A. An atrial tachycardia is now present with a regular atrial rate of 164. The ventricular rhythm exclusive of the premature ventricular contractions is perfectly regular at a rate of 31. There is no constant relation between the QRS and the preceding P wave, indicating a complete heart block. The QRS complexes are of normal configuration, indicating that the second pacemaker is in the A-V node. A ventricular bigeminy is present. All of the above resulted from digitalis intoxication.

B. Five days after (A). Digitalis has been discontinued and potassium given. The rhythm is again regular sinus.

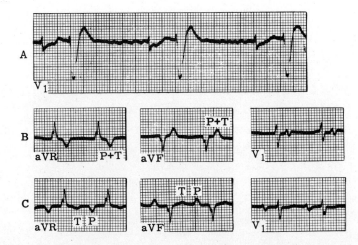

Digitalis Toxicity. Atrial Fibrillation, Complete A-V Block, and Ventricular Bigeminy. Prior to (A) the rhythm had been regular sinus. The patient was receiving increasing doses of digitalis in an attempt to improve the degree of congestive failure.

A. The atrial rhythm is that of fibrillation. The ventricular rhythm is regular; the rate exclusive of the premature ventricular beats is 37. Since the ventricular rhythm is regular, the ventricles are responding not to the atrial fibrillation but to an independent pacemaker in the A-V node. A premature ventricular contraction follows each nodal beat, i. e., ventricular bigeminy is present. All of the above has been produced by digitalis intoxication.

B. Four days after (A); digitalis withheld. The rhythm is now a first degree A-V block with a P-R interval of 0.52 sec. The P waves are fused with the T waves. This is not a nodal rhythm since the P waves are inverted in aVR and upright in aVF, i. e., the pattern is normal, indicating sinus origin.

C. Three days after (B); digitalis still withheld. First degree A-V block; the P-R interval reduced to 0.25. P and T waves are now separated and prove the interpretation made in (B).

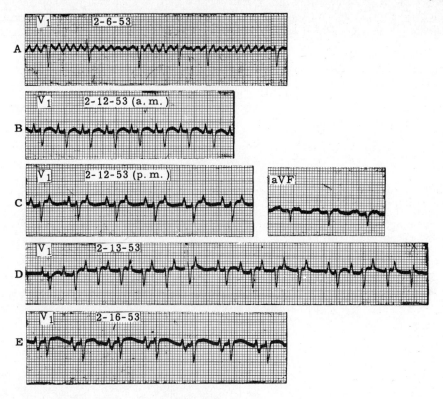

Digitalis Toxicity Producing Atrial Tachycardia.

A. 2-6-53: Atrial fibrillation.   The patient is receiving digitalis.

B. 2-12-53 a.m.: An atrial tachycardia with 1:1 conduction has appeared; the rate is 160.   This sudden appearance of an atrial tachycardia during digitalis therapy for atrial fibrillation (in the absence of quinidine therapy) should always make one suspicious of digitalis intoxication. This was not appreciated, and more digitalis was given.

C. 2-12-53 p.m.: Four hours after the last dose of digitalis.   The extra digitalis has increased the A-V block, producing atrial tachycardia (or flutter) with 2:1 block.   The direct effect of digitalis on atrial conduction has increased the atrial rate to 200.   The P′ waves are upright in aVF, indicating a high atrial ectopic focus.

D. 2-13-53: Digitalis has been discontinued and potassium and quinidine therapy begun.   The atrial rhythm remains regular at a rate of 177, but the ventricular response is irregular. One notices a progressive increase in the P-R interval and finally a failure of ventricular response.   Thus this is an atrial tachycardia with a Wenckebach type of A-V block.

E. 2-16-53: Further quinidine therapy.   The rhythm has been reverted to regular sinus.   The sinus P waves are diphasic in contrast to the tall, upright P′ waves of the tachycardia.

QUINIDINE

Quinidine produces ST segment depression and flattening of the T waves in leads reflecting a left ventricular epicardial complex.   These changes are similar to those produced by digitalis. However, in contrast to digitalis, quinidine produces a lengthening of the $Q-T_c$ interval.   The major therapeutic action of quinidine in the treatment of ectopic arrhythmias is initially a slowing of the rate of the ectopic discharge and then elimination of the ectopic discharge, allowing a re-sumption of normal rhythm.   In addition quinidine has a vagolytic action, thus increasing the ability of the A-V node to conduct impulses.   When quinidine is administered to a patient with atrial fibrillation, the initial slowing of the ectopic atrial rhythm results in atrial flutter and tachycardia.   This slower and regular atrial rhythm combined with increased conductivity through the A-V node produces a "paradoxic" increase in the ventricular rate.   This explains the neces-sity of prior administration of digitalis in order to obtain the vagotonic (i.e., blocking) action of digitalis on the A-V node.   With continued quinidine effect, the atrial ectopic discharge is completely eliminated, allowing for resumption of sinus rhythm. Quinidine is equally efficacious in the elimination of ventricular ectopic rhythms, i.e., ventricular premature contractions and ventricular tachycardia.

Toxic manifestations of quinidine are as follows: (1) first degree A-V block, (2) second degree A-V block, (3) third degree (complete) A-V block, (4) A-V dissociation, (5) A-V nodal rhythm with any associated atrial rhythm including atrial standstill, (6) widening of the QRS complex to 50% or more of the prior QRS interval, (7) idioventricular rhythm, (8) ventricular premature beats, (9) ventricular tachycardia, (10) ventricular fibrillation, and (11) cardiac standstill. The appearance of any of the above, with the exception of a first degree heart block, is an absolute contraindication to continuation of quinidine therapy.

Effect of Quinidine (case of mitral stenosis with chronic atrial fibrillation).
A. V_1: Atrial fibrillation; prior to administration of quinidine.
B. II and V_1: During quinidine therapy; A-V nodal rhythm is present; retrograde P′ waves are seen following each QRS complex. This rhythm is an indication of quinidine toxicity and hence the drug was discontinued.
C. V_1: Four hours after (B), the A-V nodal rhythm persists; a ventricular bigeminy is also present. This also could be the result of quinidine toxicity.
D. V_1: 24 hours after (B), the rhythm is now regular sinus. Quinidine administration was resumed in a smaller maintenance dosage, and regular sinus rhythm was maintained.

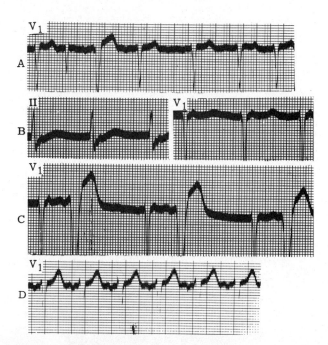

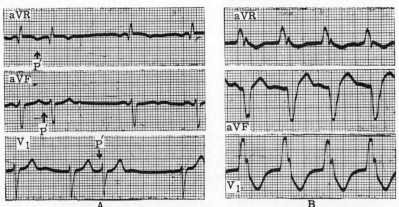

Toxic Effect of Quinidine.
A. The rhythm is basically regular sinus. Premature atrial contractions are present, as indicated by the arrows. The P′ wave is inverted in aVR and upright in aVF, indicating a high atrial ectopic focus.
B. During quinidine therapy (given because of a mistaken clinical diagnosis of atrial fibrillation). The QRS complexes have become widened and bizarre. No definite atrial activity can be identified. The ventricular rate is 90. This is a "slow" ventricular tachycardia. Twenty-four hours after quinidine was discontinued, the rhythm returned to regular sinus.

EMETINE

Emetine occasionally produces the following electrocardiographic changes:
1. ST segment depression and/or T wave inversion in epicardial leads.
2. Prolongation of the P-R interval.

These changes may persist for days to weeks after emetine is discontinued. They do not necessarily contraindicate continuation of emetine if clinically necessary. More serious toxic effects can produce intraventricular conduction disturbances.

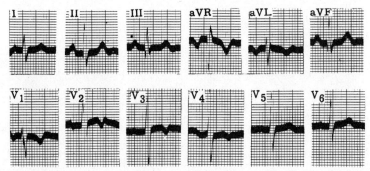

Effect of Emetine on the Electrocardiogram. Standard Leads. Right axis deviation. **Extremity Leads:** Vertical heart. The standard and extremity leads are normal. **Precordial Leads:** Clockwise rotation; the T waves are inverted in V_{1-4}. These changes are nonspecific, but could be the result of coronary artery disease or right heart strain. **Clinical Diagnosis:** Amebiasis treated with emetine. The electrocardiogram became normal after treatment had been discontinued.

TARTAR EMETIC

All patients receiving a full course of this drug (as in the therapy of schistosomiasis) will develop electrocardiographic abnormalities. Most commonly this is T wave inversion in epicardial leads. These electrocardiographic changes alone are not a contraindication to continuation of therapy.

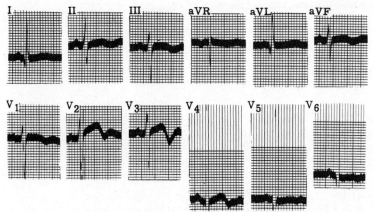

Effect of Tartar Emetic on the Electrocardiogram. Standard Leads: Left axis deviation; low amplitude T in I. **Extremity Leads:** Horizontal heart; low amplitude T in aVL. **Precordial Leads:** Inverted T waves in V_{2-4} and flat T waves in V_{5-6}. These changes are nonspecific and could result from coronary artery disease. **Clinical Diagnosis:** Schistosomiasis. The changes seen in the electrocardiogram invariably occur as the result of therapy with tartar emetic. The electrocardiogram became normal after therapy had been discontinued.

NICOTINE (SMOKING)

Nicotine is known to produce varying degrees of vasoconstriction. Nicotine may produce atrial premature beats, atrial fibrillation, and ventricular premature beats in some individuals with apparently normal hearts. In patients with coronary artery disease, nicotine may precipitate further coronary insufficiency which can be manifested clinically by anginal pain or electrocardiographically by the pattern of coronary insufficiency (myocardial anoxia). A smoking test has been used in which an electrocardiogram is taken before and after the smoking of one or two cigarettes. However, in most instances this is less reliable than an exercise test.

For the reasons given above, some physicians advise patients with known coronary artery disease to refrain from smoking.

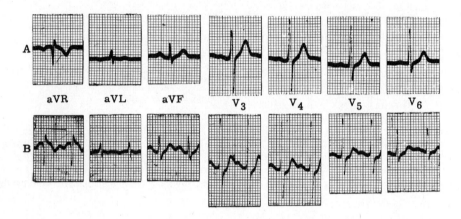

Effect of Smoking. The patient was a 58-year-old male whose clinical diagnosis was arteriosclerotic heart disease with coronary insufficiency. Leads aVR, aVL, aVF, and V_{3-6} are illustrated.
A. Resting electrocardiogram is within normal limits. The rate is 80 (this cannot be determined from the single complex tracing).
B. After smoking two cigarettes. The rate has increased to 130. There is no other significant change in extremity leads. ST segment depression has appeared in the precordial leads, a maximum of 1.5 mm. in V_3. These changes are consistent with myocardial anoxia. The patient experienced no symptoms during the test.

PROCAINAMIDE

Procainamide (Pronestyl®) can produce the same electrocardiographic changes as those produced by quinidine, but is much less effective than quinidine in the therapy of the atrial arrhythmias.

CEREBRAL DISEASE

Abnormal electrocardiograms may be seen in association with cerebral disease, especially cerebral and subarachnoid hemorrhage. These changes are ST depression, flat to inverted T waves, marked prolongation of the $Q-T_C$ interval, and prominent U waves in leads which reflect a left ventricular epicardial complex (I, aVL, V_{4-6}). In such cases autopsy examination has shown the absence of myocardial disease.

EFFECTS OF ELECTROLYTE DISTURBANCES
ON THE ELECTROCARDIOGRAM

HYPERKALEMIA

The first electrocardiographic evidence of an elevated extracellular potassium level is the appearance of tall, slender, "tented" T waves, usually best seen in precordial leads. Although this pattern strongly suggests hyperkalemia it is not absolutely diagnostic since patients with posterior wall infarction and even normal individuals may show a similar pattern.

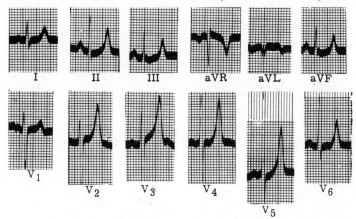

Hyperkalemia (chronic glomerulonephritis with uremia). Tall slender T waves are seen in I, II, III, aVF, and V_{2-6}. The rhythm is regular sinus; QRS interval = 0.09 sec. Serum potassium = 7.2 mEq./L.

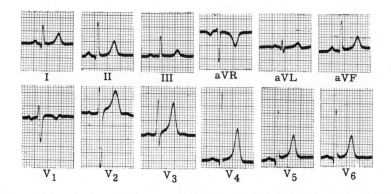

Normal Electrocardiogram Simulating a Hyperkalemia Pattern. Note the tall slender T waves in leads I, II, aVF, and V_{2-6}. This finding is strongly suggestive of hyperkalemia. However, this record was taken on a normal young adult with no clinical evidence of heart disease or electrolyte disturbance. The serum potassium at the time of this record was 4.7 mEq./L. Serial electrocardiograms over the course of many months showed no change.

With further elevation of the serum potassium level the atria can go into standstill with the development of an idioventricular rhythm and wide, slurred, bizarre QRS complexes. As the level rises, ventricular fibrillation or asystole may result.

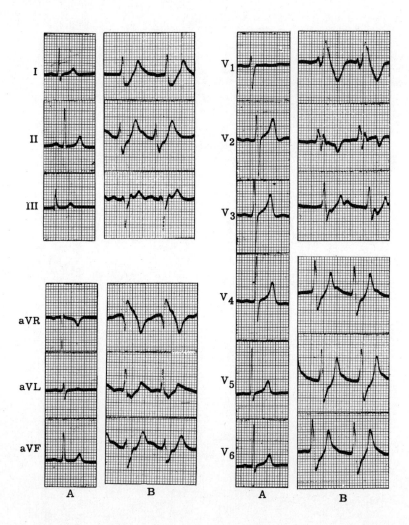

Hyperkalemia. The above tracings were taken on a patient with glomerulonephritis.
  A. Taken one year before death. The tracing is normal. Serum potassium = 5 mEq./L.
  B. Taken terminally; serum potassium = 8.9 mEq./L. There is no definite evidence of regular atrial activity. The QRS interval has increased to 0.16 sec. The QRS complexes simulate a right bundle branch block. The T waves are tall and peaked in I, II, and V_{4-6}.

ST segment elevation may be seen in association with hyperkalemia. In experimental studies in which the surface of the heart is bathed with a potassium solution, ST segment elevation is produced. It is likely that one reason for ST segment elevation in acute myocardial infarction is the leakage of potassium from damaged myocardial cells into the interstitial fluid, resulting in "localized" hyperkalemia. However, the clinical finding of ST elevation in association with hyperkalemia is uncommon.

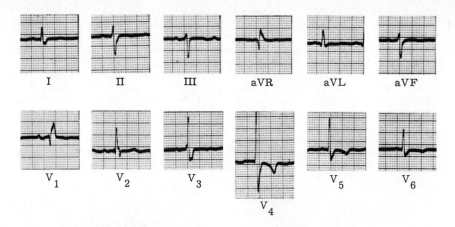

A. The above tracing was taken on a 70-year-old male with carcinoma of the prostate and coronary artery disease. A right bundle branch block is present - as evidenced by a QRS interval of 0.12 sec., wide s waves in leads I, V_5, and V_6, and wide R′ in V_1. The T wave inversion in V_{4-6} indicates additional anterior wall disease. At this time the serum potassium = 4.6 mEq./L.

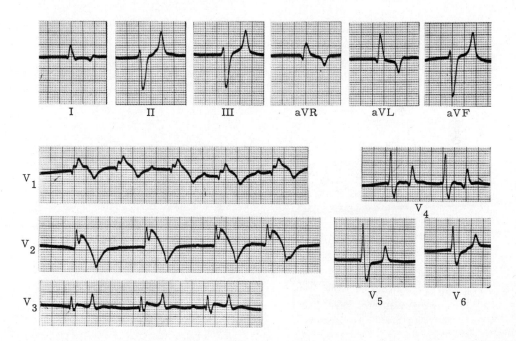

B. Several weeks after tracing A. Azotemia has developed; serum potassium = 9.3 mEq./L. Only occasional P waves are seen, and the rhythm is probably an incomplete A-V dissociation. The QRS interval has widened to 0.14 sec. The T waves are tall and peaked in II, III, aVF, and V_{3-6}. Marked ST elevation is seen in V_{1-2} and to a lesser degree in V_3. The patient was given hypertonic glucose and insulin intravenously, and 20 minutes later the electrocardiogram reverted to that seen in A. above, at which time the serum potassium equaled 6.1 mEq./L.

HYPOKALEMIA

Typically one may see prolongation of the P-R interval and ST segment depression in epicardial leads. Formerly it was stated that prolongation of the Q-T interval was a significant electrocardiographic finding. This is now known to be incorrect. For some unknown reason a prominent U wave occurs in hypokalemia. This is frequently superimposed upon the T wave and therefore produces the appearance of a prolonged Q-T interval. However, if the T and U waves are separated, both the Q-T and the Q-U intervals are of normal duration.

The electrocardiographic findings are therefore ST segment depression and at times T wave inversion in epicardial leads, prominent U waves, and prolongation of the P-R interval. It can be seen that these changes are nonspecific and can be produced by a variety of conditions.

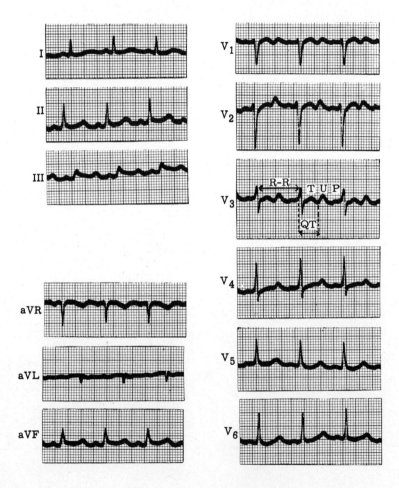

Hypokalemia. An apparently upright T wave is seen in leads II, III, aVF, V_5, and V_6. If this deflection were the T wave, the Q-T interval would be 0.4 sec. (corrected for R-R interval of 0.66 sec., the $Q-T_C$ = 0.50 sec.) and therefore prolonged. In leads V_{1-4} separate T and U waves are clearly evident. The true Q-T interval in V_3 is 0.29 sec. ($Q-T_C$ = 0.36 sec.), which is normal. The above tracing was taken on a 51-year-old male who had had persistent vomiting. The serum potassium = 2.3 mEq./L.

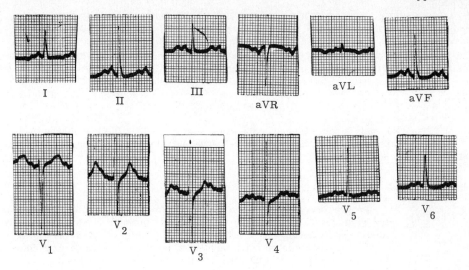

Hypokalemia. In the precordial leads a clear distinction can be made between T and U waves. The $Q\text{-}T_C$ interval is normal. The U wave is more prominent than the T in V_{4-6}, and slight ST depression is present in V_{4-6}. In the frontal plane leads only a single wave is seen between the QRS and P. If this were interpreted as a T wave, it would lead to a mistaken determination of a long Q-T interval. Instead, it is a U wave. This patient had been on corticoid therapy for rheumatoid arthritis, with more recent thiazide administration for attempted control of edema. The serum potassium = 2.6 mEq./L.

Postextrasystolic U Wave:

On occasion the normal sinus (basic) beat which follows a ventricular ectopic beat will show an abnormal U wave when such a wave is not evident in other complexes. In the illustration below, the sinus beat which follows the first ventricular ectopic beat shows a large, abnormal U wave. U waves are visible in the other sinus beats, but these are small and normal. The postextrasystolic U wave was therefore the only electrocardiographic clue to hypokalemia in this patient, who was on digitalis and thiazide therapy. Serum potassium = 3.1 mEq./L.

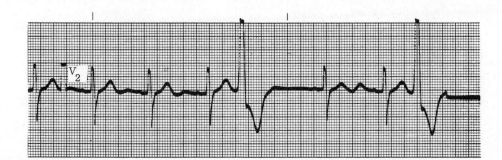

ELECTROCARDIOGRAM AS A GUIDE TO POTASSIUM LEVELS

The electrocardiogram serves as a reasonably satisfactory guide to serum potassium levels when actual determination of the serum potassium is not available.

Normal Tracing (serum potassium 4 to 5.5 mEq./L.). P-R interval = 0.16 sec.; QRS interval = 0.06 sec.; Q-T interval = 0.4 sec. (normal for an assumed heart rate of 60).

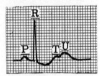

Hypokalemia (serum potassium ±3.5 mEq./L.). P-R = 0.2 sec.; QRS interval = 0.06 sec.; ST segment depression. A prominent U wave is now present immediately following the T. The actual Q-T interval remains 0.4 sec. If the U wave is erroneously considered a part of the T, a falsely prolonged Q-T interval of 0.6 sec. will be measured.

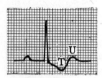

Hypokalemia (serum potassium ±2.5 mEq./L.). The P-R is lengthened to 0.32 sec.; the ST segment is depressed; the T wave is inverted; a prominent U wave is seen. The true Q-T interval remains normal.

Hyperkalemia (serum potassium ±7.0 mEq./L.). The P-R and QRS intervals are within normal limits. Very tall, slender, peaked T waves are now present.

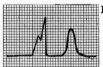

Hyperkalemia (serum potassium ±8.5 mEq./L.). There is no evidence of atrial activity; the QRS complex is broad and slurred and the QRS interval has widened to 0.2 sec. The T waves remain tall and slender. Further elevation of the serum potassium will result in ventricular tachycardia and ventricular fibrillation.

Correlation of Serum Potassium Level and the Electrocardiogram. (Assuming serum calcium is normal.) The diagrammed complexes are left ventricular epicardial leads.

HYPERCALCEMIA

Elevated serum calcium levels may produce a shortening of the Q-T_C interval similar to the effect of digitalis. However, the electrocardiogram is usually of little diagnostic value in this condition.

HYPOCALCEMIA

A low serum calcium level does produce a prolongation of the Q-T_C interval. There is no abnormality in the T wave. The Q-T prolongation results from a lengthening of the ST segment. A similar pattern may be seen in patients with severe liver disease. This cannot be correlated with the level of the total serum calcium. The reason for this finding is not known.

Hypocalcemia. The T waves are upright, but the Q-T interval is prolonged. This is 0.4 sec. (corrected for R-R of 0.66 sec., Q-T_C = 0.48 sec.) and is abnormal. The lengthening of the Q-T interval is due to a lengthening of the ST segment and not to any abnormality in the T wave itself. Blood calcium at time of above record was 8 mg./100 ml.

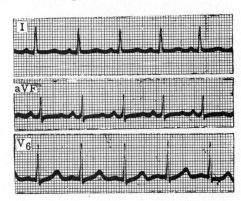

Hypocalcemia may be associated with hypokalemia, in which case epicardial leads will show ST segment depression, T wave inversion, prominent U waves, and a prolonged Q-T_C interval.

Hypocalcemia with hyperkalemia is commonly seen in patients with renal insufficiency.

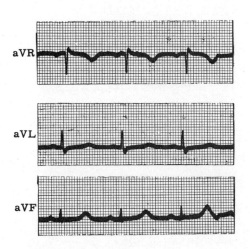
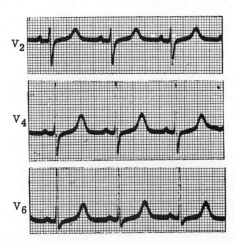

Hypocalcemia and Hyperkalemia. The ST segment is prolonged, resulting in a Q-T_C of 0.52 sec. Although not diagnostic, the T waves are tall in aVF and V_{2-6}. **Clinical Diagnosis:** Chronic glomerulonephritis; serum calcium = 7 mg./100 ml.; serum potassium = 7.1 mEq./L.

ELECTRICAL ALTERNANS

This produces an electrocardiographic pattern in which the height of the R wave (and at times also the T) alternates every other beat. Except when associated with paroxysmal tachycardia, it is an indication of organic heart disease. Electrical alternans should not be confused with the clinical sign of pulsus alternans; the two have no relationship.

Electrical Alternans. The rhythm is regular sinus. The QRS complexes are of two differing amplitudes. This occurs in an alternating pattern. **Clinical Diagnosis**: Arteriosclerotic heart disease.

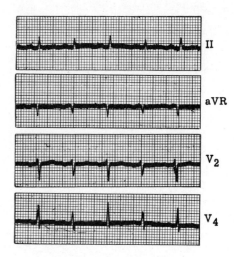

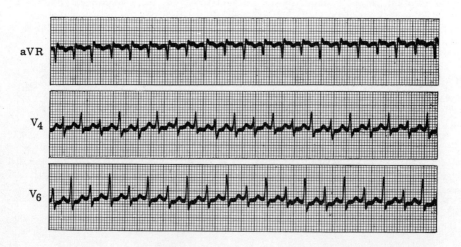

Electrical Alternans. The rhythm is a paroxysmal atrial tachycardia with a rate of 200. There is an alternating amplitude of the QRS complexes. In the presence of paroxysmal tachycardia electrical alternans has no special clinical significance.

LEFT VENTRICULAR CONDUCTION DEFECTS

As stated on p. 40, the left bundle branch divides shortly after its origin into two divisions: (1) the superior division, which extends anteriorly and superiorly over the subendocardial surface of the left ventricle; and (2) the inferior division, which extends inferiorly and posteriorly. Peripherally these two divisions are connected by the intertwining fibers of the Purkinje system.

Normally, conduction spreads simultaneously through both divisions. This results in a normally directed QRS vector, between −30° and +110° in the frontal plane (see p. 35). However, if one division of the left bundle is damaged by a pathologic process, conduction will first proceed through the undamaged division, thus altering the direction of the mean QRS vector. Since the speed of conduction through the bundle tissues and Purkinje system is rapid, this lesion will not produce a prolongation of the QRS interval.

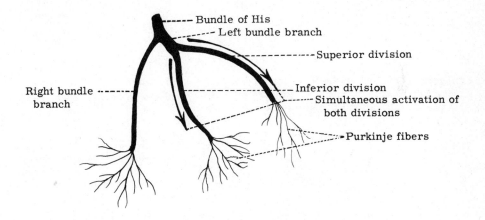

Diagram of the Conduction System, Illustrating Normal Left Ventricular Activation by Simultaneous Activation of Both Divisions of the Left Bundle

LEFT INTRAVENTRICULAR BLOCK
(Anterolateral Parietal Block)

A left intraventricular (anterolateral parietal) block is the result of a lesion in the superior division of the left bundle. Therefore, left ventricular conduction spreads through the inferior division of the left bundle, resulting in initial activation of the inferior and posterior portions of the left ventricle with late activation of the anterior and lateral portions of the left ventricle. Thus the mean QRS vector is directed superiorly, to the left, and slightly anteriorly. This will be manifested in frontal plane leads by an abnormal degree of left axis deviation, i.e., greater than −30°. There is no widening of the QRS interval.

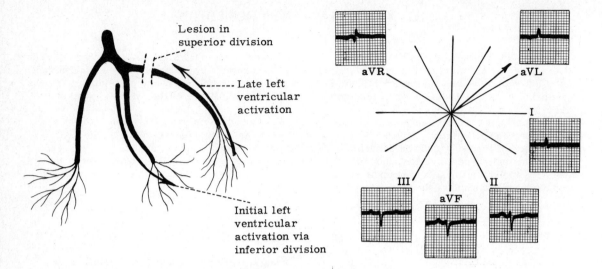

Diagram of a Block in the Superior Division of the Left Bundle Resulting in Initial Left Ventricular Activation Via the Inferior Division

Anterolateral Parietal Block. Mean QRS frontal plane vector = −40°.

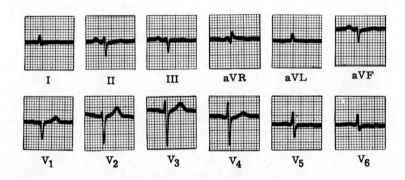

Anterolateral Parietal Block. An abnormal degree of left axis deviation is present (−40°). The T waves are flat in leads I, aVL, and V_{5-6}. **Clinical Diagnosis**: Arteriosclerotic heart disease with anginal syndrome. There was no clinical evidence for left ventricular hypertrophy or pulmonary emphysema.

The above electrocardiographic pattern is seen in the following clinical conditions:

1. Coronary artery disease - The abnormal degree of left axis deviation may be the only electrocardiographic finding. On occasion there may be associated ST segment depression and T wave inversion, thus simulating the pattern of left ventricular strain (see p. 106).

2. Left ventricular hypertrophy - The abnormal degree of left axis deviation is probably not due to the hypertrophied muscle mass per se, but is due to associated subendocardial fibrosis involving the superior division of the left bundle. One cannot make an electrocardiographic diagnosis of left ventricular hypertrophy from this finding alone. There must be increased voltage and/or prolongation of the V.A.T. (see p. 98).

3. Pulmonary emphysema - The mean QRS vector is commonly along the vertical axis and is usually directed inferiorly, i.e., close to the +90° frontal plane axis. Uncommonly, as a result of abnormal electrical conduction from the surface of the heart to the body surface caused by the diseased lungs and deformed thorax, this same vertical axis may be directed superiorly, i.e., close to the −90° frontal plane axis, resulting in an abnormal left axis deviation. The voltage of the QRS complexes is low, thus aiding in differentiation from an otherwise similar electrocardiographic pattern produced by coronary artery

. disease. However, the correct differential diagnosis will depend on proper clinical evaluation of the patient.
4. Peri-infarction block (see below).
5. Various myocarditides and myocardopathies.

Theoretically, an electrocardiographic pattern could be derived for a block in the inferior division of the left bundle. Left ventricular conduction would spread initially through the superior division and thus result in a mean QRS vector directed inferiorly, to the right, and posteriorly. The resulting electrocardiographic pattern would be that of right axis deviation. The author is unaware of any clinical and pathologic description of such an entity in the absence of infarction.

PERI-INFARCTION BLOCK

Peri-infarction block is the descriptive term for the electrocardiographic pattern resulting from infarction plus an interruption in conduction through one of the divisions of the left bundle. The electrocardiographic characteristics are:
1. Abnormality of the initial 0.04 sec. QRS vector, i.e., abnormal Q waves as evidence of infarction.
2. Abnormality of the terminal 0.04 sec. QRS vector, usually directed 110° or more from the initial 0.04 sec. QRS vector.
3. Little or no prolongation of the QRS interval, unless there is additional disturbance in peripheral I-V conduction resulting from myocardial disease or drug toxicity.

Anterolateral Peri-infarction Block:
Since the superior division of the left bundle traverses the subendocardial surface of the anterior and lateral walls of the left ventricle, it is understandable that an anterolateral wall infarct can involve the superior division. The resulting electrocardiographic pattern will be that of abnormal left axis deviation (as described for anterolateral parietal block) plus abnormal Q waves in leads I, aVL, and/or left precordial leads. Admittedly, one can only be certain that the infarction has been the cause of the superior division block if a preinfarction electrocardiogram is available which does not demonstrate the abnormal left axis deviation.

As stated above, the terminal QRS vector forces are oriented to the left and superiorly (greater than −30° in the frontal plane). These terminal forces may also be directed anteriorly, thus producing small r′ waves in right precordial leads V_{1-3}. This precordial lead pattern may resemble that of a right ventricular conduction defect (incomplete right bundle branch block or right ventricular hypertrophy). However, in the latter the terminal QRS vector is directed to the right, and an S wave will therefore be seen in lead I. In anterolateral peri-infarction block the terminal vector is oriented to the left and so no S wave will be seen in lead I.

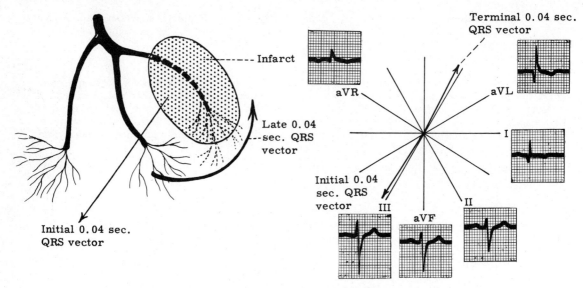

Anterolateral Peri-infarction Block Illustrating Orientation of Initial and Late QRS Vectors in the Frontal Plane

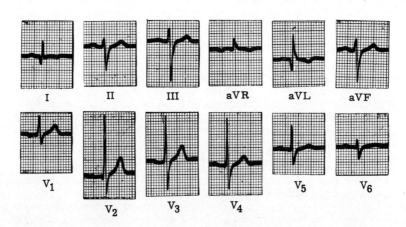

Anterolateral Peri-infarction Block. A deep and wide (0.04 sec.) Q wave is seen in leads I and aVL as evidence of anterolateral wall infarction. This indicates an initial 0.04 sec. QRS vector oriented to the right. This same QRS vector produces the r waves in leads II, III, and aVF, which indicates that this vector is directed at a +120° axis in the frontal plane. The late 0.04 sec. QRS vector, producing the R wave in lead I and the S wave in leads II, III, and aVF, results in the terminal QRS vector directed at a −63° axis. The tall initial R waves in V_{1-2} are the result of associated posterior-lateral wall infarction.

Diaphragmatic Peri-infarction Block:

Since the inferior division of the left bundle traverses the subendocardial surface of the diaphragmatic wall of the left ventricle, it may be damaged in association with inferior wall infarction. The resulting electrocardiographic pattern will be: (1) abnormal Q waves in leads II, III, and aVF, resulting from the superior orientation of the initial 0.04 sec. QRS vector; and (2) abnormal direction of the terminal QRS vector (as described above for the theoretical pattern of a block in the inferior division), i.e., orientation to the right, inferiorly, and posteriorly, producing an S wave in lead I and an R wave in leads III and aVF. The S wave in I may cause one to consider the presence of an incomplete right bundle branch block. However, in the latter the terminal QRS vector is oriented anteriorly, producing r′ waves in right precordial leads; whereas in diaphragmatic peri-infarction block the terminal QRS vector is directed posteriorly and no r′ waves can be recorded in right precordial leads.

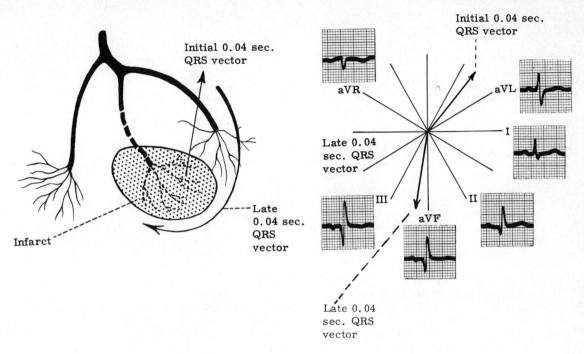

Diaphragmatic Peri-infarction Block Illustrating Orientation of Initial and Late QRS Vectors in the Frontal Plane

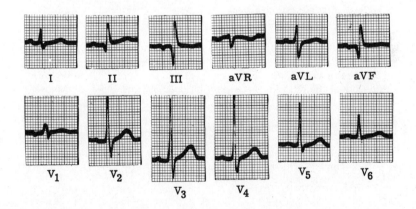

Diaphragmatic Peri-infarction Block. Deep and wide (0.04 sec.) Q waves are seen in leads II, III, and aVF, as evidence of inferior wall infarction. This indicates an initial 0.04 sec. QRS vector oriented superiorly. This same QRS vector produces the R wave in lead I, which indicates that this vector is also oriented to the left. This initial superior and left vector force is directed at a −50° axis in the frontal plane. The late 0.04 sec. QRS vector, producing the R waves in leads II, III, and aVF and the S wave in lead I, results in a late QRS vector directed at a +100° axis. The prominent R waves in V_{1-2} are the result of associated posterior wall infarction.

As a result of multiple lesions it is possible to have a combination of infarction with a block of either division of the left bundle, e.g., inferior wall infarction plus anterolateral parietal block.

ELECTRICAL DEPOLARIZATION OF THE HEART

Electrical depolarization of the heart is a valuable clinical means of therapy which by now has become commonplace. Its major uses include (1) cardiac pacing for control of rate and rhythm and (2) countershock for correction of an arrhythmia. It is beyond the scope of this text to discuss this field in detail, but it will suffice to outline the indications and technics and the appearance of the electrocardiographic tracings of the patient before and after electrical depolarization.

Electrical Pacing of the Heart:

This is indicated in any situation when an uncontrolled reduction in heart rate diminishes cardiac output sufficiently to result in syncope or other serious symptoms. The prime example is the patient with Stokes-Adams syndrome. Three methods of pacing follow:

A. External pacing is effective in an emergency situation but becomes ineffective after several hours. It is painful to the conscious patient.

B. Internal pacing with the power source external to the body can be accomplished by inserting an electrode into the heart by way of a neck or arm vein or by direct puncture of the myocardium through the chest wall. These technics are effective for emergency situations and short-term therapy.

C. Internal pacing with power source implanted in body:

1. Electrodes are sutured into the myocardium, and the power source is imbedded in the abdominal wall. This type of unit (asynchronous pacemaker) generally has a fixed ventricular rate. If sinus rhythm and A-V conduction are still possible, the ventricles can respond to the normal sinus pacemaker and the artificial electrical pacemaker, thereby producing a parasystolic rhythm (see p. 253). At an opportune time, the electrical pace could discharge in the supernormal period of the heart cycle (see p. 19) and produce a serious ventricular arrhythmia. To avoid this and to permit the physiologic control of heart rate in patients with sinus rhythm, synchronous pacemakers are available in which the patient's own P wave triggers the electrical pace.

2. An electrode is introduced into the right ventricle by way of a neck vein, and the unit is implanted in the pectoral-axillary area. This is preferable in the patient for whom a thoracotomy is too hazardous.

Many problems arise in the management of patients with pacemakers. These are primarily (1) technical problems - such as breakage of wires; coating of an electrode contact, with reactive tissue changes; or failure of one of the components of the power unit, usually the battery - and (2) parasystolic rhythm and the danger of ventricular arrhythmias, as mentioned above.

Electrocardiographic Pattern:

The electrical pace will produce a sharp, brief deflection. The ventricular excitation will mimic a ventricular ectopic beat. If the pace is in the left ventricle, the electrocardiogram will record a complex simulating a right bundle branch block. If the pace is in the right ventricle, what appears to be a left bundle branch block (see p. 242) will occur.

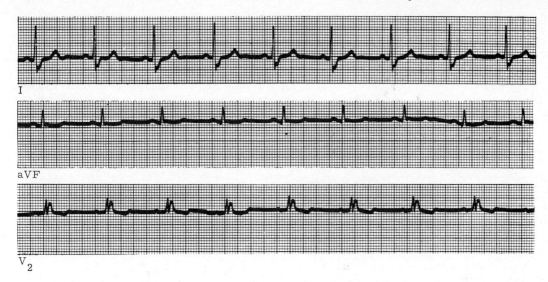

I

aVF

V$_2$

The above electrocardiogram is that of a 75-year-old male with repeated episodes of syncope. This tracing reveals a right bundle branch block. The rhythm is normal sinus; the rate = 65.

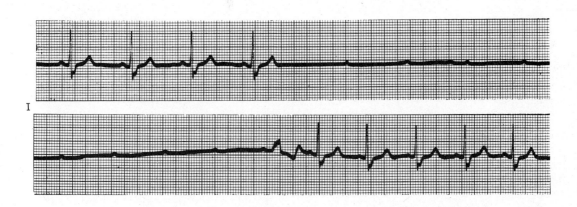

I

The above is a continuous recording of lead I in the same patient. Ventricular asystole (with continuing atrial activity) is present for 8.3 sec.

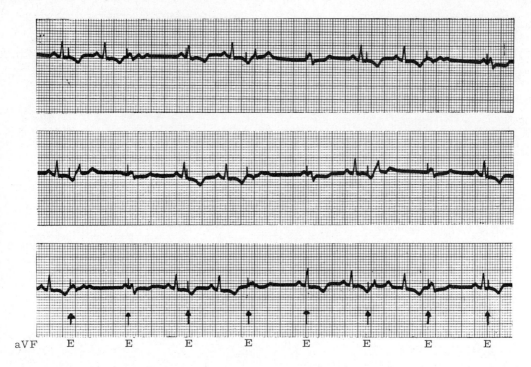

This is an electrocardiogram of the same patient after the insertion of an asynchronous implanted pacemaker. The electrical pace (E) discharges regularly at a rate of 65. A parasystolic rhythm is present. The ventricle responds to the normal sinus pacemaker or the electrical pacemaker.

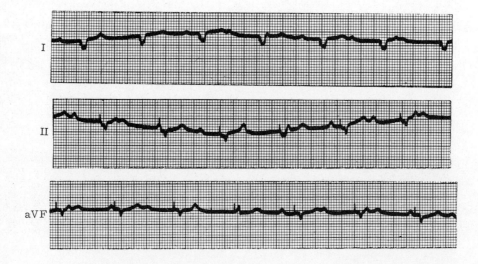

This is an electrocardiogram of the same patient several weeks later. Ventricular activation is now completely controlled by the pacemaker, which is firing at a rate of 65. Independent atrial activity continues at a rate of 85 but never results in ventricular capture. QS complexes in leads I and aVF indicate that the ventricular activation wave (i.e., vector) is oriented toward the right and superiorly due to the electrode placement in the lower portion of the left ventricle.

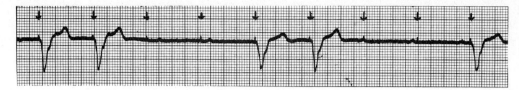

Example of Pacemaker Failure. Regular pacemaker activity (indicated by arrows) is seen at a rate of 73. However, each pace does not produce ventricular activation. The 3rd, 4th, 7th, and 8th paces do not excite the ventricle. In this patient there were also longer periods of ventricular asystole with resulting syncope. This was corrected by replacement of the power unit.

Electrical Countershock:

An electrical charge can be introduced into the myocardium which is sufficient to depolarize the entire heart and permit the normal cardiac rhythm to be reestablished. This countershock is usually delivered externally, but it can be applied internally during intrathoracic surgery. Its major life-saving function is in the elimination of ventricular fibrillation as part of the resuscitation therapy of cardiac arrest. It is also of great value in the treatment of ventricular tachycardia. When clinical judgment indicates the need for reversion of atrial flutter or atrial fibrillation, countershock may be preferable to drug therapy. Two types of units for the administration of countershock follow:

A. The AC defibrillator introduces a charge for approximately 0.25 sec. Because of this relatively long duration the charge could fall within the supernormal phase of excitability in any rhythm other than ventricular fibrillation and thereby produce a serious ventricular arrhythmia, such as fibrillation.

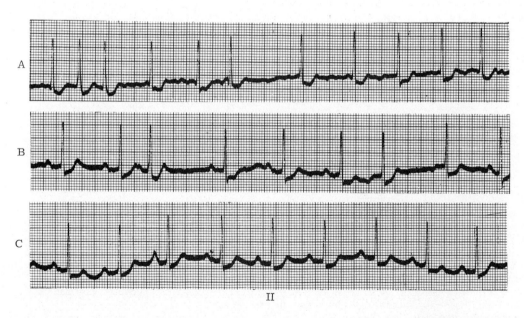

II

Electrical Cardioversion of Chronic Atrial Fibrillation in a Patient With Mitral Stenosis.
A. Immediately prior to cardioversion. The rhythm is atrial fibrillation. Digitalis therapy had been purposely withheld for three days.
B. Immediately after delivery of a 200 watt-sec. charge from a synchronized DC defibrillator.
C. Five minutes later. B and C indicate reversion to sinus rhythm, with occasional atrial premature beats.

B. The DC defibrillator introduces a charge for 0.0025 sec. Most units are now coupled with a synchronizing device that prevents discharge in the critical phase of the heart cycle and thus largely eliminates the danger of producing a more serious arrhythmia.

Caution must be used in countershock therapy for elective reversion of arrhythmias (i.e., atrial) in patients who are receiving digitalis, since serious ventricular arrhythmias can follow its use. A similar problem may occur in patients who are receiving quinidine.

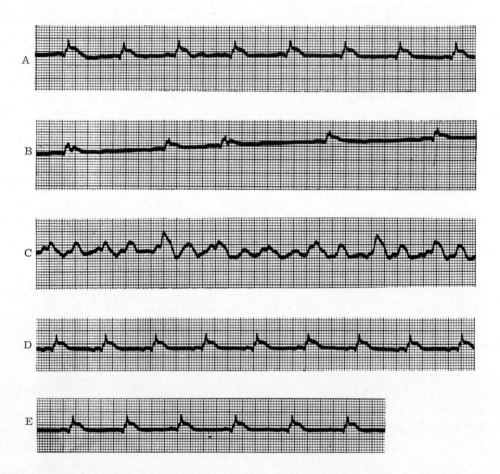

Therapy of Ventricular Fibrillation:

The above are selected strips of lead II taken during constant oscilloscopic monitoring of a patient with acute myocardial infarction.

A. Vital signs stable; sinus rhythm, rate = 72; small q and marked ST elevation indicate recent infarction.

B. One minute after A. The blood pressure has fallen; the ventricular rhythm has become irregular and slower; atrial activity cannot be identified.

C. One minute after B. Cardiac arrest has occurred; ventricular fibrillation is present. Immediate measures for cardiac resuscitation are instituted (cardiac compression, ventilation, and intravenous sodium bicarbonate). A DC countershock of 400 watt-sec. is given. (This is not recorded on the electrocardiogram.)

D. Fifteen seconds after defibrillation. A regular ventricular rhythm has been restored; the rate = 78; QRS-T complexes are similar to A. The P waves are inverted, indicating a low atrial or A-V nodal pacemaker.

E. Two minutes after D. Reversion to sinus rhythm. Following this, the patient made an uneventful recovery.

Chapter 18

AN INTRODUCTION TO
SPATIAL VECTORCARDIOGRAPHY

Vectorcardiography and electrocardiography must not be considered different sciences. They are both methods of recording the varying electrical potentials which result during the cardiac cycle. With the use of cathode ray oscilloscopes, the spatial vectorcardiogram can be recorded stereoscopically or in its projection in the frontal, sagittal, and horizontal planes. Whereas any electrocardiographic lead records the electrical potentials (i.e., the instantaneous vectors) in one single axis (see p. 34), a loop recording (i.e., vectorcardiogram) records the same electrical events simultaneously in two perpendicular axes. The frontal plane loop records simultaneous events in the right-left (X) axis and the head-foot (Y) axis. The sagittal plane loop records simultaneous events in the head-foot (Y) axis and the anterior-posterior (Z) axis. The horizontal plane loop records simultaneous events in the right-left (X) axis and the anterior-posterior (Z) axis.

In a simplified fashion the derivation of the spatial vectorcardiogram can be illustrated by the following diagrams. (The propagation of the electrical impulse through the ventricular myocardium has been described on p. 41.)

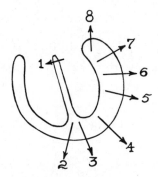

(a) The initial vector (1) is the septal activation from left to right. Next (2) is the activation of the anteroseptal region of the myocardium. Then follows the activation of the remainder of the myocardium (3-8).

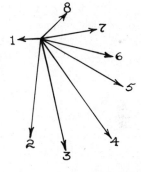

(b) By connecting all the vectors to one starting point the diagram above can be constructed.

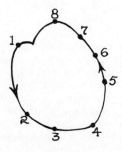

(c) A loop can now be drawn connecting the tips of all the vectors. This represents the vectorcardiogram in the frontal plane.

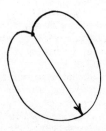

(d) The average direction and magnitude of all the instantaneous QRS vectors is the mean QRS vector. The maximal QRS vector is drawn from the starting point to the farthest point of the loop.

The major problem in electrocardiography and vectorcardiography is to determine the most accurate method by which the electrical potentials of the heart (i.e., the cardiac vector) can be recorded from the surface of the body. Vector analysis, based initially on the Einthoven triangle and modified to include unipolar electrocardiography (see p. 32), is based on the following hypotheses: (1) the heart "generator" acts as a dipole; (2) this generator is centrally located in the chest; (3) the standard leads (I, II, and III) are all equidistant from the center of the heart generator; (4) the shape of the human torso can be assumed to be a sphere; and (5) all body tissues are homogeneous electrical conductors. At the present time the dipole hypothesis is accepted, at least as a means of explaining 95% of the electrical potentials of atrial and ventricular depolarization as recorded from the body surface,* and all advancements now being made in modern vectorcardiography are based on acceptance of the dipole hypothesis. However, it is now known that the other hypotheses listed above are unwarranted: the origin of electrical activity is not centrally located in the chest, the standard leads are not all equidistant from the center of electrical activity, the human torso is by no means a perfect sphere, and all body tissues are not equally good conductors. If all this were true, electrocardiographic recording would be simple: lead I would represent the horizontal axis (right to left axis or X axis); VF would represent the long axis (head to foot axis or Y axis); and V_2 would approximate the transverse axis (anteroposterior axis, or Z axis).

The diagrams below show X, Y, and Z axes in a theoretically perfect sphere, homogeneous in conductivity with the origin of electrical activity in the center of the sphere.

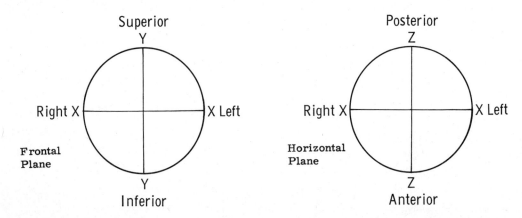

The tetrahedron vector system utilizes the standard leads with a fourth lead placed on the back; the cube vector system utilizes four different electrode positions. However, neither of these systems offers major revisions of the invalidated hypotheses discussed above and so neither is mathematically accurate. Primarily as a result of the interdisciplinary cooperation of physiologists, physicists, mathematicians, electrical engineers, and physicians in electrocardiographic research, electronic technics and equipment have been devised in an attempt to compensate for the errors in these hypotheses. The result has been the development of the "**corrected**" **orthogonal lead systems** of which the systems of Frank and Schmitt are most popular at the present time.

The vectorcardiograms to be illustrated in this chapter have been recorded with the Frank system. Although it is felt by many that the Schmitt system is slightly superior, the Frank system has the advantage of being easier to use on a patient since it requires fewer electrodes.

One result of the greater mathematical accuracy of a corrected orthogonal lead system is that it is necessary to modify the space relationships of the axes of the frontal plane electrocardiographic leads to conform to the corrected lead system. For the Frank system the frontal planes can be illustrated in the following diagrams: (The necessary corrections for the horizontal plane remain to be accurately described in a similar fashion.)

---

*The significance of the possible remaining 5% remains to be determined.

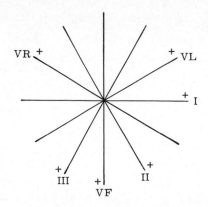

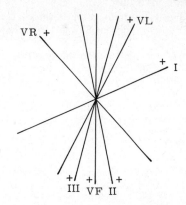

**Hexaxial Reference System Used in
Conventional Electrocardiography**

**Corrected Reference Lead System
for the Frank Technic**

Technic of the Frank System:

Seven electrodes, designated as H, F, I, E, C, A, and M, are applied to the body at the following locations:

H: Forehead or neck.

F: Left leg.

I, E, C, A, and M are located along the same transverse level: the fourth intercostal space
if the patient is supine; the fifth intercostal space if the patient is sitting.

I: Right anterior axillary line.

E: Center of sternum.

A: Left anterior axillary line.

C: At a 45° angle between E and A.

M: Center of spine.

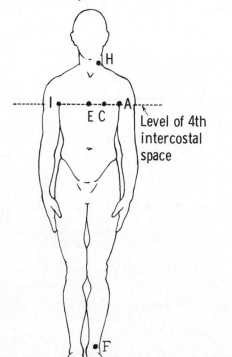

Level of 4th intercostal space

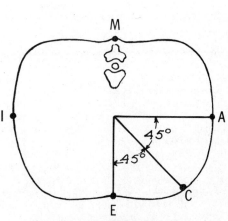

Transverse section of body
at level of 4th intercostal
space

Electrode Positions for the Frank System

For detailed information on the electronic circuitry and resistance networks of this system, the reader is referred to Frank's original articles.

The beam visualized on the oscilloscope screen is interrupted by an electrical tuning fork at a fixed rate of 500 cycles per second. This produces a series of dashes, each representing 2 milliseconds (0.002 seconds). Each dash is comma-shaped, the tail indicating the direction in which the beam is travelling. The direction of inscription of the loop is described as either clockwise or counterclockwise in the usual meaning of these terms. (This description is not to be confused with the electrocardiographic terminology used in reference to rotation on the long axis. See p. 64.)

The Value of Spatial Vectorcardiography in Clinical Medicine:

At present spatial vectorcardiography is used only in medical centers and by specialty medical groups. For routine clinical practice its value is limited (1) because of the expense of the equipment and the time involved; (2) because definite standards for the normal and abnormal vectors have not been established; and (3) because no complete uniformity of opinion exists as to the best lead system to be used.

Vectorcardiography is of little value in the recording of arrhythmias unless moving photographic equipment is used. It is of distinct value in the study and diagnosis of the hypertrophies, bundle branch blocks, and myocardial infarction.

Vectorcardiography serves its most useful purpose in the teaching and understanding of the propagation of the electrical events in the cardiac cycle.

This chapter has been entitled "An Introduction to Spatial Vectorcardiography" because it is beyond the scope of this text to present the many theoretical, mathematical, and electrophysical principles involved. The limited discussion offered here is intended only to give the beginner an insight into the subject and its present place in the field of clinical medicine.

ORIENTATION OF THE VECTORCARDIOGRAPHIC ILLUSTRATIONS

The vectorcardiographic illustrations, as recorded in the frontal, sagittal, and horizontal planes, are oriented in space as shown in the following diagrams:

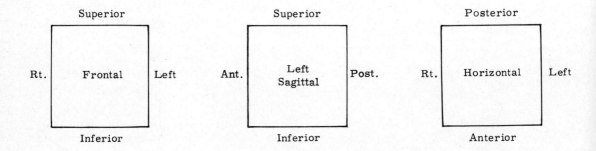

Thus, right to left movement is seen in the frontal and horizontal views; superior-inferior movement is seen in the frontal and sagittal views; and anterior-posterior movement is seen in the sagittal and horizontal views.

If accurate records are obtained, only two views are necessary (e.g., frontal and horizontal) to envision the spatial orientation. However, the third view is of value in checking the accuracy of the other two views.

The direction of the vector is defined by the angle it forms with an imaginary 360° circle surrounding each projection. The left sagittal rather than the right sagittal view was selected by the Committee on Electrocardiography of the American Heart Association. This explains the discrepancy in the degree markings of the sagittal in comparison with the frontal and horizontal views.

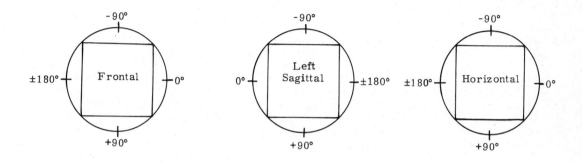

THE NORMAL ADULT SPATIAL VECTORCARDIOGRAM

Each spatial vectorcardiogram consists of three loops:

A. The P Loop: Depolarization of the atria produces a small initial loop, the P vector. It is usually oriented inferiorly, to the left and slightly anteriorly. A great deal of investigative work remains to be done in the evaluation of this spatial vector loop.

B. The QRS Loop: Depolarization of the ventricles produces the large QRS vector loop. Most of the studies in spatial vectorcardiography to date have been devoted to this vector. The normal spatial orientation of the QRS vector in the adult is to the left, inferiorly, and somewhat posteriorly.

1. Frontal plane - A small initial deflection may be seen extending to the right and occasionally superiorly. The major portion of the loop is oriented downward and to the left in the 0° to 85° range. The loop may be inscribed in either a clockwise or counterclockwise direction or may be a "figure-of-eight."
2. Left sagittal plane - A small initial deflection appears anteriorly and occasionally superiorly, with the major portion of the loop extending inferiorly and somewhat posteriorly. The normal QRS loop is always inscribed in a counterclockwise direction.
3. Horizontal plane - An initial small deflection is inscribed anteriorly and to the right. The major portion of the loop extends to the left and somewhat posteriorly in the +35° to −45° segment. The normal loop is always inscribed in a counterclockwise direction.

C. The T Loop: Repolarization of the ventricles produces a small final loop, the T vector. It is usually larger than the P loop but is considerably smaller than the QRS loop. The normal T vector is usually slightly anterior, inferior, and to the right of the QRS vector by 0° to 30°.

The periods in the cardiac cycle during which there is no electrical activity (corresponding to the isoelectric P-R, S-T, and T-P intervals of the electrocardiogram) will not be evident in the stationary record of the spatial vectorcardiogram.

SEQUENCE DIAGRAM SHOWING CORRELATION OF THE NORMAL ADULT SPATIAL VECTORCARDIOGRAM AND THE RESULTING ELECTROCARDIOGRAM *

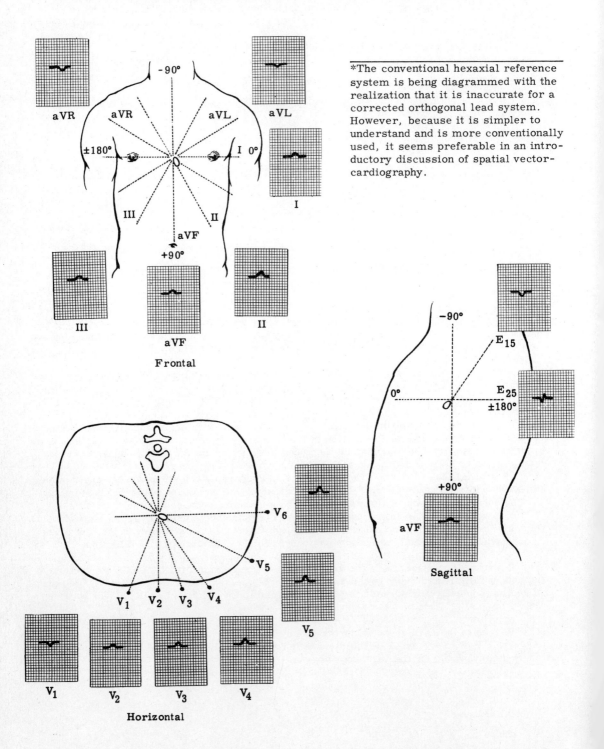

*The conventional hexaxial reference system is being diagrammed with the realization that it is inaccurate for a corrected orthogonal lead system. However, because it is simpler to understand and is more conventionally used, it seems preferable in an introductory discussion of spatial vectorcardiography.

A. The P Loop: This is produced by atrial depolarization. Since the spread of excitation in the atria is in a head-to-foot direction (see p. 56), the vector is directed inferiorly. It is also oriented to the left and anteriorly.

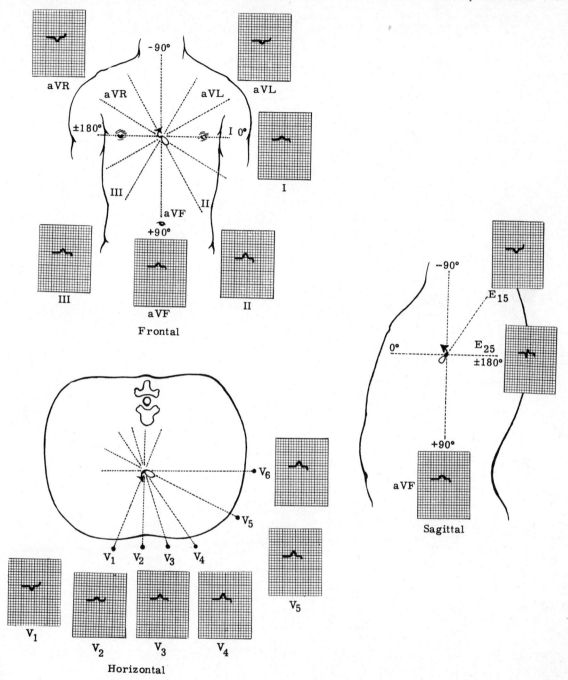

Frontal

Horizontal

Sagittal

B. Ventricular Depolarization:

1. Initial spatial QRS loop - The initial septal activation is from left to right (see p. 58), hence the initial QRS vector is oriented to the right. The early activation of the antero-septal region of the myocardium (see p. 59) contributes to this initial right direction and also results in an anterior and slightly superior orientation.

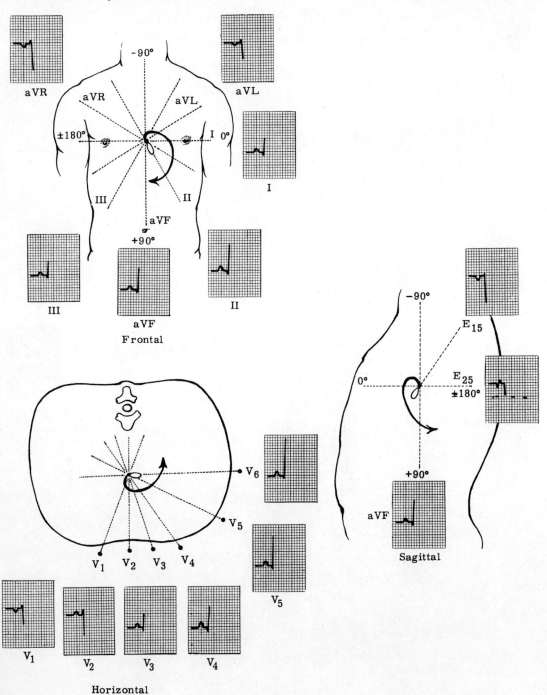

aVR

aVL

I

III

aVF

II

Frontal

Horizontal

Sagittal

B. Ventricular Depolarization:
   2. Major activation of the left and right ventricles - Since the major electromotive forces are generated in the larger muscle mass of the left ventricle (see p. 60), the major portion of the QRS vector is directed to the left, inferiorly and slightly posteriorly.

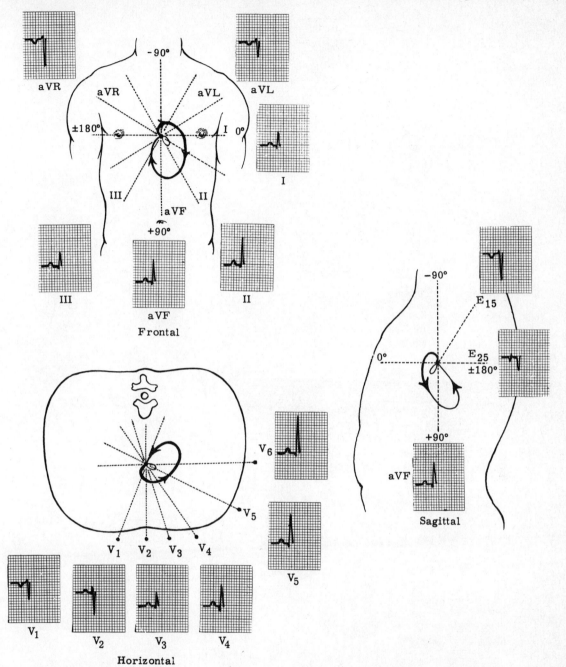

B. Ventricular Depolarization:
   3. Completion of ventricular depolarization - The loop returns to the center point. It is in-
      scribed in a clockwise direction in the frontal plane, counterclockwise in the sagittal
      plane, and counterclockwise in the horizontal plane.   The direction of inscription in the
      sagittal and horizontal planes is an absolute feature of the normal QRS loop.
          In this illustration the mean QRS vector is approximately + 90° in the frontal plane,
      +110° in the sagittal plane, and -20° in the horizontal plane.

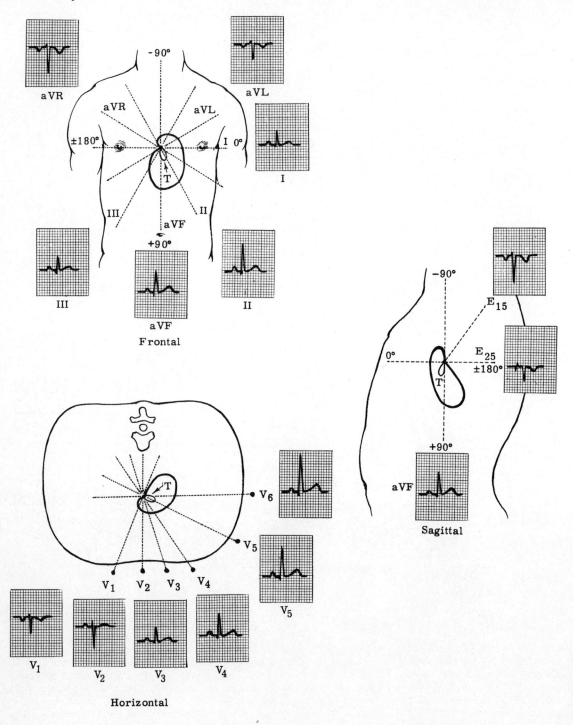

C. The T Loop: This is produced by ventricular repolarization (see p. 62). This loop is oriented in the same general direction as the QRS loop, but may be oriented anteriorly, inferiorly,
and to the right of the QRS vector by 0° to 30°. (The P loops are not illustrated.)

NORMAL ADULT VECTORCARDIOGRAM

[S = superior; I = inferior; R = right; L = left; A = anterior; P = posterior. The symbols
(×2), (×4), (×5), and (×8) in this and subsequent illustrations indicate the photographic magnification of the vector loop, (×8) being the greatest magnification.]

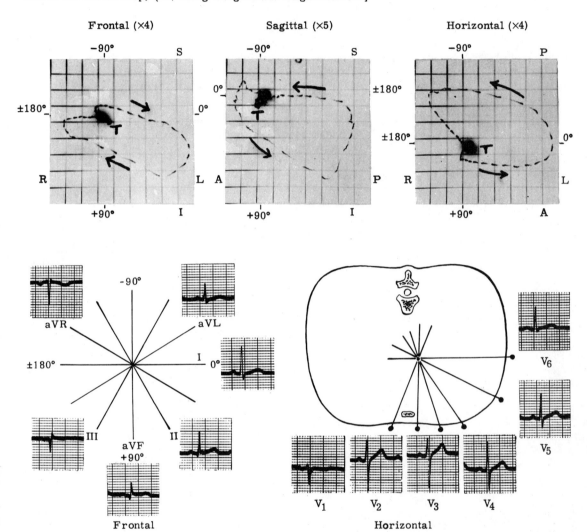

The P loop is not readily identified since it is small and buried in the larger T loop. The
initial QRS vector is oriented to the right (see frontal and horizontal views), anteriorly (see
sagittal and horizontal views), and superiorly (see frontal and sagittal views). The major portion
of the QRS loop is then inscribed inferiorly (frontal and sagittal), to the left (frontal and horizontal),
and at first anteriorly and later posteriorly (sagittal and horizontal). The last portion of the QRS
vector is oriented to the right (frontal and horizontal) and posteriorly (sagittal and horizontal). The
loop is inscribed in a clockwise direction in the frontal plane, and in a counterclockwise direction
in the sagittal and horizontal planes. The major QRS vector is approximately +40° in the frontal
plane, +120° in the sagittal plane, and −20° in the horizontal plane. The T loop is oriented to the
left and inferiorly and slightly anterior to the QRS loop.

The electrocardiogram is within normal limits. There is no abnormal axis deviation since
the mean frontal plane QRS vector is +15°; the heart position is intermediate. The small s waves
in leads I and aVL and the small r′ wave in aVR are due to the late right orientation of the QRS
vector.

LEFT VENTRICULAR HYPERTROPHY

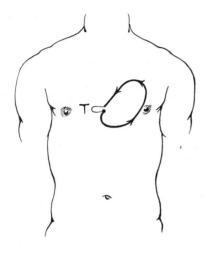

Frontal:
There is the normal initial orientation of the QRS loop to the right. The major portion of the loop is then oriented to the left and is usually inscribed in a counterclockwise direction. There is often superior orientation of the loop, resulting in a mean QRS angle of −30° or more. The QRS loop may fail to close (i.e., return to the center point before inscription of the T loop), thus explaining the ST segment change seen in the electrocardiogram. The T loop is opposite the mean QRS vector.

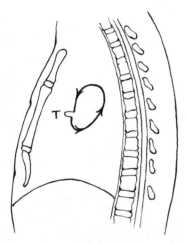

Sagittal:
The QRS loop is inscribed in a normal counterclockwise direction. There is a small initial anterior deflection, and then the major portion of the QRS loop is oriented posteriorly and at times superiorly. The QRS loop fails to close, and the T loop is opposite the mean QRS vector.

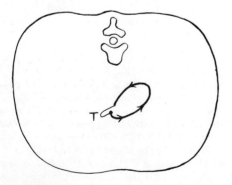

Horizontal:
The QRS loop is inscribed in the normal counterclockwise direction. There is the normal initial deflection to the right and anteriorly. The major portion of the loop is oriented to the left and posteriorly, the mean axis being more posterior than normal, usually in the -30° to -90° range. The QRS loop may fail to close, and the T loop is opposite the mean QRS vector.
Rarely, the QRS loop is inscribed in a clockwise direction, simulating anterior wall infarction. The counterpart in the electrocardiogram is the finding of QS complexes in V_{1-4} (see p. 191).

Typical Features:
The QRS loop is inscribed in a normal direction but is oriented more posteriorly, to the left, and often superiorly. The QRS loops fail to close and the T loops are oriented opposite the mean QRS vector. (The P loops are not illustrated.)

LEFT VENTRICULAR HYPERTROPHY

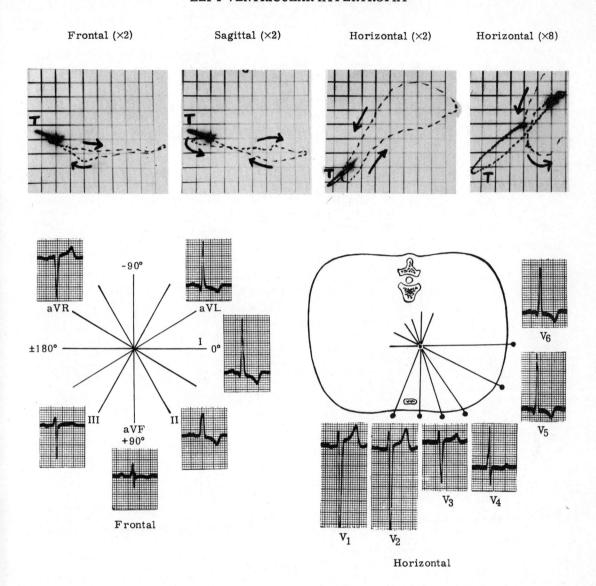

The initial portion of the QRS vector is normally oriented to the right, anteriorly, and slightly inferiorly. The major portion of the QRS loop is oriented to the left and posteriorly. The magnitude is greater than normal as indicated by the large size of the loops in a ×2 magnification. The QRS loop is inscribed in a clockwise direction in the frontal plane, in a "figure-of-eight" in the sagittal plane, and in the normal counterclockwise direction in the horizontal plane. The terminus of the QRS loop fails to return to the zero point before the T loop is inscribed (best seen in horizontal ×8). This results in an open ST vector which is oriented to the right and anteriorly. The T loop is oriented to the right, anteriorly, and slightly superiorly.

The electrocardiogram reveals a typical pattern of left ventricular hypertrophy. The frontal plane axis = 0°; the heart position is horizontal. The QRS interval = 0.1 sec.; V.A.T. = 0.07 sec.; the R in aVL = 19 mm.; there is ST depression and T wave inversion in leads I, aVL, aVF, and V_{5-6}.

Clinical and Autopsy Diagnosis: Rheumatic heart disease with aortic incompetency.

LEFT BUNDLE BRANCH BLOCK

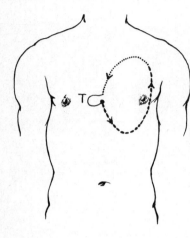

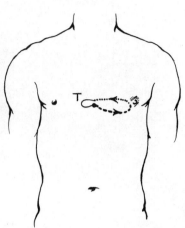

Frontal:

Since initial septal activation is from right to left (see p. 128), the initial QRS vector will be oriented to the left. The loop is usually inscribed in a counterclockwise direction with the major orientation to the left and often superiorly. There is a conduction delay in the latter part of the loop, as evidenced by the increased proximity of the time dashes (so that they appear as dots). The QRS loop fails to close and the T loop is opposite the mean QRS vector by 180°.

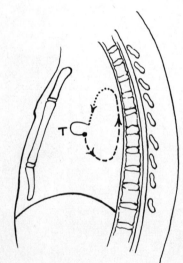

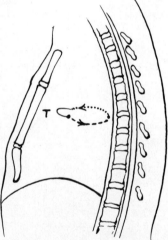

Sagittal:

The QRS loop is inscribed in the normal counterclockwise direction. It is directed posteriorly and often superiorly. There is late conduction delay, failure of closure of the QRS loop, and the T loop is inscribed opposite to the mean QRS vector.

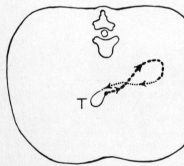

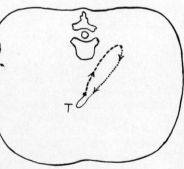

Horizontal:

There is no initial deflection to the right. The entire loop is inscribed in a clockwise direction or forms a "figure-of-eight" in which the larger distal loop is clockwise. The loop is oriented to the left and posteriorly. There is late conduction delay, failure of closure of the QRS loop, and the T loop is inscribed opposite the mean QRS vector.

Typical Features:

The QRS loop is oriented to the left and posteriorly; the normal initial orientation to the right does not occur; the entire loop in the horizontal plane is inscribed in a clockwise direction or forms a "figure-of-eight" in which the distal loop is clockwise. There is evidence of conduction delay in the latter portion of the loop, as evidenced by increased proximity of the time markings. The QRS loops fail to close, and the T loops are opposite the mean QRS vector. (The P loops are not illustrated.)

LEFT BUNDLE BRANCH BLOCK

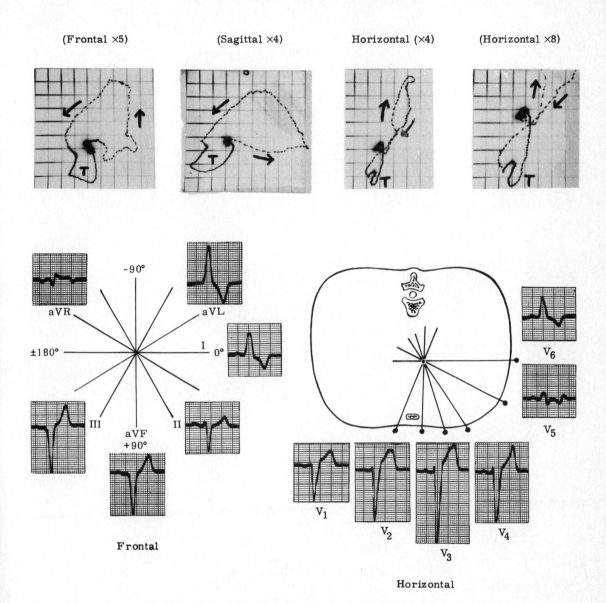

(Frontal ×5)   (Sagittal ×4)   Horizontal (×4)   (Horizontal ×8)

aVR   aVL   ±180°   I 0°   -90°   III   II   aVF +90°

Frontal

V6   V5   V1   V2   V3   V4

Horizontal

There is no initial deflection of the QRS loop to the right. The major portion of the QRS loop is directed superiorly, to the left, and posteriorly. There is increased proximity of the time markings in the latter portion of the loop. In the horizontal plane the typical "figure-of-eight" loop is seen in which the distal loop is inscribed in a clockwise direction. The QRS loop fails to close, resulting in an open ST vector to the right and anteriorly. The T loop is oriented inferiorly, anteriorly, and to the right.

The electrocardiogram reveals the typical pattern of a left bundle branch block: left axis deviation; QRS = 0.16 sec.; V.A.T. = 0.1 sec.; wide slurred R waves in I, aVL, and V_6; ST depression in I, aVL, and V_{5-6}.

Clinical Diagnosis: Arteriosclerotic heart disease.

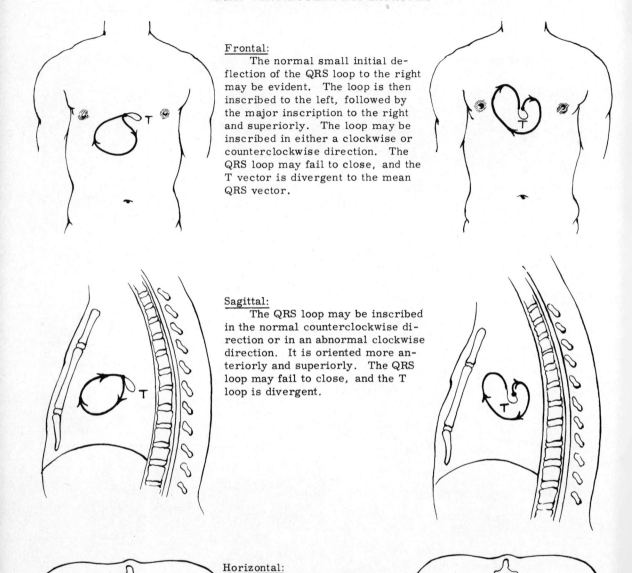

Frontal:
The normal small initial deflection of the QRS loop to the right may be evident. The loop is then inscribed to the left, followed by the major inscription to the right and superiorly. The loop may be inscribed in either a clockwise or counterclockwise direction. The QRS loop may fail to close, and the T vector is divergent to the mean QRS vector.

Sagittal:
The QRS loop may be inscribed in the normal counterclockwise direction or in an abnormal clockwise direction. It is oriented more anteriorly and superiorly. The QRS loop may fail to close, and the T loop is divergent.

Horizontal:
The initial right deflection of the QRS loop is followed by an inscription to the left. The major portion of the QRS loop is then inscribed in a clockwise direction, extending to the right and anteriorly. The QRS loop may fail to close, and the T loop is divergent.

Typical Features:
The spatial orientation of the QRS loop is to the right, anteriorly and usually superiorly. The loop is inscribed in a clockwise direction in the horizontal plane and may be inscribed in a clockwise direction in the sagittal plane. The QRS loop may fail to close, and the T loop is divergent.

RIGHT VENTRICULAR HYPERTROPHY

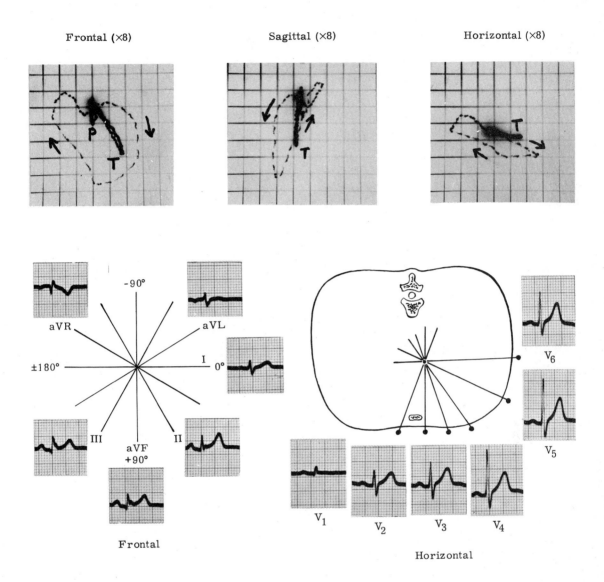

Frontal (×8)   Sagittal (×8)   Horizontal (×8)

Frontal

Horizontal

The initial portion of the QRS loop is oriented to the left, anteriorly, and slightly superiorly. The major portion of the QRS loop is oriented abnormally anteriorly, and the latter half is deviated to the right. The loop is inscribed in a clockwise (abnormal) direction in the horizontal plane. The T loop is oriented to the left and inferiorly.

The electrocardiogram is indicative of right ventricular hypertrophy. The frontal plane axis is +90°, which is normal. The only definite electrocardiographic evidence of right ventricular hypertrophy is the qr complex in V_1 (see p. 109).

Clinical Diagnosis: Cor pulmonale.

RIGHT BUNDLE BRANCH BLOCK

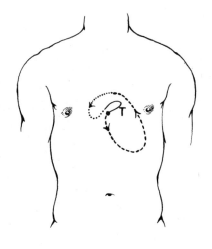

Frontal:
    The major portion of the QRS loop is inscribed in a normal fashion, with initial orientation to the right and inferiorly followed by inscription to the left and inferiorly. A terminal deflection is present which is oriented to the right and shows increased proximity of the time markings as evidence of the intraventricular conduction delay. The QRS loop may fail to close, and the T loop is opposite the terminal QRS deflection.

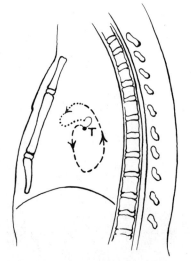

Sagittal:
    The major portion of the QRS loop is inscribed in a normal manner and in a counterclockwise direction. A terminal QRS deflection is present which is oriented anteriorly and has increased proximity of the time markings. The QRS loop may fail to close, and the T loop is opposite the terminal QRS deflection.

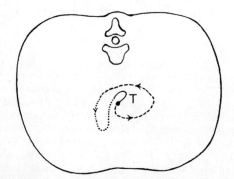

Horizontal:
    The major portion of the QRS loop is inscribed in a normal fashion, with initial deflection to the right and anteriorly followed by inscription in a counterclockwise direction to the left. The characteristic vectorcardiographic feature of right bundle branch block is a terminal deflection oriented to the right and anteriorly which shows increased proximity of the time markings. The QRS loop may fail to close, and the T loop is opposite the terminal QRS deflection.

Typical Features:
    The major portion of the QRS loop is inscribed in a normal direction. An abnormal terminal deflection is present which is oriented to the right and anteriorly. This terminal deflection is inscribed slowly (increased proximity of time markings), indicating the intraventricular conduction delay. The QRS loop may fail to close, and the T loop is opposite the direction of the terminal QRS deflection. (The P loops are not illustrated.)

RIGHT BUNDLE BRANCH BLOCK

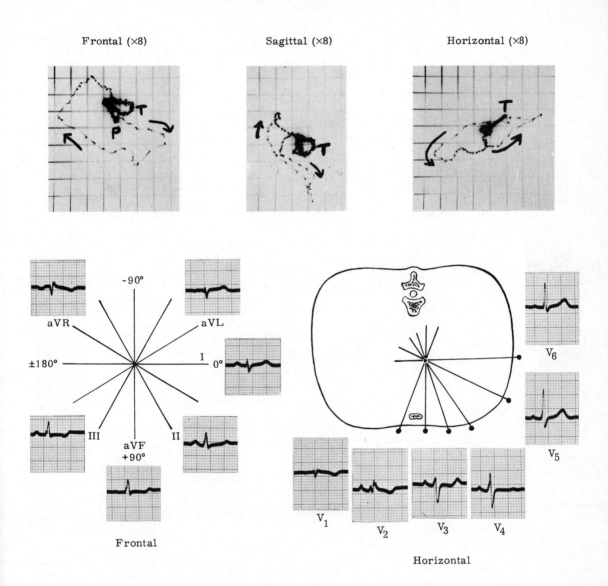

Frontal (×8) Sagittal (×8) Horizontal (×8)

Frontal

Horizontal

The first half of the QRS loop is inscribed in a normal fashion with its major orientation being to the left, inferiorly, and slightly posteriorly. However, the latter half of the QRS loop is oriented to the right, anteriorly, and superiorly. The terminal portion demonstrates conduction delay as evidenced by the increased proximity of the time markings. The loop is inscribed in a normal counterclockwise direction in the horizontal plane. The T loop is oriented to the left, posteriorly, and slight inferiorly, i.e., opposite to the terminal portion of the QRS loop.

The electrocardiogram reveals a right bundle branch block: QRS = 0.12 sec. (in V_2); rsR' with wide R' in V_2; inverted T waves in V_{1-2}.

Clinical Diagnosis: Interatrial septal defect.

RIGHT BUNDLE BRANCH BLOCK VS. RIGHT VENTRICULAR HYPERTROPHY

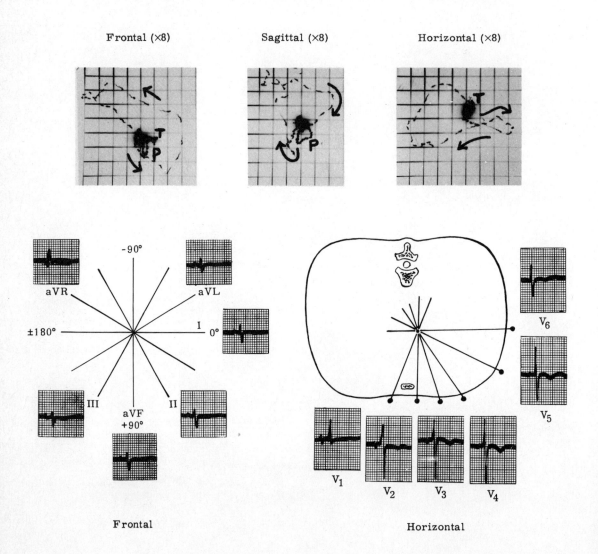

Frontal (×8) Sagittal (×8) Horizontal (×8)

Frontal Horizontal

A readily visible large P loop is seen oriented inferiorly, at a 90° angle in the frontal plane. This is consistent with right atrial hypertrophy. The initial portion of the QRS loop is oriented to the left, inferiorly, and anteriorly. The major portion of the QRS loop is then oriented to the right, superiorly, and at first anteriorly and then posteriorly in the terminal stage. The loop is inscribed in a clockwise (abnormal) fashion in the horizontal plane, and there is no terminal conduction delay. The vectorcardiogram is therefore indicative of right atrial and right ventricular hypertrophy.

The electrocardiogram reveals the following: the spiked, diphasic P wave in V_1 is suggestive of right atrial hypertrophy (however, the P waves are not abnormal in frontal plane leads); right axis deviation (frontal plane axis = +110°); an rsR′ complex in V_1; QRS = 0.09 sec. The pattern is that of an incomplete right bundle branch block and is only indirectly suggestive of right ventricular hypertrophy.

Clinical and Autopsy Diagnosis: Right atrial and right ventricular hypertrophy secondary to chronic pulmonary disease.

ACCELERATED CONDUCTION

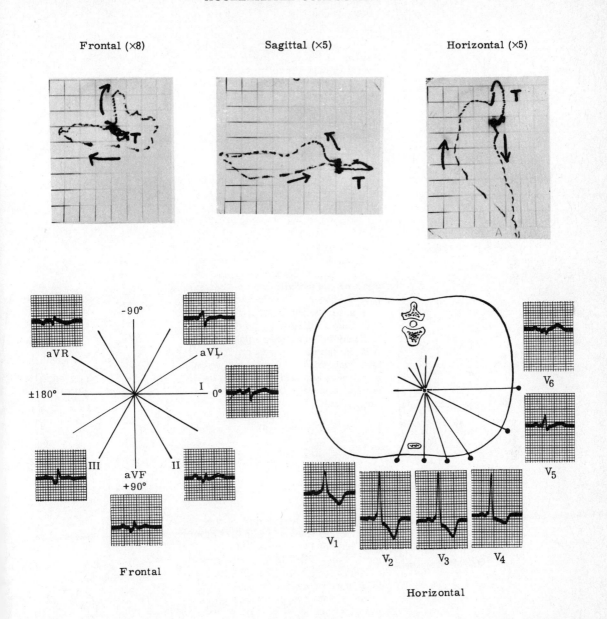

Frontal (×8)   Sagittal (×5)   Horizontal (×5)

Frontal

Horizontal

The initial portion of the QRS loop is oriented superiorly and anteriorly. The time markings are very closely recorded, indicating a conduction delay in the early phase of the QRS cycle. The major portion of the QRS loop is oriented anteriorly, at first to the left and then to the right. The ST vector and the T loop are oriented posteriorly.

The electrocardiogram is typical of accelerated conduction (W-P-W syndrome). The P-R interval = 0.09 sec.; QRS = 0.14 sec.; a wide q wave is seen in leads II, III, and aVF. However, in the presence of abnormal I-V conduction, as exists in this condition, a diagnosis of inferior wall infarction must not be made from this finding. The slurring of the q waves in II, III, and aVF and of the R waves in I, aVL, and V_{1-4} is due to the early QRS conduction delay.

ANTERIOR MYOCARDIAL INFARCTION

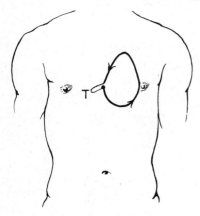

Frontal:

In localized antero-septal infarction the normal initial deflection of the QRS loop to the right is absent. The QRS loop fails to close (early stage of infarction), and the T loop becomes oriented to the right (late stage of infarction).

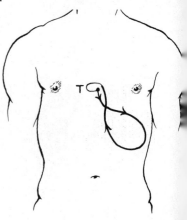

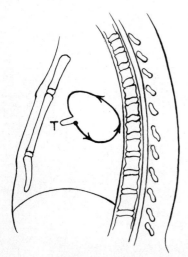

Sagittal:

In localized antero-septal infarction the initial anterior deflection is absent. With more extensive anterior infarction, the entire QRS loop is displaced posteriorly and may be inscribed in a clockwise (abnormal) direction. The QRS loop fails to close (early stage of infarction), and the T loop becomes posterior (late stage of infarction).

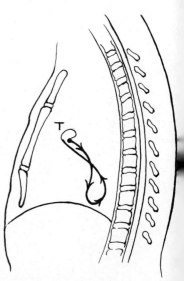

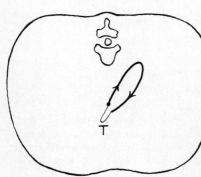

Horizontal:

The initial deflection of the QRS loop to the right and anteriorly is absent in antero-septal infarction. With more extensive anterior infarction the QRS loop is oriented posteriorly and inscribed either entirely in a clockwise (abnormal) direction or as a "figure-of-eight," or in a normal counterclockwise direction but with concavity of the centrifugal loop. The QRS loop fails to close (early stage of infarction), and the T loop becomes posterior (late stage of infarction).

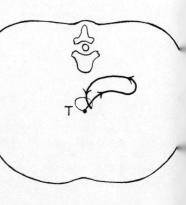

Typical Features:

The loss of electromotive forces resulting from anterior myocardial infarction causes the QRS loop to be deviated posteriorly. In localized antero-septal infarction the normal initial deflection to the right and anteriorly does not occur. Instead the initial deflection is to the left and posteriorly. With more extensive anterior infarction the QRS loop may be inscribed in a clockwise direction in the sagittal plane. In the horizontal plane the QRS loop, in addition to being oriented posteriorly, is inscribed either entirely in a clockwise direction or as a "figure-of-eight," or entirely counterclockwise but with a marked concavity of the centrifugal limb. The QRS loop will remain open in the early stage of infarction (ST change), and the T loop will become posterior in the later stage. (The P loops are not illustrated.)

ANTERIOR MYOCARDIAL INFARCTION

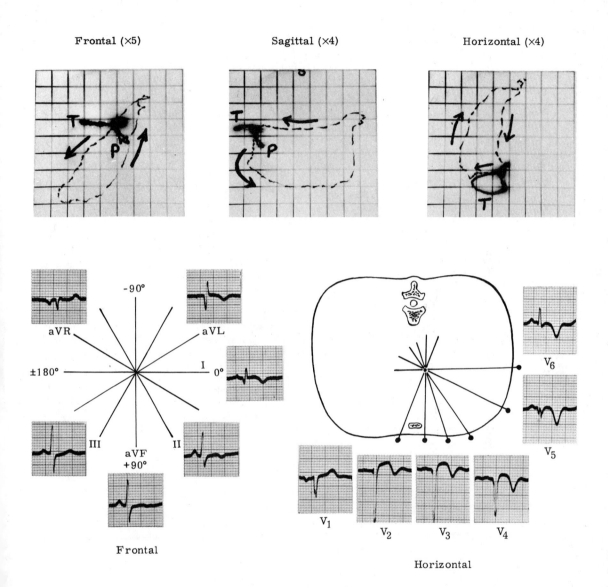

Frontal (×5)   Sagittal (×4)   Horizontal (×4)

Frontal

Horizontal

A normal P loop can be seen in the frontal and sagittal views. It is normally oriented to the left and inferiorly. The QRS loop is inscribed in a grossly abnormal direction. The initial portion is oriented far to the right and inferiorly. Almost the entire loop is oriented posteriorly, and in the horizontal plane the QRS loop is inscribed in a clockwise (abnormal) direction. The T loop is oriented to the right and anteriorly.

The electrocardiogram is indicative of anterior myocardial infarction: deep Q waves in I and aVL; QS complexes from V_2 through V_5; inverted T waves in I, aVL, and V_{2-6}.

Autopsy Diagnosis: Extensive anterior wall infarction.

INFERIOR MYOCARDIAL INFARCTION

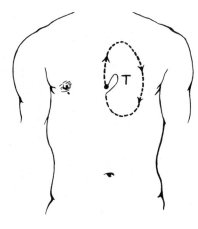

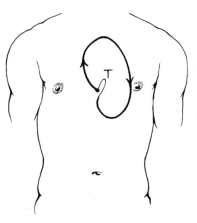

Frontal:
The initial deflection of the QRS loop is directed superiorly. The duration of the vector from onset to the maximum superior point is at least 0.02 sec. (10 dashes). The duration from onset to return to the 0°-180° axis is at least 0.04 sec. (20 dashes). The remainder of the QRS loop is inscribed in a normal fashion. The QRS loop remains open in the early stage of infarction, and the T loop is directed superiorly in the late stage.

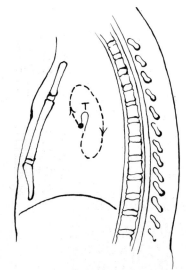

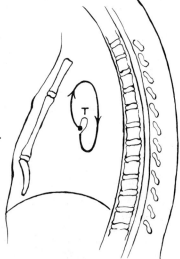

Sagittal:
The initial deflection of the QRS loop is directed superiorly in the -65° to -150° segment. The duration of this vector is as described for the frontal plane. The entire QRS loop may be inscribed in a clockwise direction (abnormal). The QRS loop remains open in the early stage of infarction, and the T loop is directed superiorly in the late stage.

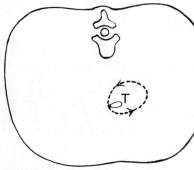

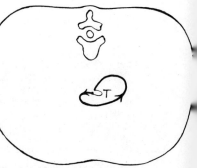

Horizontal:
In uncomplicated inferior myocardial infarction, the horizontal plane loops are inscribed in a normal manner. If there is associated lateral wall infarction, the initial portion of the QRS loop will be oriented far to the right (this will also be evident in the frontal plane).

Inferior Infarction

Inferior-lateral Infarction

Typical Features:
As a result of the loss of electromotive forces caused by inferior myocardial infarction, the QRS loop is deviated superiorly. This will be evident in the frontal and sagittal planes. The initial vector in these two planes is oriented superiorly (in the -65° to -150° segment in the sagittal plane) and to a magnitude much greater than normal. The duration of this initial superior orientation is at least 0.02 sec. (10 dashes), and the total duration before the inscription returns to the 0°-180° axis is at least 0.04 sec. (20 dashes). The QRS loop will remain open in the early stage of infarction, and the T loop will be directed superiorly in the late stage. (The P loops are not illustrated.)

INFERIOR AND POSTERIOR MYOCARDIAL INFARCTION

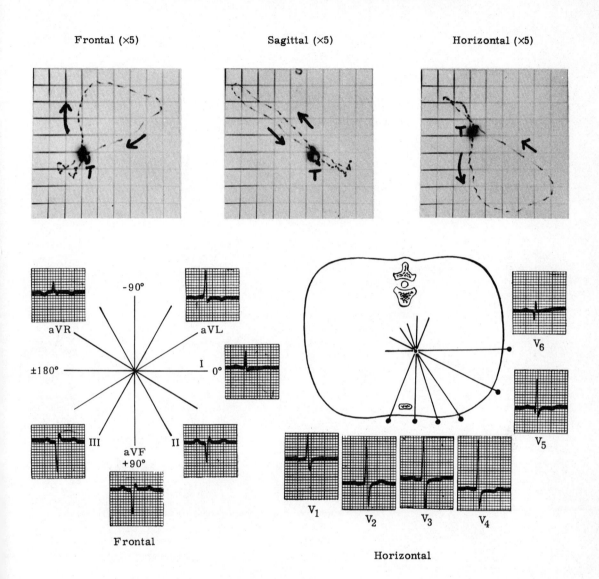

Frontal (×5) Sagittal (×5) Horizontal (×5)

There is a marked superior orientation of the QRS loop. There are 22 dashes from the onset of the QRS loop (in the frontal and sagittal planes) to the point where the QRS loop recrosses the 0° to 180° axis (22 × 0.002 = 0.044 sec.; this should equal the width of the Q wave in aVF). This is diagnostic of inferior wall infarction. In addition, practically the entire QRS loop is oriented markedly anteriorly, with only a very small terminal orientation posteriorly (and to the right and inferiorly). This unusual degree of anterior displacement is indicative of true posterior wall infarction.

The electrocardiogram reveals deep and wide (0.04 sec.) Q waves in II, III, and aVF indicative of inferior wall infarction. The prominent q wave in V_6 indicates associated lateral wall infarction. Abnormally tall R waves are seen in V_{1-3}. This is the result of the marked anterior orientation of the QRS vector as the result of posterior wall infarction.

Autopsy Diagnosis: Extensive infarction involving the inferior and posterior portions of the left ventricle.

INFERIOR WALL INFARCTION VS. NORMAL RECORD

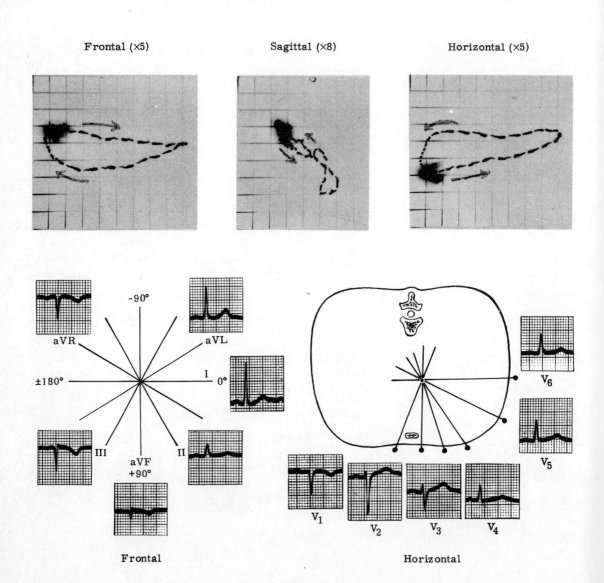

Frontal (×5)   Sagittal (×8)   Horizontal (×5)

Frontal

Horizontal

The electrocardiogram reveals a prominent Q wave and inverted T in aVF. This is strongly suggestive of inferior wall infarction. A deep Q is seen in III, but the absence of a Q in II could be reason to question the diagnosis of inferior wall infarction.

The vectorcardiogram reveals no evidence of any superior orientation in the frontal and sagittal planes. The vectorcardiogram reveals no evidence of infarction.

Clinical Findings: The patient had Laennec's cirrhosis. There was no clinical evidence of heart disease. Five electrocardiograms and vectorcardiograms taken over a one-year period remain unchanged from those illustrated.

Autopsy Findings: Normal heart; death due to cirrhosis.

In this instance the vectorcardiogram offered more correct information than the electrocardiogram.

VENTRICULAR GRADIENT

As explained in Chapter 2, the activation of a myocardial cell involves two major phases: depolarization and repolarization. If repolarization begins at the same point as depolarization and spreads in the same direction and at the same uniform rate as depolarization (see pp. 23-24), the area of the wave of repolarization (T wave) will equal the area of the wave of depolarization (R wave) but will be of opposite polarity. Expressed as vectors, these two forces will be equal but 180° apart. This does not hold true when one analyzes the waves of depolarization (QRS) and repolarization (T) of the entire ventricular myocardium. It is apparent that the R wave and the T wave are normally in the same direction in lead I (an approximate right to left axis) and that the area of the QRS does not necessarily equal the area of the T wave. The vector which represents the net effect of the QRS vector and the T vector is the ventricular gradient. By definition, this vector has magnitude, polarity, and direction in space (three-dimensional). In clinical unipolar electrocardiography the determination of the ventricular gradient has been limited to the frontal plane. The determination is quite time-consuming and is not popular as a routine measurement in clinical electrocardiography.

The ventricular gradient in the frontal plane can be determined in the following manner: The net areas of the QRS complexes and T waves are measured in two frontal plane leads, such as I and III (see p. 35). The QRS and T vectors are thereby determined and plotted. The resultant of the QRS and T vectors can be geometrically determined by the law of the parallelogram, and will represent the frontal plane ventricular gradient. Since this is a reflection of the QRS vector and the T vector, the concept of primary and secondary T wave changes has been proposed. When the changes in repolarization (T wave) are associated with changes in depolarization (QRS complex), as in bundle branch block and infarction, the T changes are termed secondary. T wave changes are termed primary if there are changes in repolarization with apparently normal depolarization.

With the advent of corrected orthogonal leads, an accurate determination of the spatial ventricular gradient is possible. It is quite time-consuming, and it is questionable that this determination will offer valuable information that cannot be obtained by the more routine evaluation of the record.

Chapter 19

INTERPRETATION OF THE
ELECTROCARDIOGRAM

Ideally, the person best qualified to read and interpret the electrocardiogram is the physician who is taking care of the patient. Since this is not always possible, the individual reading the record must have the following data as a minimum:

History Accompanying Record:

A. Age: Remember that the normal pattern in infants or children is considerably different from that in adults.

B. Race: Young adult Negroes may show a pattern which would be abnormal in a white person of the same age.

C. Height, Weight, and Body Build: Obese and thick-chested individuals will have reduced amplitude of the complexes.

D. Associated Pulmonary Disease: Marked emphysema, pleural effusion, and previous chest surgery may affect the heart position and voltage of the complexes.

E. Medication, Especially Digitalis: Remember that digitalis leaf and digitoxin can affect the electrocardiographic pattern for as long as three weeks after the drug has been discontinued.

F. Blood pressure and clinical impression.

G. Tentative diagnosis and/or pertinent cardiorespiratory findings.

Technic of Reading the Record:

It is preferable to read the tracing before it is cut and mounted since in arrhythmias it is frequently essential to study long strips of any one lead in order to reach the proper diagnosis (see, for example, pp. 254 and 257). Furthermore, isolated abnormalities may be present which are unintentionally omitted when small segments of the tracing are mounted. One sequence that can be followed is:

A. Scan the entire record to make sure it is technically good, i.e., free of electrical interference, good skin contact, and leads properly taken. Check the standardization; this should be 10 mm.

B. Determine the rhythm. If an arrhythmia is present, check the leads which best illustrate it (usually V_1).

C. Determine the heart rate. If the rhythm is not of sinus origin, determine both the atrial and ventricular rates.

D. Determine the P-R, QRS, and Q-T_C intervals. By custom this is done from the standard leads, but this is not essential.

E. Study of Standard Leads (I-III): Many authorities feel that these leads are now superfluous since they merely reflect the pattern seen in the extremity leads. However, they do serve as a check on the interpretation of the extremity leads. Note any axis deviation; note any abnormalities of the P wave, QRS complex, ST segment, and T wave.

F. Study of Extremity Leads: Note the heart position; note any abnormalities of the P, QRS, ST, and T.

G. Study of Precordial Leads: Note the degree of rotation on the long axis; note any abnormalities of the P and T waves, QRS complexes, and ST segments.

Electrocardiographic Interpretation:
The following types of conclusions can be made.
A. The tracing is normal.

B. Borderline record; there are minor changes (enumerate) the significance of which will depend on the clinical findings and serial electrocardiograms if clinically indicated.

C. Abnormal record typical of (name of condition).

D. Abnormal record consistent with (names of conditions).

E. Abnormal record not characteristic of any specific entity.

In all the above instances one must remember that a normal electrocardiogram does not imply a normal heart and that an abnormal electrocardiogram does not necessarily imply organic heart disease. The tracing must be interpreted in the light of clinical findings and serial tracings and additional leads taken as indicated.

ELECTROCARDIOGRAMS FOR INTERPRETATION

In order that the reader of this text might gain some practical experience in the interpretation of the electrocardiogram, the following electrocardiograms are included. It is suggested that the reader interpret these tracings himself before reading the text, and then compare his interpretation with that of the author.

In most of the following electrocardiograms it will not be possible to determine the heart rate and the Q-T_c since only single complexes are shown. However, in the tracings selected this does not affect the interpretation.

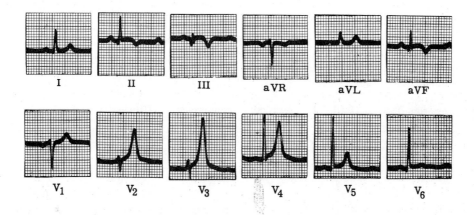

Regular sinus rhythm; P-R = 0.14 sec.; QRS = 0.06 sec.; small q waves with ST elevation and T wave inversion in leads II, III, and aVF. There are very tall symmetrical T waves in V_{2-4}.

Interpretation: (See p. 173.) Inferior-posterior myocardial infarction.

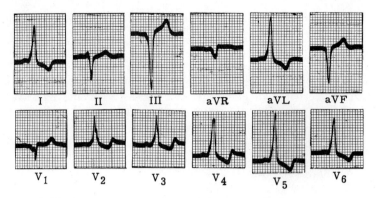

Regular sinus rhythm; P-R = 0.1 sec.; QRS = 0.12 sec. There is left axis deviation and a horizontal heart position. The initial portion of the R is slurred in leads I, aVL, and V_{2-6}. There is ST depression and T wave inversion in the latter leads. The voltage of the R in lead aVL = 15 mm. Ordinarily this would indicate left ventricular hypertrophy, but in the presence of the abnormal conduction pattern, this is invalid.

Interpretation: (See p. 261.) Accelerated conduction (Wolff-Parkinson-White syndrome).

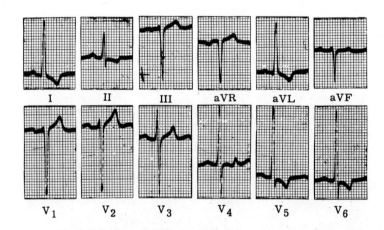

Regular sinus rhythm; P-R = 0.18 sec.; QRS = 0.08 sec.; frontal plane axis = -18°. There is ST depression and T wave inversion in leads I and II. The heart position is horizontal. R in aVL = 18 mm. There is ST depression and T wave inversion in aVL. $SV_1 + RV_5$ = 49 mm. There is ST depression and T wave inversion in V_{5-6}.

Interpretation: (See p. 100.) Left ventricular hypertrophy. **Clinical Diagnosis:** Hypertensive cardiovascular disease.

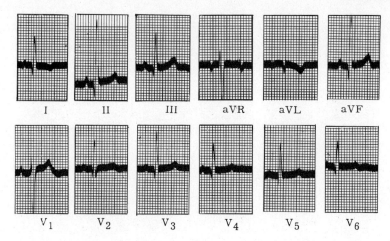

Regular sinus rhythm; P-R = 0. 16 sec. ; QRS = 0. 08 sec. There is no abnormal axis deviation. The T in lead I is inverted. The heart position is vertical. The T is inverted in aVL as a
manifestation of normal left ventricular cavity potential. Precordial leads show counterclockwise
rotation.

Interpretation: (See p. 83.) Abnormal electrocardiogram as evidenced by inverted T in lead
I. No clinical diagnosis can be made from the electrocardiogram. In view of the clinical finding
of dextroversion and the absence of other evidence of cardiovascular disease, one is justified in
considering this electrocardiogram normal for this individual. The counterclockwise rotation is
also consistent with the clinical diagnosis. **Clinical Diagnosis:** Heart displaced to the right; bronchiectasis; sinusitis.

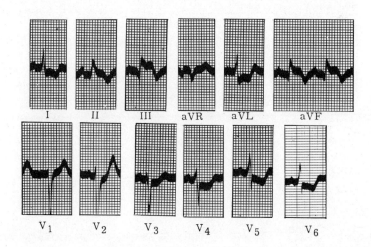

Regular sinus rhythm; rate = 107; P-R = 0. 14 sec.; QRS = 0. 08 sec.; intermediate heart
position. There is ST elevation with T wave inversion in leads II, III, and aVF; ST depression in
leads I, aVL, and V_{2-6}.

Interpretation: (See p. 189.) The pattern is consistent with early inferior wall infarction.
However, since this pattern has persisted for three months, a ventricular aneurysm must be considered. Cardiac fluoroscopy and subsequent autopsy confirmed the diagnosis of ventricular
aneurysm involving the inferior and posterior walls of the left ventricle.

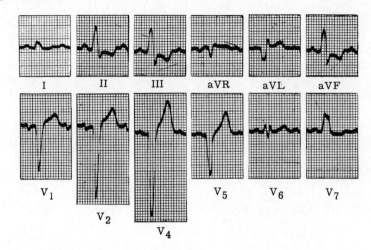

Regular sinus rhythm; P-R = 0.16 sec.; QRS = 0.15 sec.; depressed ST with T wave inversion in leads II and III; vertical heart position; wide R with depressed ST and inverted T in aVF. There is an rsr′ complex in V_6 and a wide, notched R in V_7. V.A.T. = 0.1 sec. in V_6.

Interpretation: (See p. 135.) Left bundle branch block. **Clinical and Autopsy Diagnosis:** Hypertensive and arteriosclerotic heart disease; no evidence of myocardial infarction:

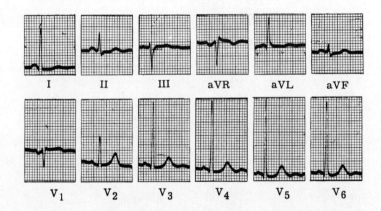

Regular sinus rhythm; P-R = 0.14 sec.; QRS = 0.08 sec.; frontal plane axis = 0°; slight ST depression with low amplitude T in lead I. The heart position is semi-horizontal: the T is of low amplitude in aVL. Precordial leads reveal counterclockwise rotation. There are tall R waves in V_{3-6}; R in V_5 = 28 mm.

Interpretation: (See p. 104.) Left ventricular hypertrophy. **Clinical Diagnosis:** Hypertensive cardiovascular disease.

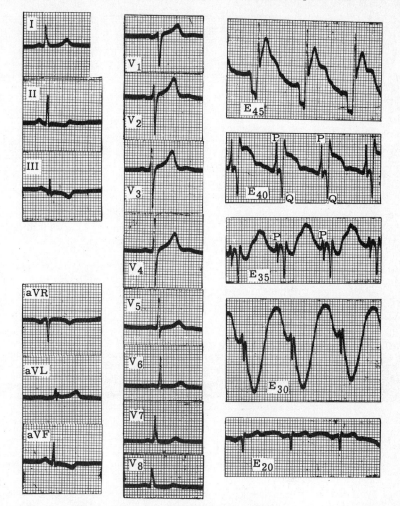

Regular sinus rhythm; rate = 80; P-R = 0.14 sec.; QRS = 0.06 sec. The heart position is semi-vertical. There is slight ST depression with T wave inversion in leads III and aVF. Esophageal leads over the left ventricle reveal abnormal Q waves and ST elevation.

Interpretation: (See p. 178.) Posterior myocardial infarction, early pattern. Clinical Diagnosis: Myocardial infarction with typical history and physical findings, including a transitory pericardial friction rub.

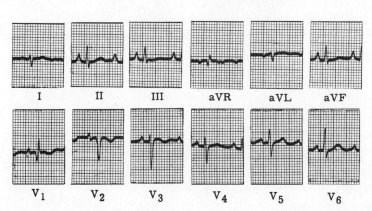

Regular sinus rhythm; P-R = 0.14 sec.; QRS = 0.06 sec.; right axis deviation; tall slender P waves in leads II and III. The heart position is vertical; tall slender P in aVF. A qR complex is seen in V_1; the T waves are inverted in V_{1-3}.

Interpretation: (See p. 111.) Right ventricular hypertrophy; right atrial hypertrophy. Clinical Diagnosis: Pulmonary emphysema with right heart failure. Autopsy Diagnosis: Right ventricular hypertrophy.

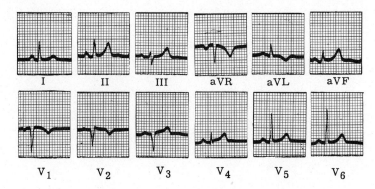

Regular sinus rhythm; P-R = 0.14 sec.; QRS = 0.06 sec.; frontal plane axis = +30°; intermediate heart position. QS complexes are seen in V_{1-3} with an abrupt transition to a left ventricular epicardial complex in V_4. The T is inverted in aVL, V_{1-2}.

Interpretation: (See p. 168.) Anteroseptal myocardial infarction. In view of the inverted T in aVL it would be advisable to take third interspace leads to investigate the possibility of higher anterolateral wall infarction. **Clinical and Autopsy Diagnosis:** Old anteroseptal infarction.

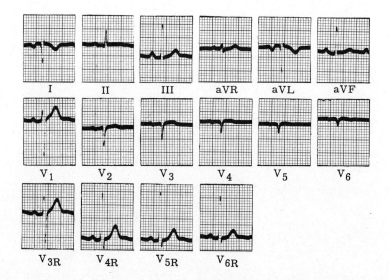

Regular sinus rhythm; P-R = 0.16 sec.; QRS = 0.06 sec. The entire pattern of lead I is inverted. Lead aVL resembles a normal aVR. Leads V_{1-6} never reflect left ventricular epicardial potential. However, leads V_{4R-6R} do reflect the epicardial surface of the left ventricle.

Interpretation: (See p. 84.) Dextrocardia (complete transposition). **Clinical Diagnosis:** 30-year-old male with dextrocardia and situs inversus; no evidence of heart disease.

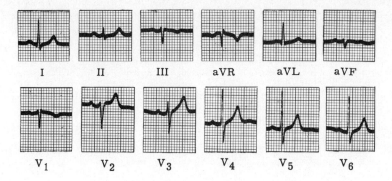

Regular sinus rhythm; P-R = 0.16 sec.; QRS = 0.08 sec.; frontal plane axis = -10°; semi-horizontal heart position; clockwise rotation; normal rsr′ in V_1.

Interpretation: (See p. 74.) Within normal limits.

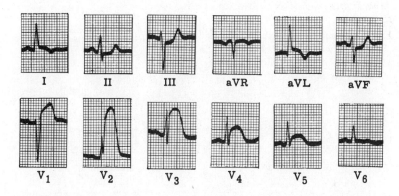

Regular sinus rhythm; P-R = 0.14 sec.; QRS = 0.06 sec.; frontal plane axis = -10°; horizontal heart position. There is ST elevation with an upward convexity in leads I, aVL, and V_{2-5}. There is ST depression in leads II, III, and aVF. The T wave is inverted in leads I and aVL, and flat in V_6.

Interpretation: (See p. 163.) Early anterior wall infarction. **Clinical Diagnosis:** Recent **(six** hours) myocardial infarction.

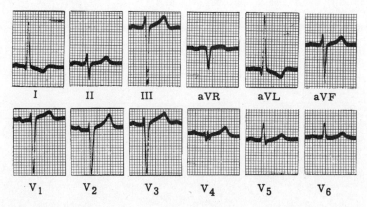

Regular sinus rhythm; P-R = 0.16 sec.; QRS = 0.08 sec.; left axis deviation (−38°), ST depression and T wave inversion in lead I. The heart position is horizontal; R in aVL = 19 mm.; ST depression and T wave inversion in aVL. Precordial leads are normal.

Interpretation: (See p. 101.) Left ventricular hypertrophy.

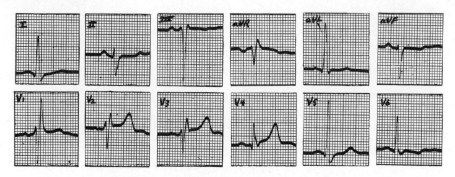

Regular sinus rhythm; P-R = 0.18 sec.; QRS = 0.16 sec.; left axis deviation; low amplitude T in lead I; horizontal heart position; R in aVL = 17 mm.; T of low amplitude in aVL; rSR' complexes in V_{1-3}; V.A.T. in V_1 = 0.1 sec.; wide S waves in V_{5-6}; inverted T in V_6.

Interpretation: (See p. 126.) Right bundle branch block; left ventricular hypertrophy
Clinical Diagnosis: Hypertensive cardiovascular disease.

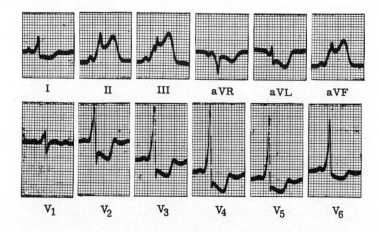

| | | | | | |
| I | II | III | aVR | aVL | aVF |

| | | | | | |
| V_1 | V_2 | V_3 | V_4 | V_5 | V_6 |

The P-R interval = 0.1 sec.; QRS = 0.12 sec. There is slurring of the upstroke of the R in leads I, II, III, aVF, and all precordial leads. There is marked ST elevation in II, III, and aVF, with ST depression in I, aVL, and all precordial leads.

Interpretation: (See pp. 174 and 258.) Recent inferior wall infarction; accelerated conduction (Wolff-Parkinson-White syndrome).

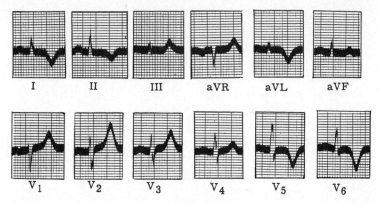

Regular sinus rhythm; P-R = 0.18 sec.; QRS = 0.08 sec.; semi-horizontal heart position. The T waves are deeply and symmetrically inverted in leads I, II, aVL, V₅, and V₆. No abnormal Q waves are present.

Interpretation: (See p. 183.) Abnormal electrocardiogram consistent with subendocardial infarction involving the anterior and lateral walls of the left ventricle. **Autopsy Diagnosis:** Myocardial infarction involving the anterior and lateral walls.   The area of infarction is not transmural but involves the inner half of the myocardium.

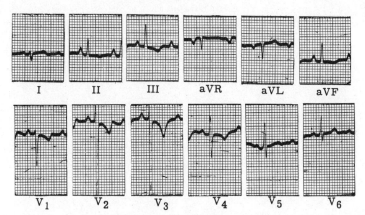

Regular sinus rhythm; P-R = 0.14 sec.; QRS = 0.06 sec.; right axis deviation; slight ST depression and T wave inversion in leads II and III.   The heart position is vertical; the T is inverted in aVF.   There is ST depression in V₁₋₃ and T wave inversion in V₁₋₄.

Interpretation: (See p. 114.) Abnormal electrocardiogram consistent with cor pulmonale (right ventricular strain). **Clinical Diagnosis:** Pulmonary sarcoidosis with right heart failure.

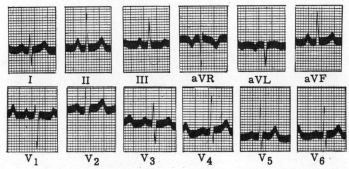

This tracing was taken after cortisone treatment of the above patient with resultant clinical improvement.

Interpretation: (See p. 114.) The present tracing is within normal limits.

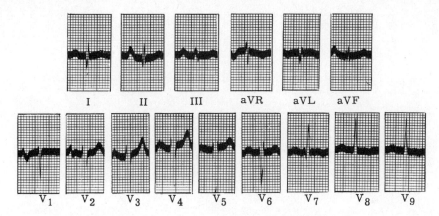

Regular sinus rhythm; P-R = 0.2 sec.; QRS = 0.08 sec.   The heart position is vertical. There are rsr' complexes in leads I, II, aVL, and aVF.   Small r waves are present in V_{1-4}. rSr' complexes are present in V_{5-6}, and an rsR' complex is present in V_7.   There is shallow inversion of the T in V_{7-9}.

Interpretation: (See p. 165.) Abnormal electrocardiogram of nonspecific pattern.   In view of the clinical findings it is consistent with the pattern of late anterior wall infarction with remaining viable muscle fibres in the epicardium.

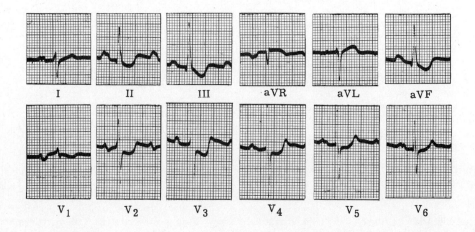

Regular sinus rhythm; P-R = 0.24 sec.; QRS = 0.08 sec.; right axis deviation; notched P waves of the P mitrale type in leads I and II.   There is ST depression with some T wave inversion in leads II and III.   The heart position is vertical.   There is ST depression and T wave inversion in aVF.   A diphasic P with wide negative deflection is seen in V_1.   A prominent r is present in V_1 and a deep S is present in V_6.   There is ST depression in the precordial leads, most marked in V_{2-3}.

Interpretation: (See p. 92.) Right ventricular hypertrophy; left atrial hypertrophy; first degree A-V block; some of the ST-T changes could be the result of digitalis.   Clinical Diagnosis: Mitral stenosis.

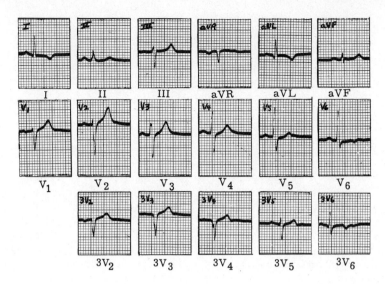

Regular sinus rhythm; P-R = 0.14 sec.; QRS = 0.06 sec.; frontal plane axis = 0°; semi-horizontal heart position. A small but wide q is seen in aVL. T waves are inverted in leads I, aVL, and V_6. Third interspace leads reveal QS complexes in the V_{2-4} positions.

Interpretation: (See p. 170.) High anterior and lateral myocardial infarction. **Clinical Diagnosis:** Arteriosclerotic heart disease; history of myocardial infarction one year previously.

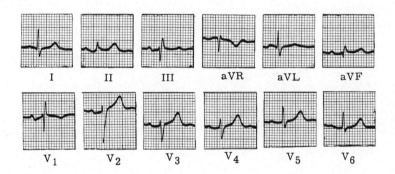

Regular sinus rhythm; P-R = 0.18 sec.; QRS = 0.08 sec.; frontal plane axis = +5°; horizontal heart position. An rSR´ complex is present in V_1; V.A.T. in V_1 = 0.04 sec.

Interpretation: (See p. 128.) Incomplete right bundle branch block. This is not necessarily indicative of organic heart disease. The significance of this must be decided by the clinical evaluation of the patient.

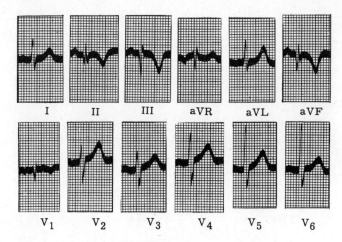

Regular sinus rhythm; P-R = 0.14 sec.; QRS = 0.08 sec.; intermediate heart position; clockwise rotation.   There are abnormal Q waves with deep, symmetrically inverted T waves in leads II, III, and aVF.

Interpretation: (See p. 177.) Inferior myocardial infarction, late pattern. **Clinical Diagnosis:** Myocardial infarction, four weeks old.

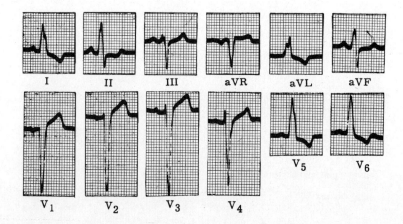

Regular sinus rhythm; P-R = 0.16 sec.; QRS = 0.12 sec.; frontal plane axis = 0°. The heart position is horizontal. There are wide notched R waves in lead I, aVL, V_{5-6}. V.A.T. in aVL = 0.1 sec. ST segments are depressed and the T waves inverted in these leads.

Interpretation: (See p. 134.) Left bundle branch block. **Clinical Diagnosis:** Hypertensive and arteriosclerotic heart disease.

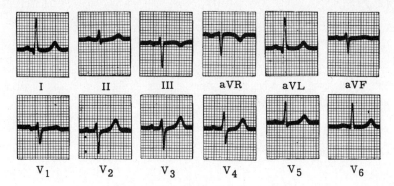

Regular sinus rhythm; P-R = 0.14 sec.; QRS = 0.08 sec.; frontal plane axis = -20°; horizontal heart position; voltage of R in aVL = 10.5 mm.

Interpretation: (See p. 68.) Within normal limits.

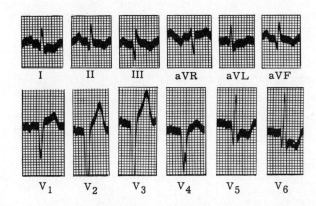

Regular sinus rhythm; P-R = 0.18 sec.; QRS = 0.1 sec.; intermediate heart position. There are abnormal Q waves in leads I, II, III, aVL, aVF, and V_{5-6}. QS complexes are seen in V_{1-4}. T waves are inverted in leads I, II, III, aVF, and V_{5-6}. There is ST depression in leads I, aVL, and V_{5-6}.

Interpretation: (See p. 187.) Inferior wall infarction, recent; anterior wall infarction, old. **Clinical Diagnosis:** Recent myocardial infarction; old myocardial infarction (by history, ten months previously). **Autopsy Diagnosis:** Old anterior wall infarction; recent posterior and inferior wall infarction; occlusion of left anterior descending and left circumflex arteries.

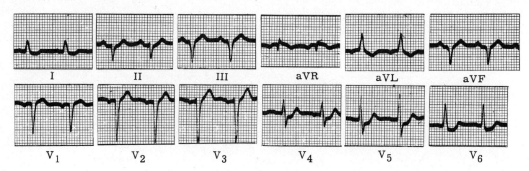

Regular sinus rhythm; P-R = 0.14 sec.; QRS = 0.08 sec.; left axis deviation; ST depression in lead I. The heart position is horizontal. The P and T are inverted, and there is ST depression in aVL. A QS complex is present in aVF. There is ST depression in V_{4-6}.

Interpretation: (See p. 106.) Abnormal electrocardiogram of nonspecific pattern. The QS complex in aVF can be a normal finding in a horizontal heart; yet an old inferior wall infarct cannot be excluded. The ST-T changes are not diagnostic of any specific entity. **Clinical and Autopsy Diagnosis:** Left ventricular hypertrophy.

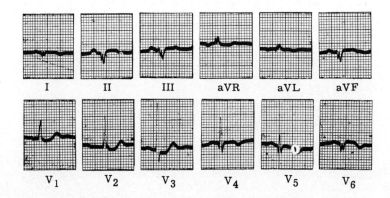

Regular sinus rhythm; P-R = 0.14 sec.; QRS = 0.08 sec.; semi-vertical heart position. There are notched QS complexes with inverted T waves in leads I, II, aVF, and V_6. T is also inverted in V_{4-5}. There are tall R waves with no S waves in V_{1-2}. V.A.T. in V_1 = 0.03 sec.

Interpretation: (See p. 180.) Inferior and lateral myocardial infarction. **Clinical Diagnosis:** Recent myocardial infarction; no clinical evidence of right ventricular hypertrophy. **Autopsy Diagnosis:** Inferior and lateral wall infarction; normal size right ventricle; occlusion of left circumflex coronary artery.

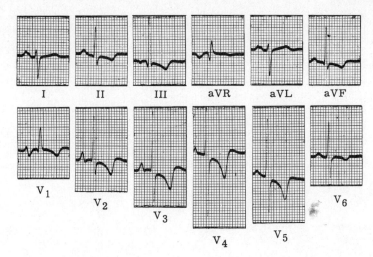

Regular sinus rhythm; P-R = 0. 18 sec.; QRS = 0. 08 sec.; right axis deviation; notched P in lead I; ST depression and T wave inversion in leads II and III.   A qR complex with ST depression and T wave inversion is seen in aVF which is a reflection of right ventricular epicardial potential. A wide diphasic P with qR complex is present in V_1.   V. A. T. in V_1 = 0. 06 sec.   There is a deep S in V_6.   The T waves are inverted in all precordial leads.   There is ST depression in V_{2-5}.

Interpretation: (See p. 110.) Right ventricular hypertrophy; left atrial hypertrophy.   **Clinical Diagnosis:** Mitral stenosis.

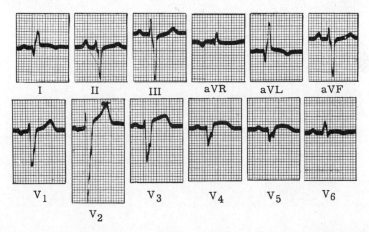

Regular sinus rhythm; P-R = 0. 2 sec.; QRS = 0. 12 sec.; left axis deviation; horizontal heart position.   Abnormal Q waves are seen in leads I and aVL.   QS complexes are seen in V_{4-5}.   There is ST elevation in leads I, aVL, and V_{2-5}.   T waves are inverted in leads I, aVL, and V_6.

Interpretation: (See p. 169.) Anteroapical myocardial infarction; intraventricular conduction defect (anterolateral peri-infarction block).

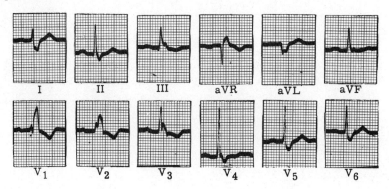

Regular sinus rhythm; P-R = 0.24 sec.; QRS = 0.14 sec. The heart position is vertical. A wide s wave is present in leads I, V_{4-6}; a wide r in aVR; an rsR' (with a very small s) in V_1; notched and wide R in V_{2-3}; ST depression and T wave inversion in V_{1-3}; V.A.T. in V_1 = 0.11 sec.

Interpretation: (See p. 195.) Posterior wall infarction; right bundle branch block; first degree A-V block. **Clinical Diagnosis:** Myocardial infarction.

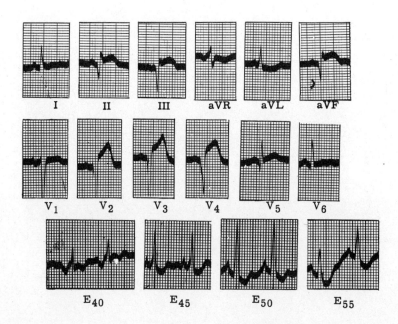

Regular sinus rhythm; P-R = 0.14 sec.; QRS = 0.08 sec. There are abnormal Q waves in leads II, III, and aVF. QS complexes are present in V_3 and V_4. There is convex ST elevation in leads II, III, aVF, and V_{4-5}. Esophageal leads over the left ventricle show ST depression but no abnormal Q waves.

Interpretation: (See p. 166.) Early anterior wall infarction. The pattern in leads II, III, and aVF suggests inferior wall infarction but is a reflection of the anterior wall infarct due to backward rotation of the apex. **Clinical Diagnosis:** Recent (two days) myocardial infarction.

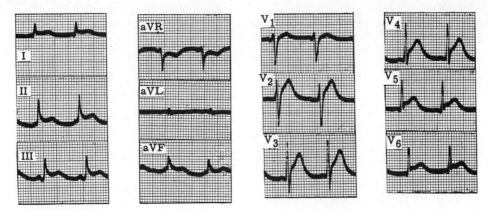

Regular sinus rhythm; P-R = 0.1 sec.; QRS = 0.06 sec.; semi-vertical heart position. There is concave ST elevation in leads I, II, III, aVF, and V_{2-6}; ST depression in aVR.

Interpretation: (See p. 269.) Early pattern of pericarditis; possible accelerated conduction rhythm. **Clinical and Autopsy Diagnosis:** Carcinoma of the esophagus, with rupture; secondary mediastinitis and pericarditis.

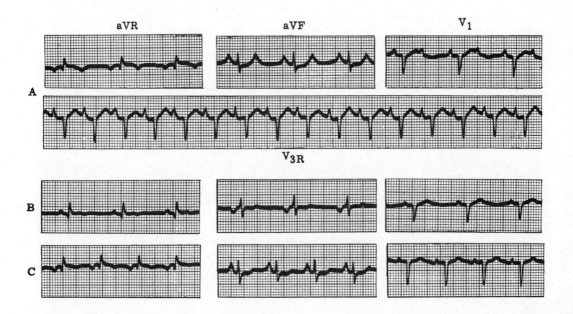

A: There is 2:1 A-V conduction with an atrial rate of 142 and a ventricular rate of 71. In lead V_{3R} 1:1 conduction is present at a rate of 127.

B: 1:1 conduction at a rate of 75. The P wave is upright in aVR and inverted in aVF.

C: Sinus rhythm, rate = 100.

Interpretation: (See p. 279.) **A:** Atrial tachycardia with 2:1 and 1:1 conduction due to digitalis toxicity. **B:** Two days after A (digitalis discontinued): A-V nodal rhythm, still indicating digitalis toxicity. **C:** Sinus rhythm reestablished one week after A and one week after discontinuation of digitalis.

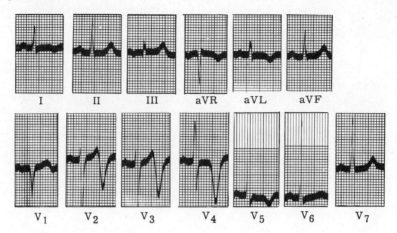

Regular sinus rhythm; P-R = 0.16 sec. QRS = 0.08 sec.; intermediate heart position. There is T wave inversion in leads I and aVL; very deep, symmetrically inverted T waves in V_{2-4}. No abnormal Q waves are present. There are tall R waves in V_{5-6}. R in V_5 = 30 mm.

Interpretation: (See p. 184.) Abnormal electrocardiogram consistent with subendocardial infarction of the anterior wall of the left ventricle; left ventricular hypertrophy. **Autopsy Diagnosis:** Anterior wall infarction, not transmural but involving the endocardial half of the myocardium. The major area of infarction is anteroseptal.

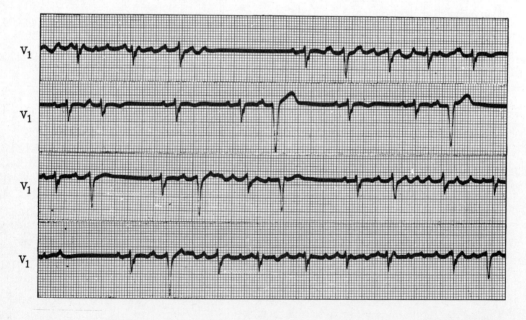

The above are portions of a continuous strip of lead V_1. Occasional regular sinus-conducted beats are seen (fourth ventricular complex in first strip; first, third, fourth, sixth, and seventh ventricular complexes in second strip, etc.). Frequent atrial ectopic beats are present, many with aberrant interventricular conduction (as second, fifth, and eighth ventricular complexes in second strip). In addition there are periods of atrial flutter-fibrillation.

Interpretation: (See p. 219.) Regular sinus rhythm with atrial ectopic beats and atrial flutter-fibrillation. This illustration emphasizes the validity of the unitarian concept of the atrial arrhythmias.

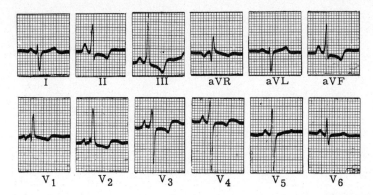

Regular sinus rhythm; P-R = 0.14 sec.; QRS = 0.08 sec.; right axis deviation; ST depression and T wave inversion in leads II and III.   There is ST depression and T wave inversion in aVF as a reflection of right ventricular epicardial potential.   There is an rsR complex in V_1.   V.A.T. in V_1 = 0.05 sec.   There is ST depression and T wave inversion in V_{1-4}.

Interpretation: (See p. 127.) Incomplete right bundle branch block.   In view of the clinical diagnosis of pulmonary sarcoidosis and right heart failure, this electrocardiogram could be indicative of right ventricular hypertrophy or strain.

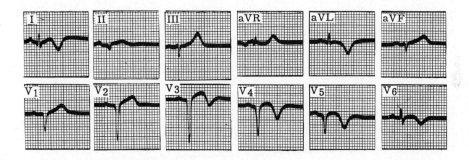

Regular sinus rhythm; P-R = 0.16 sec.; QRS = 0.06 sec.; left axis deviation; horizontal heart position.   There are QS complexes in V_{1-5}.   T waves are inverted in leads I, aVL, and V_{3-6}.

Interpretation: (See p. 185.) Anterior myocardial infarction, late pattern.

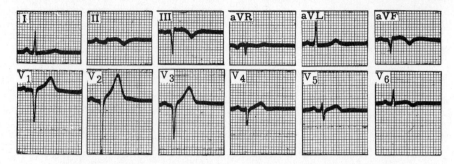

In comparison with the tracing at bottom of p. 333, a QS complex with slight ST elevation and T wave inversion is now present in aVF. The previously inverted T waves are now upright in leads I, aVL, and V_{3-5}.

Interpretation: (See p. 186.) Recent inferior wall infarction; old anterior wall infarction.

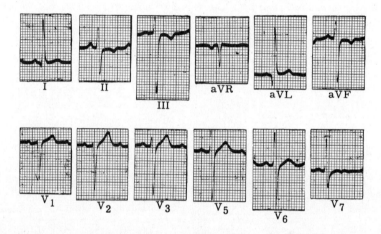

Regular sinus rhythm; P-R = 0.14 sec.; QRS = 0.09 sec.; left axis deviation. ST depression with inverted T is present in leads II and III. The heart position is horizontal. R in aVL = 17 mm. Precordial leads show evidence of clockwise rotation. The T is diphasic in V_7.

Interpretation: (See p. 103.) Left ventricular hypertrophy. **Clinical Diagnosis:** Hypertensive cardiovascular disease.

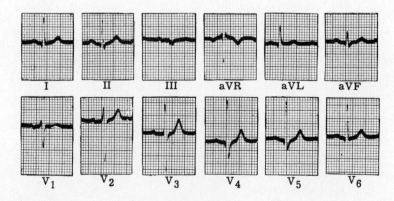

Regular sinus rhythm; P-R = 0.16 sec.; QRS = 0.08 sec.; intermediate heart position.

Interpretation: (See p. 70.) Within normal limits.

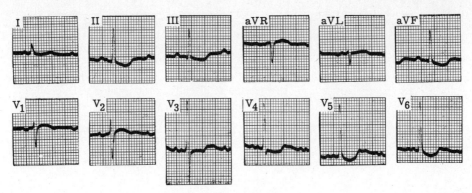

Regular sinus rhythm; rate = 80; P-R = 0.19 sec.; QRS = 0.07 sec.; vertical heart position. The P waves are notched in leads II and V_{3-6}. There is rounded ST depression in leads I, II, III, aVF, and V_{4-6}.

Interpretation: (See p. 275.) Abnormal electrocardiogram; the ST changes are consistent with digitalis effect; the P waves are consistent with left atrial hypertrophy (P mitrale).

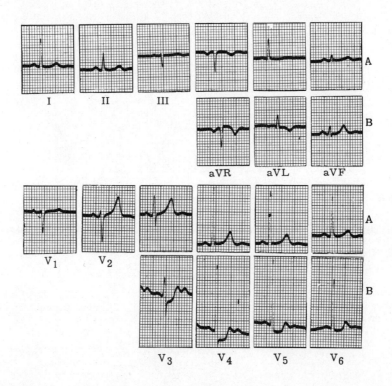

A: Regular sinus rhythm; P-R = 0.14 sec.; QRS = 0.06 sec.; frontal plane axis = +5°; semi-horizontal heart position. The T is flat in aVL. Precordial leads are normal.

B: After exercise, there is horizontal ST depression in V_{3-6}; this is 4 mm. in V_4; there is slight ST elevation in aVR; the T has become inverted in aVL.

Interpretation: (See p. 147.)

A: Borderline electrocardiogram; the flat T in aVL may be evidence of some lateral wall abnormality.

B: The changes after exercise are consistent with coronary insufficiency (myocardial anoxia).

Clinical Diagnosis: Arteriosclerotic heart disease; anginal syndrome.

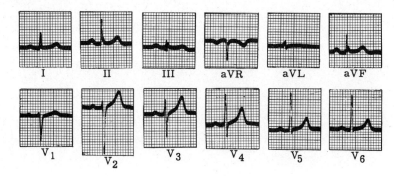

Regular sinus rhythm; P-R = 0.16 sec.; QRS = 0.06 sec.; semi-vertical heart position.

Interpretation: (See p. 72.) Within normal limits.

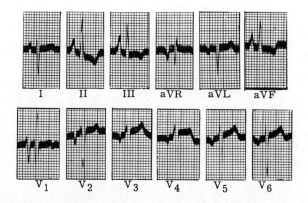

Regular sinus rhythm; P-R = 0.12 sec.; QRS = 0.06 sec.; right axis deviation. There are tall, slender P waves in leads II and III; ST depression and T wave inversion in leads II and III. A tall, slender P with depressed ST and inverted T is present in aVF. A prominent diphasic P is present in V_1. An rSR' complex is seen in V_1 and a deep S in V_6. V.A.T. in V_1 = 0.06 sec.

Interpretation: (See p. 93.) Right atrial hypertrophy; incomplete right bundle branch block which is probably indicative of right ventricular hypertrophy. **Clinical Diagnosis:** Pulmonary fibrosis with right heart failure.

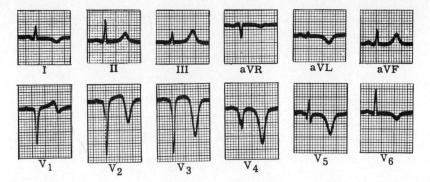

Regular sinus rhythm; P-R = 0.14 sec.; QRS = 0.08 sec.; the frontal plane axis = +60° (semi-vertical heart position). There are QS complexes in V_{1-4}. There are deep, symmetrically inverted T waves in I, aVL, V_{2-6}.

Interpretation: (See p. 164.) Anterior wall infarction, late pattern (clinically 6 months old).

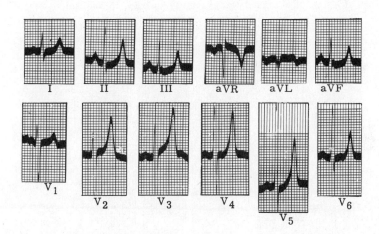

Regular sinus rhythm; P-R = 0.16 sec.; QRS = 0.06 sec.; vertical heart position. The T waves are tall and slender in leads I, II, III, aVF, and V_{2-6}.

Interpretation: (See p. 283.) The above record is consistent with hyperkalemia; however such a pattern can be a normal variant.

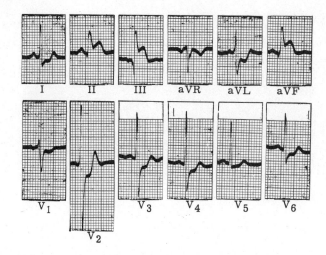

Regular sinus rhythm; P-R = 0.14 sec.; QRS = 0.08 sec. The heart position is intermediate. The small q in aVF is not necessarily abnormal. The ST segments are elevated in leads II, III, and aVF, and are depressed in leads I, aVL and V_{1-6}.

Interpretation: (See p. 176.) Early inferior myocardial infarction.

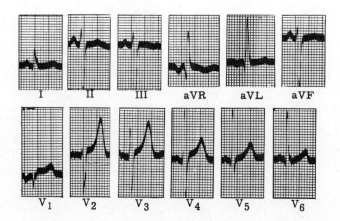

Regular sinus rhythm; P-R = 0.14 sec.; QRS = 0.08 sec.; left axis deviation. An inverted P with qR complex is present in both aVR and aVL, indicating backward rotation of the apex. R in aVL = 16 mm. The precordial leads are normal.

Interpretation: (See p. 105.) Left ventricular hypertrophy. **Clinical and Autopsy Diagnosis:** Hypertensive cardiovascular disease.

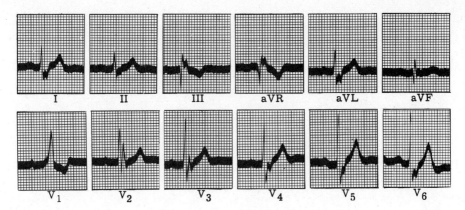

Regular sinus rhythm; P-R = 0.2 sec.; QRS = 0.15 sec.; there are wide S waves in leads I, V_{5-6}; a wide r in aVR; a wide, notched R in V_1; an RsR′ complex in V_2; V.A.T. in V_1 = 0.09 sec. The absence of an S wave in V_1 and the prominent initial R in V_2 indicate abnormally directed anterior vector forces.

Interpretation: (See p. 123.) Posterior wall infarction; right bundle branch block. **Clinical Diagnosis:** Myocardial infarction.

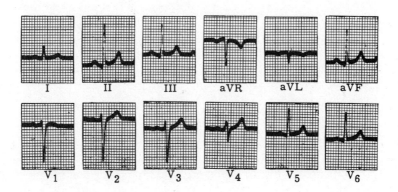

Regular sinus rhythm; P-R = 0.14 sec.; QRS = 0.08 sec.; vertical heart position.

Interpretation: (See p. 66.) Within normal limits.

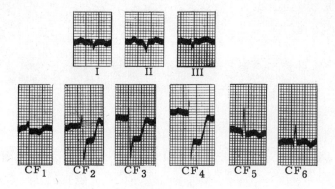

Regular sinus rhythm; P-R = 0.18 sec.; QRS = 0.08 sec.   The complexes are of low voltage in standard leads.   A prominent R is seen in CF_1.   There is marked ST depression in CF_{2-4}.   T waves are inverted in CF_{5-6}.

Interpretation: (See p. 179.)   Abnormal electrocardiogram consistent with early posterior and lateral myocardial infarction.   **Autopsy Diagnosis:**   Posterior and lateral myocardial infarction.

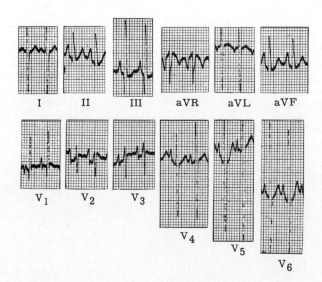

Regular sinus rhythm; rate = 177; P-R = 0.1 sec.; QRS = 0.06 sec.; right axis deviation; tall P waves in leads II and III.   aVF could be a reflection of right ventricular epicardial potential.   A qR complex is seen in V_1; this initial q wave is abnormal in a three-day-old infant.

Interpretation: (See p. 112.)   Right ventricular hypertrophy; probable right atrial hypertrophy; sinus tachycardia.   **Clinical Diagnosis:**   Tetralogy of Fallot.

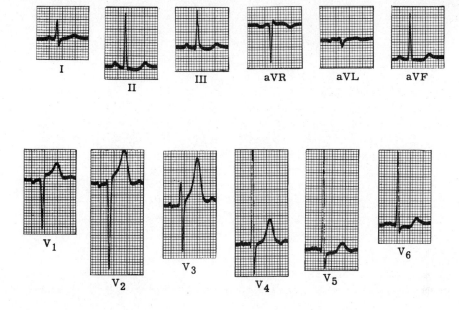

Regular sinus rhythm; P-R = 0.16 sec.; QRS = 0.09 sec.; frontal plane axis = +75°; vertical heart position. The P waves are notched in all leads. $SV_1 + RV_5 = 55$ mm. There is ST depression in leads II, III, aVF, V_{5-6}.

Interpretation: (See p. 102.) Left ventricular and left atrial hypertrophy.

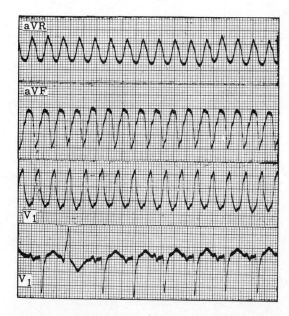

The ventricular rate is 240. The ventricular rhythm is slightly irregular. The QRS complexes are wide and slurred, upright in V_1. No definite evidence of atrial activity is seen.

Interpretation: (See p. 246.) Paroxysmal ventricular tachycardia; the ectopic focus is in the left ventricle. In the bottom record the rhythm has reverted to regular sinus with one left ventricular premature beat.

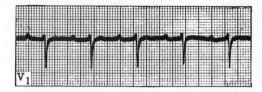

Regular sinus rhythm; P-R = 0.28 sec.; QRS = 0.08 sec.

Interpretation: (See p. 222.) First degree A-V block.

Regular sinus rhythm with atrial premature contractions. The P' waves are upright in aVR and inverted in aVF.

Interpretation: (See p. 204.) Atrial premature beats arising from a low atrial focus.

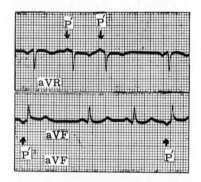

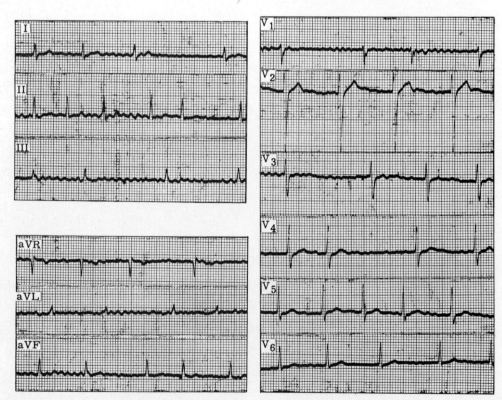

The ventricular rhythm is grossly irregular. The ventricular rate = 75. There is no regular atrial activity. The QRS-T complexes are normal. The heart position is intermediate.

Interpretation: (See p. 216.) Atrial fibrillation.

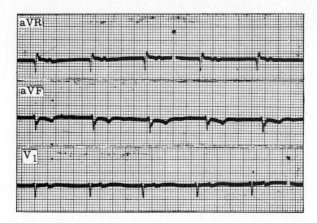

A regular ventricular rhythm is present with a rate of 70. No atrial activity precedes the QRS complexes. An atrial wave is seen following each QRS complex. The P' is upright in aVR and inverted in aVF, indicating retrograde atrial conduction.

Interpretation: (See p. 233.) A-V nodal rhythm.

A regular ventricular rhythm is present at a rate of 188. The QRS complexes are of normal configuration. P' waves are seen in V_1 and V_2. There is minimal ST depression in precordial leads which may be the result of T_a waves.

Interpretation: (See p. 208.) Paroxysmal supraventricular tachycardia.

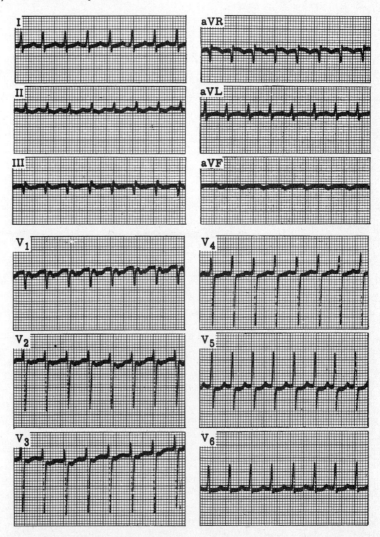

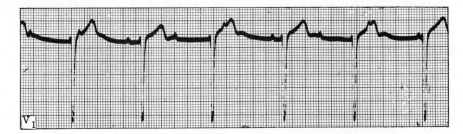

The atrial rhythm is regular at a rate of 72. The ventricular rhythm is regular at rate of 54. There is no relation between the atrial and ventricular complexes. The QRS complexes appear normal.

Interpretation: (See p. 225.) Third degree (complete) A-V block; the ventricular pacemaker is at or close to the A-V node.

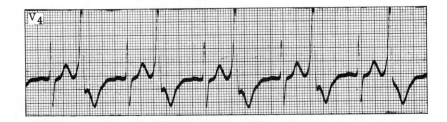

Regular sinus rhythm is present alternating with ventricular premature beats.

Interpretation: (See p. 243.) Regular sinus rhythm with ventricular bigeminy.

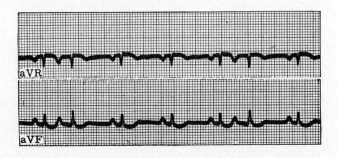

Regular sinus rhythm; rate = 75. There are premature atrial contractions. The P′ waves are inverted in aVR and upright in aVF.

Interpretation: (See p. 204.) Atrial premature beats arising from a high atrial focus.

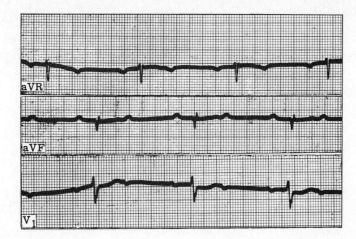

The atrial rhythm is regular at a rate of 82; the P waves are inverted in aVR and upright in aVF; the ventricular rhythm is regular at a rate of 41; there is a constant P-R interval of 0.3 seconds preceding each QRS complex.

Interpretation: (See p. 223.) Second degree A-V block (2:1).

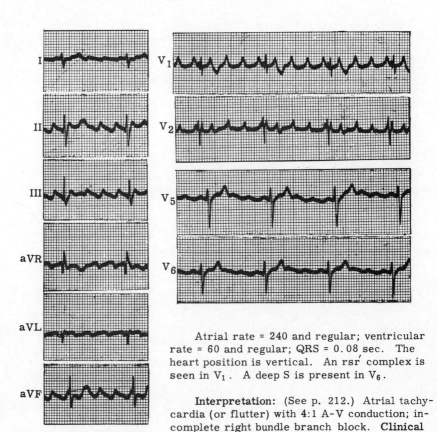

Atrial rate = 240 and regular; ventricular rate = 60 and regular; QRS = 0.08 sec. The heart position is vertical. An rsr′ complex is seen in V_1. A deep S is present in V_6.

Interpretation: (See p. 212.) Atrial tachycardia (or flutter) with 4:1 A-V conduction; incomplete right bundle branch block. **Clinical Diagnosis:** Mitral stenosis.

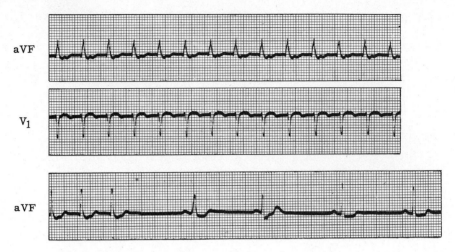

A regular ventricular rhythm is present. The rate is 150. A P wave is seen to follow each QRS complex. This could represent either a retrograde P wave from a pacemaker in the A-V node or an atrial stimulus producing ventricular activity after a P-R interval of 0.28 sec. The bottom strip illustrates reversion to regular sinus rhythm with carotid pressure.

Interpretation: (See p. 234.) Paroxysmal supraventricular tachycardia.

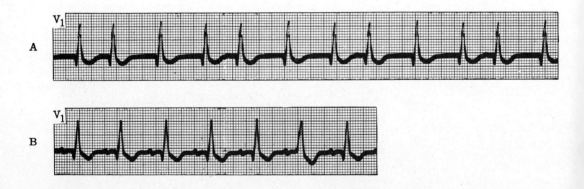

A: The basic rhythm is A-V nodal at a rate of 86. An independent atrial rhythm is present at a rate of 30. On occasion (second, fifth, eighth, and eleventh complexes) the ventricle responds to the atrial stimulus.

B: Regular sinus rhythm; rate = 86; QRS = 0.12 sec.; an initial deep q wave precedes the tall wide R wave.

Interpretation: (See pp. 256 and 192.) A: Interference dissociation (incomplete A-V dissociation). B: Right bundle branch block; anterior wall infarction.

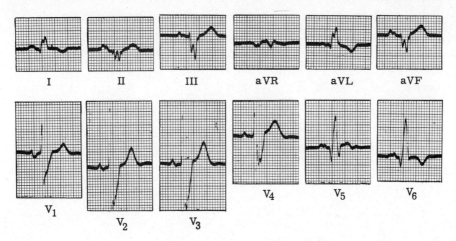

Regular sinus rhythm; P-R = 0.16 sec.; QRS = 0.17 sec. The heart position is horizontal. The R waves are notched and wide in leads I, aVL, V_5, and V_6. Initial q waves and inverted T waves are present in these leads.

Interpretation: (See p. 194.) The initial q waves in left ventricular leads indicate that this is not an uncomplicated left bundle branch block. It is consistent with an anterolateral myocardial infarction with a marked intraventricular conduction defect. If this represents a true bundle branch block it would indicate additional septal infarction. **Autopsy Diagnosis:** Extensive, diffuse myocardial fibrosis in a 35 year old male. Unfortunately, the presence or absence of a left bundle branch block was not determined by the autopsy examination.

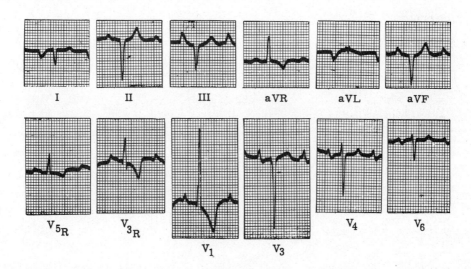

Regular sinus rhythm; P-R = 0.2 sec.; QRS = 0.08 sec. The record is technically correct. The P waves are broad and large; they are inverted in I and upright in aVR. Leads aVR and aVL would appear more nearly normal if they were reversed. There are tall R waves in V_1, V_{3R}, and V_{5R}, with ST depression and T wave inversion in these leads.

Interpretation: (See pp. 84 and 90.) Dextrocardia; right ventricular and right atrial hypertrophy. **Clinical Diagnoses:** Situs inversus; Eisenmenger complex (systolic pulmonary artery pressure = 110 mm. Hg).

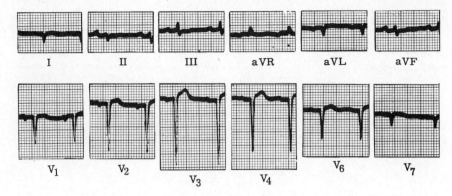

Regular sinus rhythm; P-R = 0.17 sec.; QRS = 0.06 sec.; rate = 90. QS complexes are present in leads I, aVL, and precordial leads. A prominent R is seen in aVR.

Interpretation: (See p. 191.) The pattern is consistent with anterior wall infarction. However, this could represent right ventricular hypertrophy and dilatation. Autopsy Diagnosis: Right ventricular hypertrophy and dilatation secondary to severe pulmonary emphysema; no evidence of infarction.

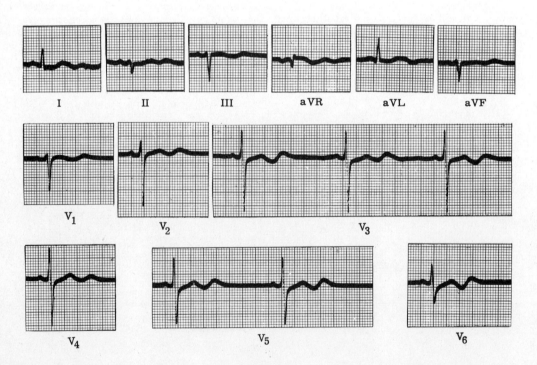

Regular sinus rhythm; P-R = 0.16 sec.; QRS = 0.1 sec. The heart position is horizontal and there is clockwise rotation. There is ST depression in leads I, aVL, and V_{3-6}. Prominent U waves are seen in all precordial leads. The measured QT interval = 0.51 sec.; but when corrected for a heart rate of 37, the QTc = 0.39 sec.

Interpretation: (See p. 286.) Hypokalemia. Clinical Diagnosis: Cushing's syndrome due to adrenal hyperplasia (serum potassium = 2.5 mEq./L.).

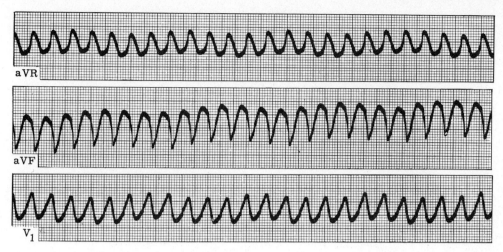

A tachycardia is present with a regular ventricular rate of 200.   The QRS complexes are wide and bizarre.   There is no definite evidence of atrial activity.

Interpretation: (See p. 249.)   Ventricular tachycardia is the most likely diagnosis.   However, in view of the absolute regularity of the ventricular complexes, a supraventricular tachycardia with aberrant intraventricular conduction must be considered (see below).

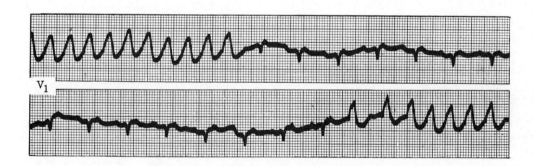

Continued record of the above patient with right carotid pressure: Carotid pressure results in the following changes: (1) slowing of the ventricular rate from 200 to 100; (2) the wide, bizarre QRS complexes of the rapid rate are changed to normal appearing complexes; (3) an atrial rate of 200 is now evident with a constant 2:1 A-V relationship.   The original pattern returns when carotid pressure is released.

Interpretation: Supraventricular tachycardia; rate = 200; 1:1 A-V conduction; aberrant intraventricular conduction.   With carotid pressure, a 2:1 atrial tachycardia is produced with a ventricular rate of 100 and loss of the aberrant intraventricular conduction.

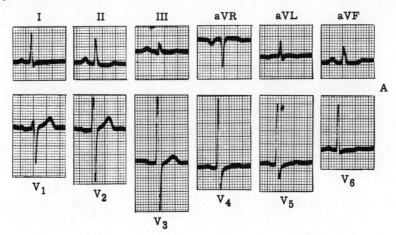

A: Regular sinus rhythm; P-R = 0.2 sec.; QRS = 0.08 sec.; the heart position is intermediate (frontal plane axis = +35°). There is minimal ST depression with flattened T waves in I, aVL, V_{4-6}.

Interpretation: Abnormal electrocardiogram indicating some abnormality of the left anterior-lateral myocardium but not diagnostic of any specific etiology.

Clinical Features: A 60-year-old male with typical angina of exertion; no evidence of previous infarction; above electrocardiogram taken when patient was asymptomatic.

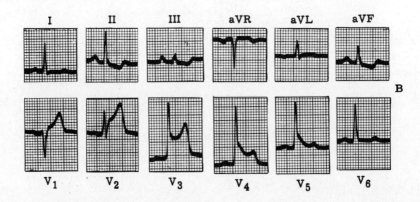

B: Nine days after A: Marked changes have occurred since A. There is marked ST elevation in leads V_{2-5} and ST depression in II, III, and aVF.

Interpretation: The electrocardiogram is consistent with very recent anterior wall infarction. However, it could represent the unusual variant of angina. The differential will be dependent upon clinical evaluation and serial electrocardiograms.

Clinical Features: The above was taken at a time when the patient was experiencing anginal pain while at rest in bed. The pain lasted for 10 minutes and was promptly relieved by nitroglycerin. A repeat electrocardiogram taken after the pain had subsided was exactly the same as illustrated in A. Serial electrocardiograms over the next 2 months showed no change from A. There were no clinical confirmatory signs of infarction. It must be concluded that electrocardiogram B represented the uncommon variant of angina (see p. 144).

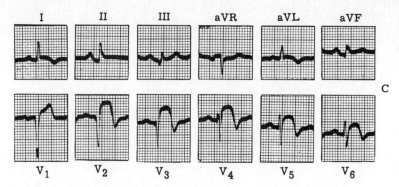

C: One year after B: QS complexes are now present in V_{1-2-3}; the ST segments are convexly elevated in I, aVL, V_{1-6} and the T waves are inverted in I, aVL and V_{2-6}.

Interpretation: Recent anterior wall infarction.

Clinical Features: The patient had suffered a myocardial infarct two days prior to the recording of the above electrocardiogram.

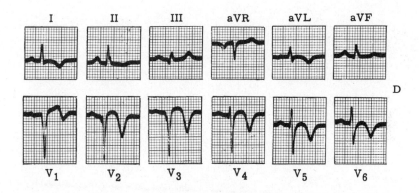

D: One month after C: QS complexes present in V_{1-3}; the ST segments are now isoelectric; the T waves are deeply and symmetrically inverted in I, aVL, and V_{2-6}.

Interpretation: Later pattern of anterior wall infarction.

Clinical Features: The patient had made an uneventful convalescence.

The above series of electrocardiograms (A, B, C, D) not only illustrate the unusual variant of angina, but point out the prognostic significance of the former, namely, that myocardial infarction developed in that area of the myocardium (anterior wall) which previously showed evidence of severe myocardial anoxia (see footnote on p. 141).

Appendix:

INTERPRETATION OF ABNORMALITIES OF THE ADULT
TWELVE-LEAD ELECTROCARDIOGRAM

The following is offered as a guide to the evaluation of electrocardiographic abnormalities. It is not intended as a complete diagnostic index since the diagnosis must always depend upon evaluation of the complete tracing in the light of the clinical findings. Even though many electrocardiographic tracings are considered "diagnostic," experience has shown that this is not always the case. The electrocardiogram is a laboratory test, and as such must be integrated with the clinical situation. Many patients are made unnecessary cardiac invalids solely on the basis of an "abnormal" or "diagnostic" electrocardiogram. This appendix is intended to be used only as an aid in suggesting possible explanations of abnormal complexes. It is hoped that the reader will refer to the text for a more detailed explanation and, finally, correlate the clinical picture with the electrocardiogram before arriving at a final diagnosis.

P Wave Abnormalities 368
    Abnormalities of P Wave Configuration and Magnitude 368
    Abnormalities of Direction of P Wave 368

QRS Complex Abnormalities 369
    Abnormal "Mean" Frontal Plane Direction With Normal
      QRS Duration 369
    Abnormal QRS Duration 369

Q Wave Abnormalities 370

QS Complex Abnormalities 371

Abnormalities of R Wave Magnitude 372

ST Segment Abnormalities 373
    Elevation of ST Segment 373
    Depression of ST Segment 374

T Wave Abnormalities 376
    Deep Inversion of T Wave 376
    T Wave Flat to Inverted 376
    Upright T Wave 377

U Wave Abnormalities 377

Abnormal Intervals 377
    P-R Interval 377
    Prolonged S-T Interval 377
    $Q-T_c$ Interval 377

Arrhythmias 378
    Sinus Arrhythmias 378
    Atrial Arrhythmias 378
    A-V Nodal Arrhythmias 379
    Ventricular Arrhythmias 380
    Pararrhythmias 380
    Accelerated Conduction 381

P WAVE ABNORMALITIES

I. Abnormalities of P Wave Configuration and Magnitude.

(1) Broad, notched P waves in leads I, aVL, and V_{4-6}. Diphasic P wave with broad negative deflection in lead V_1.

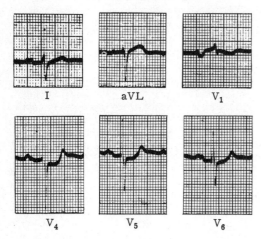

Left Atrial Hypertrophy (see p. 92)

(2) Tall, peaked P waves in leads II, III, and aVF. Tall or diphasic peaked wave in lead V_1.

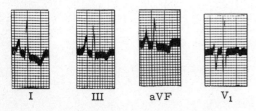

Right Atrial Hypertrophy (see p. 93)

II. Abnormalities of Direction of P Wave.

(1) Inverted P wave in lead I. Upright P wave in lead aVR.

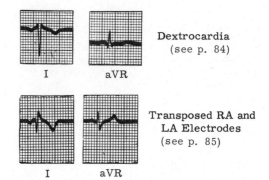

Dextrocardia
(see p. 84)

Transposed RA and
LA Electrodes
(see p. 85)

(2) Inverted P waves in lead aVF (also II and III); upright P waves in aVR.

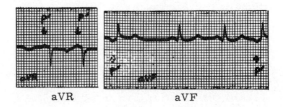

Ectopic Atrial Focus Low in Atrium or in AV Node (see pp. 203 and 204)

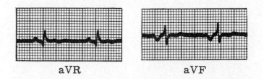

Low AV Nodal Rhythm (see p. 231)

QRS COMPLEX ABNORMALITIES

I. Abnormal "Mean" Frontal Plane Direction With Normal QRS Duration.

(1) QRS upright in lead I. QRS diphasic; S > R in lead II. (Left [or superior] axis deviation [anterolateral parietal block]).

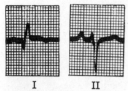

I   II

Coronary Artery Disease (see p. 292)

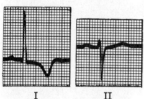

I   II

Left Ventricular Hypertrophy (see pp. 98-107)

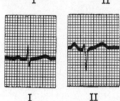

I   II

Emphysema (see p. 292)

Note: The above patterns may be seen in other myocardial diseases also.

(2) QRS upright; diphasic or inverted in lead aVF. QRS diphasic; S > R in lead I. (Right axis deviation.)

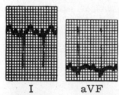

I   aVF

Infants and Children (Normal) (see pp. 81-2)

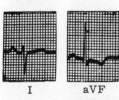

I   aVF

Right Ventricular Hypertrophy (see pp. 108-12)| **or Acute Right Ventricular Strain** (see pp. 113-6)

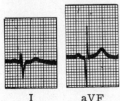

I   aVF

Diaphragmatic Peri-infarction Block (see pp. 294-5)

II. Abnormal QRS Duration (> 0.12 sec.).

(1) Wide S in leads I and V_{4-6}. Wide R' in lead V_1.

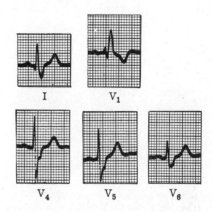

I V_1

V_4 V_5 V_6

Right Bundle Branch Block (see pp. 121-30)

(2) Wide notched RR' or RSR' in leads I and V_{4-6}, with absent q.

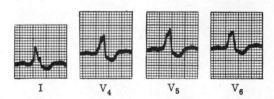

I V_4 V_5 V_6

Left Bundle Branch Block (see pp. 131-8)

(3) Wide QRS complexes in all leads.

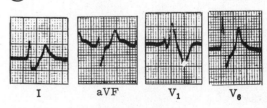

I   aVF V_1 V_6

Hyperkalemia (see p. 284)

Q WAVE ABNORMALITIES

(0.04 sec. or more in duration, or > 25% of R)

1 Abnormal Q waves in leads II, III, and aVF.

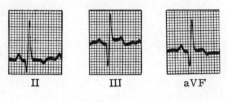

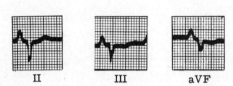

Pulmonary Emphysema or Right Ventricular Hypertrophy (see p. 191)

2 Abnormal Q waves in leads I, aVL, and V_{4-6}.

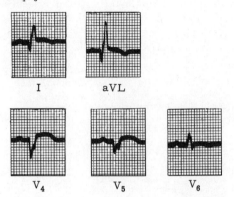

Anterior Infarction (see pp. 159-71)

3 Abnormal Q waves in leads V_{3R}-V_1, V_{1-2}, V_{1-3}, or V_{1-4}.

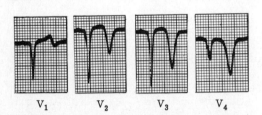

Anteroseptal Infarction (see p. 168)

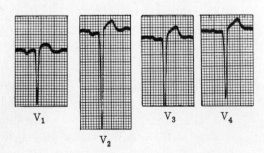

Left Ventricular Hypertrophy (see pp. 190, 191)

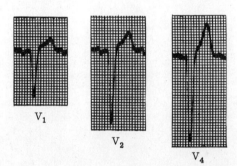

Left Bundle Branch Block (see pp. 131-8)

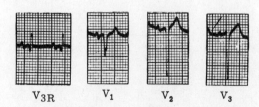

Right Ventricular Hypertrophy (see pp. 111, 191, 192)

QS COMPLEX ABNORMALITIES

(1) QS complex in leads V_{1-2}, V_{1-3}, or V_{1-4}.

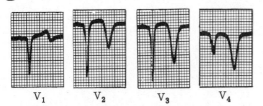

V_1　　V_2　　V_3　　V_4

Anteroseptal Infarction (see p. 167)

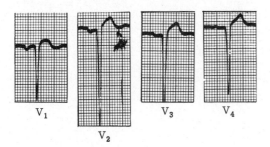

V_1　　V_2　　V_3　　V_4

Left Ventricular Hypertrophy (see pp. 190, 191)

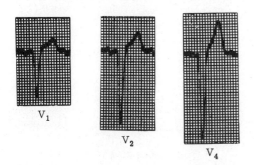

V_1　　V_2　　V_4

Left Bundle Branch Block (see p. 132)

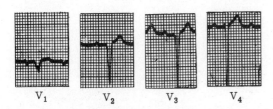

V_1　　V_2　　V_3　　V_4

Right Ventricular Hypertrophy (see pp. 191, 193)

(2) QS complex in leads I and $V_{1-3(4)}$.

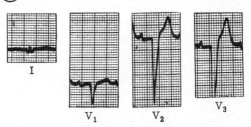

I　　V_1　　V_2　　V_3

Anterior Infarction (see pp. 159-71)

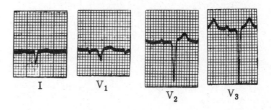

I　　V_1　　V_2　　V_3

Emphysema; Right Ventricular Hypertrophy (see pp. 191, 192)

(3) QS complex in leads II, III, and aVF.

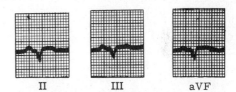

II　　III　　aVF

Inferior Infarction (see pp. 174-7)

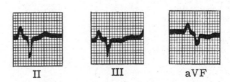

II　　III　　aVF

Emphysema or Right Ventricular Hypertrophy (see p. 191)

ABNORMALITIES OF R WAVE MAGNITUDE

(1) R wave > 13 mm. in aVL, or > 27 mm. in V_5 or V_6, or > 35 mm. in V_5 (or V_6) plus S in V_1.

aVL

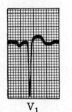 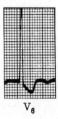

V_1 V_5 V_6

Left Ventricular Hypertrophy (with exceptions) (see p. 98)

(2) R wave > S in V_1.

V_1

Right Ventricular Hypertrophy (especially if right axis deviation is present) (see p. 108)

V_1

Posterior Infarction (see pp. 179-80)

(3) R wave > S in V_1 or V_2.

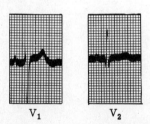

V_1 V_2

Dextroversion (see p. 83)

S WAVE ABNORMALITIES
(See QRS Complex, QS Complex, and R Wave.)

ST SEGMENT ABNORMALITIES

① **Elevation of ST Segment.** (Elevation of ST segment 1 mm. or more.)

(1) Elevation of ST segment in all leads except aVR and V_1, and in aVL in a vertical heart.

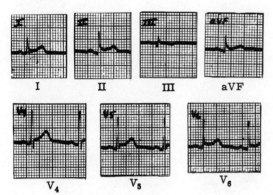

Pericarditis (see pp. 267-9)

② Elevation of ST segment in II, III, and aVF.

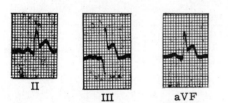

Inferior Infarction (see p. 176)

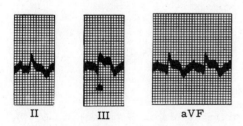

Ventricular Aneurysm (see p. 189)

③ Elevation of ST segment in I, aVL, and V_{4-6}.*

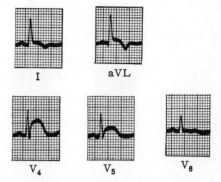

Anterior Infarction (see pp. 159-71)

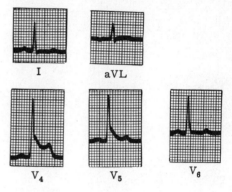

Angina (see pp. 144, 364 at bottom)

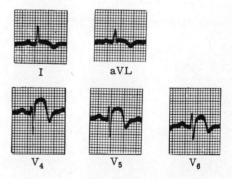

Ventricular Aneurysm (see p. 189)

*May be a normal variant (see pp. 86-7).

II. Depression of ST Segment.*

(1) Oblique or horizontal depression of ST in any lead except aVR and aVL with vertical heart.

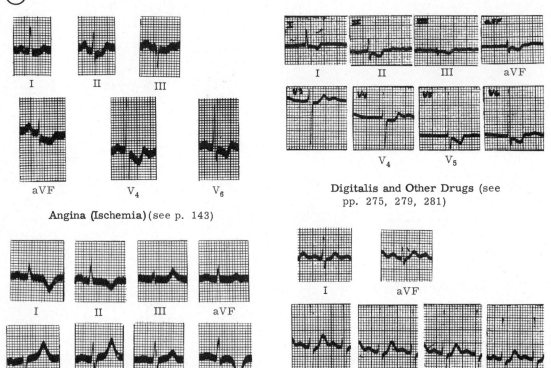

I   II   III

aVF   V₄   V₆

Angina (Ischemia) (see p. 143)

I   II   III   aVF

V₁   V₃   V₄   V₆

Subendocardial Infarction (see p. 182)

I   II   III   aVF

V₄   V₅

Digitalis and Other Drugs (see pp. 275, 279, 281)

I   aVF

V₃   V₄   V₅   V₆

Anxiety or Tobacco (see pp. 88, 282)

(2) Oblique or horizontal depression of ST segment in leads V_1, V_2, and V_3.

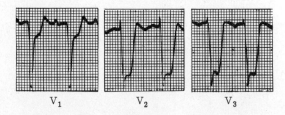

V₁   V₂   V₃

Ischemia (see p. 143)

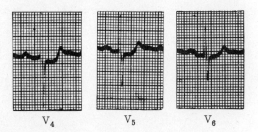

V₄   V₅   V₆

Right Ventricular Hypertrophy (see pp. 108-17)

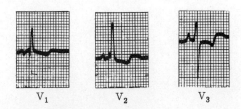

V₁   V₂   V₃

Right Bundle Branch Block (see pp. 121-30) (But need other [QRS and T] criteria for diagnosis.)

---

*0.5 mm. or more: in any lead except aVR and aVL with vertical heart. An associated QRS complex or T wave abnormality is usually required before a definitive electrocardiographic diagnosis is justified. "Scooped" depression of the ST segment in any lead except aVR and aVL with vertical heart favors a diagnosis of digitalis effect (see p. 275).

II. Depression of ST Segment (Cont'd.).

(3) Oblique or horizontal depression of ST segment in leads I, aVL, and V_{4-6}.

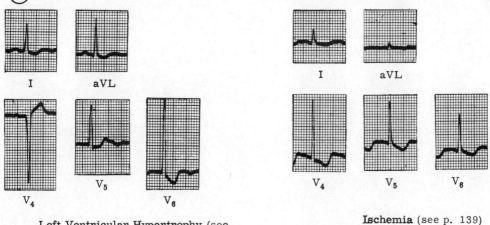

I   aVL

V_4 V_5 V_6

Left Ventricular Hypertrophy (see pp. 98-107)

I   aVL

V_4 V_5 V_6

Ischemia (see p. 139)

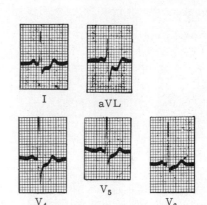

I   aVL

V_4 V_5 V_6

Left Bundle Branch Block (see pp. 131-8)
(But need other [QRS and T] criteria for diagnosis.)

Reciprocal of ST Elevation With Inferior Infarction (see p. 176)

(4) Oblique or horizontal depression of ST segment in leads II, III, and aVF.

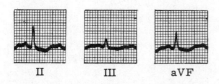

II   III   aVF

Ischemia (see p. 139)

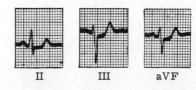

II   III   aVF

Reciprocal of ST Elevation With Anterior Infarction (see p. 163)

T WAVE ABNORMALITIES

I. Deep Inversion of T Wave.

(1) Symmetrical in any lead except aVR and aVL in vertical heart.

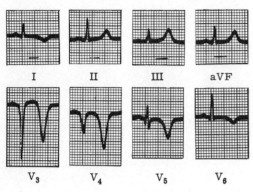

Infarction (see p. 157

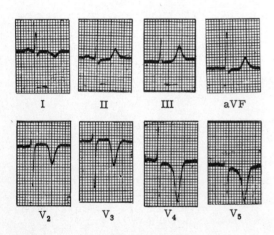

Ischemia (see p. 148)

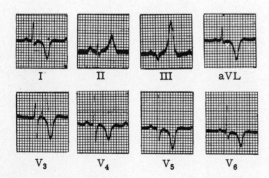

Perimyocarditis (see p. 269)

(2) Symmetrical inversion of T waves in leads I, aVL, and V_{4-6}.

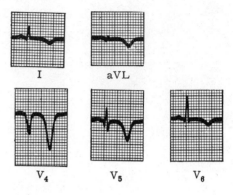

Anterior Infarction (see pp. 159-66)

(3) Symmetrical in leads II, III, and aVF.

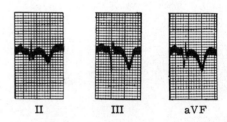

Inferior Infarction. (Diagnosis more certain if associated with abnormal Q waves; see pp. 173-7.)

II. T Wave Flat to Inverted.

(1) Asymmetrical in any lead except aVR and aVL in vertical heart. Usually not diagnostic unless associated with QRS-ST abnormalities. Possibilities same as for ST depression.

III. Upright T Wave.

(1) Tall, peaked, and slender upright T waves in all leads except aVR and aVL in vertical heart.

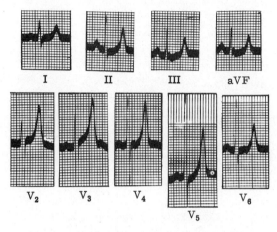

Hyperkalemia (see pp. 283-4)

(2) Tall, symmetrical T waves in leads V_{1-4}.

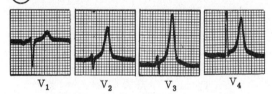

Posterior Infarction (see pp. 173, 179)

U WAVE ABNORMALITIES

Upright U Wave, Taller Than T in Same Lead, Especially in V_{2-4}.

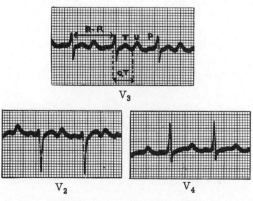

Hypokalemia (see p. 286)

ABNORMAL INTERVALS*

I. P-R Interval, > 0.21 Sec. in Any Lead.

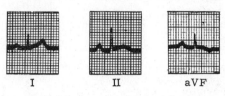

1st Degree A-V Block (see pp. 220-2)

II. Prolonged S-T Interval in Any Lead.

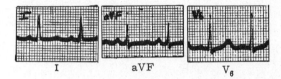

Hypocalcemia (see p. 289)
(Also seen in liver disease.)

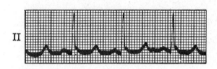

Refrigeration (see p. 274)

III. Q-T_C Interval, > 0.42-0.43 Sec. in Any Lead.

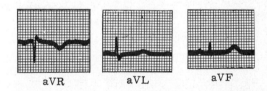

Multiple Causes. Any type of myocardial disease, quinidine effect or toxicity, hypocalcemia, refrigeration (see pp. 271, 274, 279, 280).

---

*QRS Interval: See QRS Complex.

ARRHYTHMIAS

I. Sinus Arrhythmias.

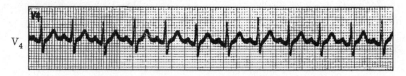

Sinus Tachycardia; Rate 100-160 (see p. 200)

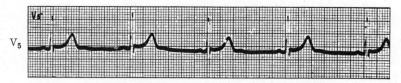

Sinus Bradycardia; Rate < 60 (see p. 201)

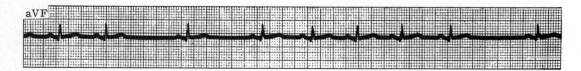

Sinus Arrhythmia (see p. 201)

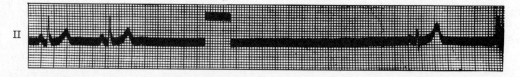

Sinus Arrest (see p. 202)

II. Atrial Arrhythmias.

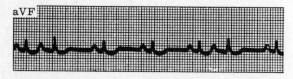

Premature Beats (see pp. 203, 204, 205)

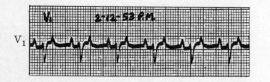

Tachycardia With A-V Block (see pp. 276, 278, 279)

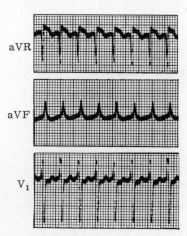

Tachycardia With 1:1 A-V Conduction (see pp. 276, 278, 279)

II. Atrial Arrhythmias. (Cont'd.)

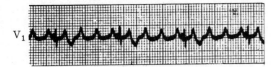

Atrial Flutter (see pp. 211-4)

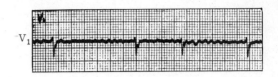

Atrial Fibrillation (see pp. 215-8)

III. A-V Nodal Arrhythmias.

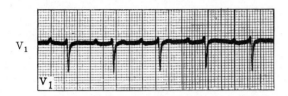

First Degree A-V Block (see pp. 221-2)

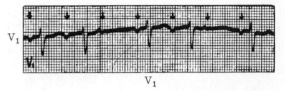

Second Degree A-V Block, Wenckebach Type (see p. 224)

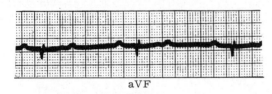

Second Degree A-V Block, Constant (see pp. 222, 223)

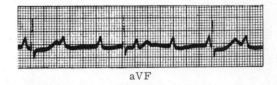

Third Degree A-V Block (see pp. 225-7)

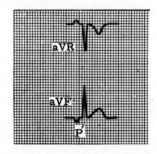

High A-V nodal focus. Note upright P′ in aVR and inverted P′ in aVF preceding the QRS complex.

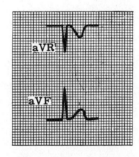

Mid A-V nodal focus. P′ buried in QRS complex.

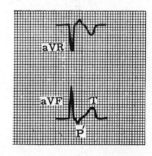

Low A-V nodal focus. Note upright P′ in aVR and inverted P′ in aVF following the QRS complex.

Premature Beats (see pp. 228-31)

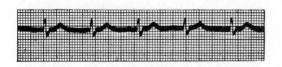

A-V Nodal Rhythm (see p. 233)

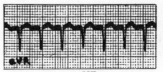

Nodal Tachycardia (see p. 234)

IV. Ventricular Arrhythmias.

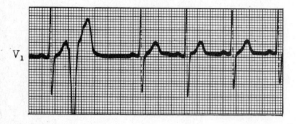

Premature Beats (see pp. 236-42)

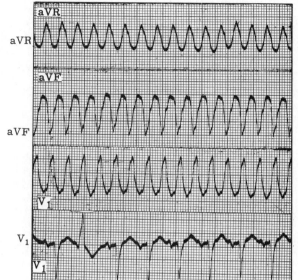

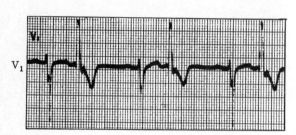

Bigeminy

Tachycardia (see pp. 245-9)

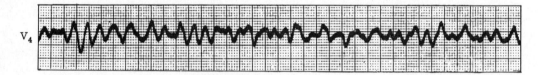

Fibrillation (see pp. 250-2)

V. Pararrhythmias.

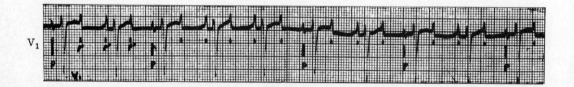

Parasystole (see pp. 253-5)

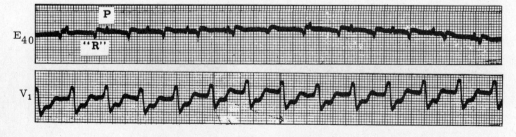

A-V Dissociation (see pp. 255-7)

VI. Accelerated Conduction..

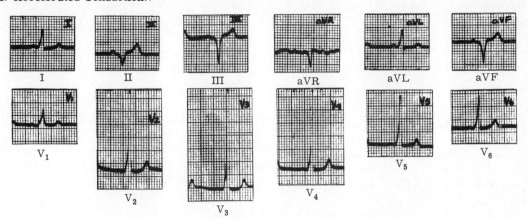

Wolff-Parkinson-White Syndrome (see p. 260)

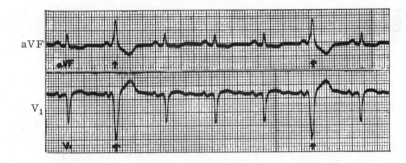

Isolated Accelerated Conduction Beats (see p. 264)

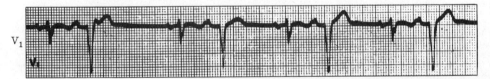

Aberrant Intraventricular Conduction With Atrial Premature Beats (see p. 265)

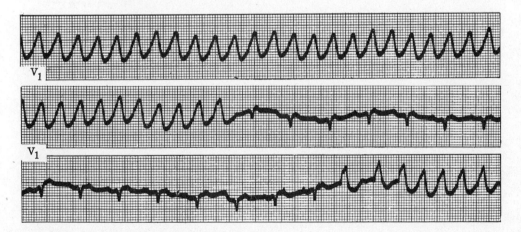

Aberrant Intraventricular Conduction With Atrial Tachycardia (see pp. 266, 363)

REFERENCES

BOOKS

Burch, G. E. , Abildskov, J. A. , and Cronvich, J. A.: Spatial Vectorcardiography. Lea & Febiger, 1953.

Cassels, D. E. , and Ziegler, R. F.: Electrocardiography in Infants and Children. Grune & Stratton, 1966.

Grant, R. P.: Clinical Electrocardiography. McGraw-Hill, 1957.

Grishman, A. , and Scherlis, L.: Spatial Vectorcardiography. Saunders, 1952.

Hoffman, B. F. , and Cranefield, P. F.: Electrophysiology of the Heart. Blakiston-McGraw, 1960.

Katz, L. N. , and Pick, A.: Clinical Electrocardiography. Part I. The Arrhythmias. Lea & Febiger, 1956.

Kossmann, C. E.: Advances in Electrocardiography. Grune & Stratton, 1958.

Lepeschkin, E.: Modern Electrocardiography, Vol. I. Williams & Wilkins, 1951.

Massie, E. , and Walsh, T. J.: Clinical Vectorcardiography and Electrocardiography. Year Book, 1960.

Prinzmetal, M. , Corday, E. , Brill, I. C. , Oblath, R. W. , and Kruger, H. E.: The Auricular Arrhythmias. Thomas, 1952.

Scherf, D. , and Schott, A.: Extrasystoles and Allied Arrhythmias. Heinemann, 1953. (Distributed in U. S. A. by Grune & Stratton.)

Simonson, E.: Differentiation Between Normal and Abnormal in Electrocardiography. Mosby, 1961.

Sodi-Pallares, D. , and Calder, R. M.: New Bases of Electrocardiography. Mosby, 1956.

Uhley, H. N.: Vector Electrocardiography. Lippincott, 1962.

ARTICLES

The Normal Electrocardiogram

Blackburn, H. W. , Jr. , and Simonson, E.: The total QRS duration. Am. Heart J. 53:699, 1957.

Brody, J. I. , Golden, L. H. , and Tobin, J. L.: A review of 3,369 electrocardiograms in young male hospitalized patients. Am. Heart J. 53:821, 1957.

Buxton, T. M. , Hsu, I. , and Barter, R. H.: Fetal electrocardiography. J. A. M. A. 185:441, 1963.

Einthoven, W.: The telecardiogram. Translated by H. W. Blackburn, Jr. Am. Heart J. 53: 602, 1957.

Einthoven, W. , Fahr, G. , and de Waart, A.: On the direction and manifest size of the variations of potential in the human heart and on the influence of the position of the heart on the form of the electrocardiogram. Translated by H. E. Hoff and P. Sekeli. Am. Heart J. 40: 163, 1950.

Gardberg, M. , and Rosen, I. L.: The effects of nonpathologic factors on the electrocardiogram. Am. Heart J. 53:494 and 711, 1957.

James, T. H.: The connecting pathways between the sinus node and A-V node and between the right and left atrium in the human heart. Am. Heart J. 66:498, 1963.

Johnston, F. D.: Reflection on electrocardiography. (Editorial.) Circulation 15:801, 1957.

Kennamer, R. , Bernstein, J. L. , Maxwell, M. H. , Prinzmetal, M. , and Shaw, C. M.: Studies on the mechanism of ventricular activity. V. Intramural depolarization potentials in the normal heart with a consideration of currents of injury in coronary heart disease. Am. Heart J. 46:379, 1953.

Kossman, C. E.: The normal electrocardiogram. Circulation 8:920, 1953.

Lamb, L. E.: The effects of respiration on the electrocardiogram in relation to differences in right and left ventricular stroke volume. Am. Heart J. 54:342, 1957.

Lepeschkin, E. L. , and Surawicz, B.: The measurement of the QT interval of the electrocardiogram. Circulation 6:378, 1952.

Prinzmetal, M. , et al.: Studies on the nature of the repolarization process. XIX. Studies on the mechanism of ventricular activity. Am. Heart J. 53:100, 1957.

Scher, A. M.: The sequence of ventricular excitation. Am. J. Cardiol. 14:294, 1964.

Symposium on cardiology in aviation. Electrocardiographic findings in 67,375 asymptomatic subjects. Am. J. Cardiol. 6:76-200, 1960.

Symposium on the U wave of the electrocardiogram. Circulation 15:68, 1957.

Tranchesi, J., et al.: Atrial repolarization, its importance in clinical electrocardiography. Circulation 22:635, 1960.

Uhley, H. N., and Rivkin, L.: Peripheral distribution of the canine A-V conduction system. Observations on gross morphology. Am. J. Cardiol. 5:688, 1960.

Van Dam, R. T., and Durrer D.: The T wave and ventricular repolarization. Am. J. Cardiol. 14:294, 1964.

Wolferth, C. C.: Clinical electrocardiography: offspring of science or empiricism? Circulation 16:321, 1957.

Hypertrophy and Bundle Branch Block

Banta, H. D., Greenfield, J. C., Jr., and Estes, E. H., Jr.: Left axis deviation. Am. J. Cardiol. 14:330, 1964.

Braunwald, E., and Morrow, A. G.: Sequence of ventricular contraction in human bundle branch block. Am. J. Med. 23:205, 1957.

Dodge, H. T., and Grant, R. P.: Mechanisms of QRS complex prolongation in man. Right ventricular conduction defects. Am. J. Med. 21:534, 1956.

Eliot, R. S., Millhon, W. A., and Millhon, J.: The clinical significance of uncomplicated marked left axis deviation in men without known disease. Am. J. Cardiol. 12:767, 1963.

Grant, R. P., and Dodge, H. T.: Mechanisms of QRS complex prolongation in man. Left ventricular conduction disturbances. Am. J. Med. 20:834, 1956.

Kennamer, R., and Prinzmetal, M.: Studies on the mechanism of ventricular activity. X. Depolarization of the ventricle with bundle branch block. Am. Heart J. 47:769, 1954.

Milnor, W. R.: Electrocardiogram and vectorcardiogram in right ventricular hypertrophy and right bundle branch block. Circulation 16:348, 1957.

Pryor, R., and Blount, S. G., Jr.: The clinical significance of true left axis deviation. Am. Heart J. 72:391, 1966.

Scott, R. C.: The correlation between the electrocardiographic patterns of ventricular hypertrophy and the anatomic findings. Circulation 21:256, 1960.

Scott, R. C.: Left bundle branch block - a clinical assessment. Am. Heart J. 70:813, 1965.

Sokolow, M., and Lyon, T. P.: The ventricular complex in left ventricular hypertrophy as obtained by unipolar precordial and limb leads. Am. Heart J. 37:161, 1949.

Sokolow, M., and Lyon, T. P.: The ventricular complex in right ventricular hypertrophy as obtained by unipolar precordial and limb leads. Am. Heart J. 38:273, 1949.

Uhley, H. N., and Rivkin, L.: Electrocardiographic patterns following interruption of main and peripheral branches of the canine right bundle of His. Am. J. Cardiol. 7:810, 1961.

Uhley, H. N., and Rivkin, L.: Electrocardiographic patterns following interruption of the main and peripheral branches of the canine bundle of His. Am. J. Cardiol. 13:41, 1964.

Walker, I. C., Jr., Helm, R. A., and Scott, R. C.: Right ventricular hypertrophy. Circulation 11:215 and 223, 1955.

Myocardial Anoxia and Infarction

Bellet, S., Deliyiannis, S., and Eliakim, M.: The electrocardiogram during exercise as recorded by radioelectrocardiography. Am. J. Cardiol. 8:385, 1961; Circulation 25:5 and 686, 1962.

Georgopoulos, A. J., et al.: Effect of exercise on electrocardiograms of patients with low serum potassium. Circulation 23:567, 1961.

Grant, R. P.: Peri-infarction block. Prog. Cardiovas. Dis. 2:237, 1959.

Lepeschkin, E.: Exercise tests in the diagnosis of coronary artery disease. Circulation 22:986, 1960.

Massumi, R. A., Goldman, A., Rakita, L., Kuramoto, K., and Prinzmetal, M.: Studies on the mechanism of ventricular activity. XVI. Activation of the human ventricle. Am. J. Med. 19:832, 1955.

Myers, G. B., Klein, H. A., and Hiratzka, T.: Correlation of electrocardiographic and pathologic findings in anteroposterior infarction. Am. Heart J. 37:205, 1949.

Myers, G. B., Klein, H. A., and Hiratzka, T.: Correlation of electrocardiographic and pathologic findings in large anterolateral infarcts. Am. Heart J. 36:838, 1948.

Myers, G. B., Klein, H. A., and Hiratzka, T.: Correlation of electrocardiographic and pathologic findings in posterior infarction. Am. Heart J. 38:547, 1949.

Myers, G. B., Klein, H. A., and Hiratzka, T.: Correlation of electrocardiographic and pathologic findings in posterolateral infarction. Am. Heart J. 38:837, 1949.

Myers, G. B., Klein, H. A., and Stofer, B. E.: Correlation of electrocardiographic and pathologic findings in anteroseptal infarction. Am. Heart J. **36**:535, 1948.

Myers, G. B., Klein, H. A., and Stofer, B. E.: Correlation of electrocardiographic and pathologic findings in lateral infarction. Am. Heart J. **37**:374, 1949.

Pearce, M. L., and Chapman, M. G.: The evaluation of Q aVF by the initial sagittal QRS vectors in 70 autopsied cases. Am. Heart J. **53**:782, 1957.

Prinzmetal, M., et al.: Studies on the mechanism of ventricular activity. VI. The depolarization complex in pure subendocardial infarction; role of the subendocardial region in the normal electrocardiogram. Am. J. Med. **16**:469, 490, 1954.

Prinzmetal, M., et al.: A variant of angina pectoris. Am. J. Med. **27**:375, 1959.

Prinzmetal, M., et al.: Angina pectoris. Clinical and experimental difference between ischemia with ST elevation and ischemia with ST depression. Am. J. Cardiol. **7**:412, 1961.

Pruitt, R. D., Dennis, E. W., and Kinard, S. A.: The difficult ECG diagnosis of myocardial infarction. Progr. Cardiovas. Dis. **6**:85, 1963.

Simonson, E.: Use of the ECG in exercise tests. Am. Heart J. **66**:552, 1963.

Sodi-Pallares, D., et al.: Unipolar QS morphology and Purkinje potential of the free left ventricular wall. Circulation **23**:863, 1961.

Arrhythmias

Chardack, W. M.: Heart block treated with implantable pacemaker. Progr. Cardiovas. Dis. **6**:507, 1964.

Culler, M. R., Boone, J. A., and Gazes, R. C.: Fibrillatory wave size as a clue to etiological diagnosis. Am. Heart J. **66**:435, 1963.

Fox, T. T.: Further remarks on the syndrome of aberrant A-V conduction (Wolff-Parkinson-White). Am. Heart J. **53**:771, 1957.

Kleiger, R., and Lown, B.: Cardioversion and digitalis. Circulation **33**:878, 1966.

Lown, B., Amarasingham, R., and Newman, J.: New method for terminating cardiac arrhythmias. Use of synchronized capacitor discharge. J. A. M. A. **182**:548, 1962.

Lown, B., and Levine, S.: The carotid sinus. Circulation **23**:766, 1961.

Marriott, H. J. L.: Interactions between atria and ventricles during interference dissociation and complete A-V block. Am. Heart J. **53**:884, 1957.

Miller, R., and Sharrett, R. H.: Interference dissociation. Circulation **16**:803, 1957.

Nathan, D. A., Samet, P., Center, S., and Wu, C. Y.: Long-term correction of complete heart block. Clinical and physiologic studies of a new type of implantable synchronous pacer. Progr. Cardiovas. Dis. **6**:538, 1966.

Pick, A., and Dominguez, P.: Nonparoxysmal A-V nodal tachycardia. Circulation **16**:1022, 1957.

Pick, A., Langendorf, R., and Katz, L. N.: Advances in the electrocardiographic diagnosis of cardiac arrhythmias. M. Clin. North America **41**:269, 1957.

Pick, A.: A-V dissociation. Am. Heart J. **66**:147, 1963.

Rosenbaum, M. B., and Lepeschkin, E. L.: The effect of ventricular systole on auricular rhythm in auriculoventricular block. Circulation **11**:240, 1955.

Runge, T. M., Oates, J. R., Herrmann, G. R., and Hejtmancik, M. R.: Extremely rapid arrhythmias and regular tachycardias in paroxysms in patients with and without accelerated A-V conduction. Am. J. M. Sc. **234**:170, 1957.

Scherf, D.: The atrial arrhythmias. New England J. Med. **252**:928, 1955.

Drugs, Electrolytes, Miscellaneous

Bellet, S.: The electrocardiogram in electrolyte imbalance. Arch. Int. Med. **96**:618, 1955.

Cropp, G. J., and Manning, G. W.: Electrocardiographic changes simulating myocardial ischemia and infarction associated with spontaneous intracerebral hemorrhage. Circulation **22**:25, 1960.

Mullican, W. S., and Fisch, C.: Postextrasystolic alternans of the U waves due to hypokalemia. Am. Heart J. **68**:383, 1964.

Pick, A.: Digitalis and the electrocardiogram. Circulation **15**:603, 1957.

Surawicz, B., Braun, H. A., Crum, W. B., Kemp, R. L., Wagner, S., and Bellet, S.: Quantitative analysis of the electrocardiographic pattern of hypopotassemia. Circulation **16**:750, 1957.

Villamil, A., et al.: Electrocardiographic changes in artificial hibernation. Am. Heart J. **53**:365, 1957.

Spatial Vectorcardiography

Brinberg, L.: The ventricular gradient in space. Am. J. Med. **23**:212, 1957.

Cosma, J., Levy, B., and Pipberger, H. V.: The spatial ventricular gradient during alterations in the ventricular activation pathway. Am. Heart J. **71**:84, 1966.

Draper, H. W., Peffer, C., Stallman, F. W., Littman, D., and Pipberger, H. V.: The corrected orthogonal electrocardiogram and vectorcardiogram in 510 normal men. Circulation **30**:853, 1964.

Frank, E.: An accurate, clinically practical system for spatial vectorcardiography. Circulation **13**:737, 1956.

Frank, E.: General theory of heart vector projection. Circulation Res. **2**:258, 1954.

Frank, E.: The image surface of a homogeneous torso. Am. Heart J. **47**:757, 1954.

Goldman, M. J., and Ferrari, L.: A simplified, inexpensive, bedside technique for recording corrected orthogonal scalar electrocardiograms. Am. J. M. Sc. **246**:212, 1963.

Helm, R. A.: An accurate lead system for spatial vectorcardiography. Am. Heart J. **53**:415, 1957.

Helm, R. A.: Vectorcardiographic notation. Circulation **13**:581, 1956.

Johnston, F. D.: The clinical value of vectorcardiography. Circulation **23**:297, 1961.

Kornbluth, A. W., and Allenstein, B. J.: The normal direct spatial vectorcardiogram. Am. Heart J. **54**:396, 1957.

Milnor, W. R., Talbot, S. A., and Newman, E. V.: A study of relationship between unipolar leads and spatial vectorcardiograms, using the panoramic vectorcardiograph. Circulation **7**:545, 1953.

Pipberger, H. V.: The normal orthogonal electrocardiogram and vectorcardiogram. Circulation **17**:1102, 1958.

Pipberger, H. V.: Current status and persistent problems of electrode placement and lead systems for vectorcardiography and electrocardiography. Progr. Cardiovas. Dis. **2**:248, 1959.

Pipberger, H. V.: Correlation and clinical information in the standard 12 lead ECG and in a corrected orthogonal 3 lead VCG. Am. Heart J. **61**:35, 1961.

Schmitt, O. H., and Simonson, E.: The present status of vectorcardiography. Arch. Int. Med. **96**:575, 1955.

Simonson, E., Tuna, N., Okamoto, N., and Toshima, H.: Diagnostic accuracy of the vectorcardiogram and electrocardiogram. Am. J. Cardiol. **17**:829, 1966.

Index

-A-

Abnormalities of Ecg. , 369
Accelerated conduction, 258-266
  beats, isolated, 264
Action potential, 18
Activation, atrial, normal, 41
  ventricular, normal, 42
Alternating current interference,
  16
Anemia, electrocardiographic
  voltage, 99
  myocardial anoxia, 139,
    148-149
Aneurysm, ventricular, 189
Angina pectoris, 139. See also
  Myocardial anoxia.
  electrocardiographic patterns,
    143-144
Anxiety state, 88
Aortic insufficiency, bundle branch
  block, 137
  electrocardiographic pattern,
    313
  ventricular hypertrophy,
    left, 98
  stenosis, myocardial anoxia,
    139
  ventricular hypertrophy,
    left, 98
Aortitis, myocardial anoxia, 139
Arrhythmia(s), 197-266
  atrial, 203-219
    bigeminy, 265
    carotid pressure, effect of,
      363
    digitalis, effect of, 198-199
      toxicity due to, 278-279
    ectopic beats, 203-205
    electrocardiographic
      patterns, 346
    fibrillation, 215-219
      electrocardiographic
        patterns, 356
      simulated by atrial
        flutter, 214
      simulating ventricular
        tachycardia, 248
      with ventricular premature
        beats, 241
    flutter, 211-215
      vs. atrial fibrillation, 217
      flutter-fibrillation, 217
    premature beats, 203-205
      aberrant intraventricular
        conduction, 265
      blocked, 205
      electrocardiographic
        patterns, 356, 358
    procainamide, effect of, 198
    quinidine, effect of, 198-199
    tachycardia, 207-209
      accelerated conduction,
        265

Arrhythmia(s), atrial,
  tachycardia, Cont'd.
    vs. atrial fibrillation, 217
    following atrial premature
      beats, 205
    electrocardiographic
      patterns, 359
    with Wolff-Parkinson-White
      syndrome, 258
  hypothermia, due to, 274
  myocardial anoxia, 139
  neuromuscular diseases, 273
  nodal, ectopic beats in sinus
    arrest, 202
  para-arrhythmias, 253-257
  sinus, 201
  supraventricular tachycardia,
    electrocardiographic pat-
      terns, 357, 360
    vs. ventricular tachycardia,
      249
  tobacco, due to, 282
  ventricular, 235-252
    digitalis toxicity, due to,
      276-278
    ectopic beats in sinus arrest,
      202
    fibrillation, 250
    hyperkalemia, 284
    intraventricular conduction
      defect, 235-236
    premature beats, due to
      digitalis toxicity, 276-
        278
    procainamide, effect of, 198
    quinidine toxicity, 279-280
    tachycardia, 245-250
      bidirectional, 247
      electrocardiographic
        patterns, 355, 363
      with Wolff-Parkinson-White
        syndrome, 258
Arteriosclerotic heart disease. See
  Coronary artery disease.
Atrial, arrhythmias, 203-219
  depolarization. See Depolari-
    zation, atrial.
  fibrillation. See Arrhythmias.
  flutter. See Arrhythmias.
  hypertrophy. See Hypertrophy,
    atrial.
  muscle, digitalis, effect of,
    198-199
  quinidine, effect of, 198-199
  vagal stimulation, effect of,
    211
  pathways, internodal, 39
  repolarization. See Repolari-
    zation, atrial.
  septal defect, 90
  standstill, 202
    hyperkalemia, due to, 284
  tachycardia, 207-209
Atrioventricular block, 220-227

Atrioventricular block, Cont'd.
  atrial flutter, 212-215
  complete. See Atrioventricu-
    lar block, third degree.
  digitalis toxicity, due to,
    276-279
  first degree, 222
    definition, 220
    electrocardiographic
      patterns, 356
    second degree A-V block,
      associated with, 222
  second degree, 222-224
    definition, 220
    electrocardiographic
      patterns, 359
  third degree, 225-227
    definition, 220
    electrocardiographic
      patterns, 358
  dissociation, 253, 255, 256
    with interference, 255
  node, 40-41
    accelerated conduction, 258-
      266
    blood supply, 158
    cardiac rhythm, 197-198
    "delay," normal, 54
    digitalis, effect of, 198-199
    myocardial infarction, caus-
      ing atrioventricular
        block, 220
    quinidine, effect of, 198-199
    sinus arrest, 202
    vagal stimulation, effect of,
      198
  premature beats, 228-231
  rhythm, 228-234. See also
    Arrhythmias, nodal.
    digitalis toxicity, due to, 277
    electrocardiographic pattern,
      357
    interference dissociation,
      253, 254-257
    electrocardiographic
      pattern, 360
  tachycardia, 234
Augmented extremity leads. See
  Leads, aVF, aVL, aVR.
Auricular. See Atrial.
Autonomic nervous system, anxiety
  state, 88
  cardiac rhythm, effect on, 198
A-V dissociation, 256
  node. See Atrioventricular node.
Axis deviation, definition of, left,
  36, 98
  normal, 36
  right, 36
  left, 98
  right, 108
  frontal plane, 35

-B-

"Back of the heart" complex, 51
Beri-beri heart disease, 271
   ventricular hypertrophy, left,
      98
Bibliography, 366-368
Bigeminal rhythm. See Rhythm,
   bigeminal.
Bigeminy, digitalis toxicity, due
   to, 276
   ventricular, electrocardio-
      graphic pattern, 358
Bipolar leads. See Leads, bipolar.
   precordial compared to unipolar
      precordial leads, 89
Block, anterolateral parietal,
   291-292
   intraventricular, left, 291-292
   peri-infarction, 293-295
Bradycardia, digitalis toxicity,
   due to, 276
   hypothermia, due to, 274
   myxedema, 272
   sinus, definition of, 201
   and sinus arrhythmia, 201
Bronchiectasis, right ventricular
   hypertrophy, 108
Bundle branch block, 120-137
   complete and incomplete,
      definition of, 120
   left, 131-138
      electrocardiographic
         patterns, 315, 332,
         340
      horizontal heart, 132, 134
      incomplete, 136-137
      intermittent, 136
      vs. left ventricular hyper-
         trophy, 137
      minimal criteria, 138
      myocardial infarction, ven-
         tricular premature
         beats, 244
      normal individuals, 131,
         132
      relation to left intraven-
         tricular block, 291
      respiration, effect of, 136
      summary of electrocardio-
         graphic criteria, 138
      transient, 132
      vectorcardiogram, 314-315
      vertical heart, 135
   myocardial infarction, 194-
      195
   right, electrocardiographic
      patterns, 319, 320, 344,
      353, 360
      horizontal heart, 125
      incomplete, 127
      vs. anterolateral peri-
         infarction block,
         293
      electrocardiographic
         patterns, 339,
         347, 359
      normal individuals, 128
      intermittent, 129
      with left ventricular hyper-
         trophy, 126
      electrocardiographic
         pattern, 336
      minimal criteria, 130

Bundle branch block, right, Cont'd.
   nodal rhythm, 233
   normal individuals, 121
   vs. right ventricular hyper-
      trophy, vectorcardio-
      gram, 320
   summary of electrocar-
      diographic criteria,
      130
   vectorcardiogram, 318-
      319
   ventricular strain, 116
   vertical heart, 122-124
   with ventricular premature
      beats, 241
   branches, 40-41
   of His, 40-41

-C-

Calcium, electrocardiogram,
   effect on, 289
Cardiac pacemaker, 197
   rhythm, 197-266
      drugs, effect of, 198-199
      normal physiology of, 197-
      198
   vector. See Vector.
Cardioscope, 2
Carotid sinus pressure, 210, 217
   atrial arrhythmias in, 211-214
   nodal rhythm, caused by, 233
   sinus arrest, caused by, 202
   ventricular tachycardia in, 248
Cavity complex, 49, 50
Cell to cell conduction, 19
Cerebral disease, 282
CF. See Leads.
Children, Ecg.'s in, 81-82
"Circus" movement in atrium, 211
Coarctation of the aorta, left
   ventricular hypertrophy, 98
Coffee, atrial premature beats,
   caused by, 205
Combined right and left ventricular
   hypertrophy, 118, 119
Compensatory pause, 236, 240
Complexes. See specific complex.
Conduction, cell to cell, 19
   system, 39-42
Congestive heart failure. See
   Heart failure.
Coronary artery (arteries),
   anatomy, 158
   disease, 139-196
      atrial fibrillation, 215
      flutter, 211
      atrioventricular block,
         caused by, 220-221
      electrocardiographic
         pattern, right bundle
         branch block,
         124
      intraventricular conduction
         defect, caused by,
         235
      left bundle branch block,
         131
      intraventricular block,
         292
      nodal rhythm, caused
         by, 233
      ventricular hypertrophy,
         98

Coronary artery (arteries),
   disease, Cont'd.
      right bundle branch block,
         121
      tobacco, effect of, 282
      ventricular premature
         beats, 236
      tachycardia, 245
      right, occlusion causing atrio-
         ventricular block, 220
   circulation. See Coronary
      arteries.
   insufficiency. See Myocardial
      anoxia.
   occlusion, myocardial infarc-
      tion, 151
   "sinus" rhythm, 233
Cor pulmonale. See Ventricular
   hypertrophy, right.
   acute. See Strain, ventricular,
      right.
   electrocardiographic patterns,
      320, 333, 337
      right ventricular hypertrophy,
         111
   myocardial anoxia, 139
   ventricular hypertrophy, right,
      108
Cortisone in treatment of pericarditis, 270
Countershock, electrical, 299
"Cove-plane" T. See T wave,
   cove-plane.
Current of injury, 140-141

-D-

Delta wave, 259
Depolarization, 17-18, 23
   atrial, 25
      vectorcardiogram, P loop,
         305-306
   electrical, of the heart, 296
   muscle strip, 18-19, 23-24
   ventricular, 25
      vectorcardiogram, QRS
         loop, 305, 307-309
Dextrocardia, complete transposition, 84
   congenital rotation, 83
   electrocardiographic patterns,
      334, 361
   technical, 85
Diabetes mellitus, coronary artery
   disease, 139
Diagnosis of Ecg. abnormalities,
   369
Digitalis, 275-279
   atrial fibrillation, effect in, 218
   flutter, effect on, 211, 215
   premature beats caused by,
      205
   atrioventricular block, caused
      by, 220
   bigeminal rhythm, caused by,
      237
   bundle branch block, left, tran-
      sient, caused by, 132
   cardiac rhythm, effect on,
      198-199
   effect, electrocardiographic
      pattern, 349
   intraventricular conduction
      defect, caused by, 236

Digitalis, Cont'd.
  nodal rhythm, caused by, 233
  sinus arrest, caused by, 202
  toxicity, 237, 276-279
  ventricular fibrillation, caused
    by, 250
    premature beats, caused by,
      236-237
    tachycardia, caused by, 245
Diphtheria, atrioventricular block
  caused by, 220-221

-E-

Ectopic beats. See Arrhythmias.
Effusion, pericardial, 267
Einthoven, equation, 3, 6
  triangle, 31-32
    relation to frontal plane
      vector, 31-32
Eisenmenger's complex, electro-
    cardiographic pattern, 361
  syndrome, right ventricular
    hypertrophy, 108
Electrical alternans, 290
  countershock, 299
  depolarization of the heart, 296
  pacing of the heart, 296
Electric shock, ventricular
  fibrillation, caused by, 250
Electrocardiogram, method of
    interpretation, 328-329
  normal, 25-30, 45-61
    "back-of-the-heart" com-
      plexes, 51
    backward rotation of heart,
      79
    children, 82
    clockwise rotation of heart,
      76
    counterclockwise rotation of
      heart, 77
    diagrammatic, 30
    forward rotation of heart, 78
    horizontal heart position,
      67-68
    infants, 81
    intermediate heart position,
      69-70
    left ventricular cavity
      complex, 49
      epicardial complex, 45-46
    relation to cardiac contrac-
      tion, 42
    respiration effect, 80
    right ventricular cavity
      complex, 50
      epicardial complex, 45,
        47
    semi-horizontal heart
      position, 73-74
    semi-vertical heart position,
      71-72
    simulating hyperkalemia
      pattern, 283
    transitional zone ventricular
      epicardial complex, 48
    vertical heart position, 65-66
  standardization, 16
  technical difficulties, 16
  voltage, 25
    measurements, 29
Electrocardiographic paper, 25
Electrocardiograph, types, 2

Electrocardiography, relation to
    vectorcardiography, 301
Electrode(s), 2
  Frank system of vectorcardi-
    ography, 303
  indifferent, 5
Electrogram, 21
Electrolyte disturbances, electro-
    cardiographic effects, 283-
    289
Electrophysiology of the heart, 17
Embolism, in atrial fibrillation,
    218
Emetine, effect of, 281
Emphysema, pulmonary, left
    intraventricular block, 292
  right ventricular hypertrophy,
    108
Epicardial complexes, 45, 48
Ergotamine, effect on electro-
    cardiogram in anxiety state,
    88
Esophageal leads. See Leads,
    esophageal.
Essential hypertension. See Hyper-
    tensive cardiovascular
    disease.
Excitation potential, 19
Exercise tests, 145-146

-F-

Fetal electrocardiography, 81
Fever, electrocardiographic,
    voltage, 99
Fibrillation. See Arrhythmias.
Flutter. See Arrhythmias.
Frank system of vectorcardiog-
    raphy, 302-303
Friedreich's ataxia, 273

-G-

Galvanometer, string, 2
Ground, 2

-H-

Heart block. See Atrioventricular
    block.
  digitalis toxicity, due to, 277
  failure, atrial tachycardia, due
    to, 210
    bigeminal rhythm, caused by,
      237
    high-output, electrocardio-
      graphic voltage, 99
    transient left bundle branch
      block, 132
    ventricular premature con-
      tractions, caused by,
      237
  position(s), 63-80
    backward rotation, 64, 79
    clockwise rotation, 64, 76
      ventricular strain, right,
        113
    counterclockwise rotation,
      64, 77
    forward rotation, 64, 78
    horizontal, 67-68
    intermediate, 69-70
    left, bundle branch block,
      132-135

Heart position(s), left, Cont'd.
    ventricular hypertrophy
      patterns, 98-105
    right, bundle branch block,
      122-125
    semi-horizontal, 73-74
    semi-vertical, 71-72
    vertical, 65-66
  rate, 26
    atrial fibrillation, 215-216
      flutter, 211
      tachycardia, 207
    atrioventricular rhythm, 233
    heart cycle length, 26
    nodal tachycardia, 234
    regular sinus rhythm, 200
    ventricular tachycardia, 245
Hemorrhage, myocardial anoxia,
    148-149
Hexaxial reference system, 33
Hormonal hypertension. See
    Hypertensive cardiovascular
    disease.
Hypercalcemia, effect on electro-
    cardiogram, 289
Hyperkalemia, 283-284
  electrocardiographic pattern,
    351
  hypocalcemia, associated with,
    289
Hypertension (systemic). See
    Hypertensive cardiovascular
    disease.
Hypertensive cardiovascular dis-
    ease, electrocardiographic
    pattern, backward
      rotation, 105
  bundle branch block, left,
    incomplete, 137
  clockwise rotation, 103
  counterclockwise rotation,
    104
  horizontal heart, 100-101
  left, bundle branch block,
    134-135
    ventricular hypertrophy,
      right bundle branch
        block, 126
  vertical heart, 102
  left atrial hypertrophy, 90
    ventricular hypertrophy, 98
      electrocardiographic pat-
        terns, 330, 332, 348,
          352, 355
  right bundle branch block, 121
    ventricular tachycardia, 245
Hyperthyroidism. See Thyrotoxi-
    cosis.
Hypertrophy, 90-119
  atrial, 90-94
    left, electrocardiogram, 92
      electrocardiographic pat-
        terns, 338, 343, 349
    right, electrocardiogram, 93
      electrocardiographic pat-
        terns, 333, 350
    P waves, 115-116
  ventricular, 95-119
    left, 98-105
      backward rotation of heart,
        105
      clockwise rotation of heart,
        103

Hypertrophy, ventricular, left,
  Cont'd.
    counterclockwise rotation
      of heart, 104
    electrocardiographic pat-
      terns, 313, 330, 332,
        335, 348, 352,
        355
    equivocal criteria, 107
    horizontal heart, 98-101
    left bundle branch block,
      131
    vs. left bundle branch
      block, 137
    and left intraventricular
      block, 292
    minimal criteria, 107
    myocardial anoxia, 139
    with right bundle branch
      block, 126
    electrocardiographic
      pattern, 336
    summary of electrocardio-
      graphic criteria, 107
    vectorcardiogram, 312-313
    vertical heart, 102
  right, 108-112
    vs. anterolateral peri-
      infarction block, 293
    electrocardiographic pat-
      terns, 317, 333, 338,
        343, 354, 361,
        362
    equivocal criteria, 117
    minimal criteria, 117
    normal infants, 81
    right bundle branch block,
      121
    vectorcardiogram, 320
    vs. right bundle branch
      block, 129
    simulated by myocardial
      infarction, 180
    simulating myocardial
      infarction, 192
    summary of electrocardio-
      graphic criteria, 117
    vectorcardiogram, 316-317
Hypocalcemia, 289
Hypokalemia, 286
  electrocardiographic patterns,
    345, 362
Hypothermia, electrocardiographic
  effect, 274
Hypoxia, ventricular fibrillation,
  caused by, 250

-I-

Idioventricular rhythm, 225-227
Indifferent electrode. See Elec-
  trode, indifferent.
Infant patterns, 81
Infarction, myocardial. See
  Myocardial infarction.
Injury current, 140-141
Interference dissociation, 253, 257
Internodal atrial pathways, 39
Interpolated beat, 240
Interpretation of Ecg., 369
Intrinsic deflect, 22, 28. See also
  Ventricular activation time.
  muscle strip, 20
Irritability. See Myocardial
  irritability.

-J-

J (RS-T junction), 28
Juvenile pattern, 81-82

-K-

Kirchoff's law, 3

-L-

Lead(s), I, II, III. See Leads,
  standard.
  aVF, 6, 8, 9, 14-15
    normal electrocardiogram,
      52
    position of heart, 75
    ventricular epicardial com-
      plex, left, 55
  aVL, 6, 8, 9, 14-15
    normal electrocardiogram,
      52
    position of heart, 75
    ventricular cavity, complex,
      left, 49
    potential, left, 55
  aVR, 6, 8, 9, 14-15
    normal electrocardiogram,
      52
    position of heart, 75
    ventricular cavity, complex,
      right, 50
    potential, right, 55
  bipolar, chest, 4
    standard, 2-3
  CF. See Leads, precordial,
    bipolar.
  E. See Leads, esophageal.
  esophageal, 4, 13
    anterior myocardial in-
      farction, 166
    atrial arrhythmias, 219
      premature beats, 203
    nodal premature beats, 228
    P waves, normal, 44
    sagittal plane vector, re-
      lation to, 38
    supraventricular tachycardia,
      234
    ventricular tachycardia, 246-
      247
  extremity, 4, 6-9
    frontal plane vector, relation
      to, 33-36
    standard leads, relation to,
      14-15
  precordial, 4, 9-10
    bipolar vs. unipolar, 89
    horizontal plane vectors,
      relation to, 37
    normal electrocardiogram, 53
  standard, 2-3, 14-15
    frontal plane vector, relation
      to, 31-36
    normal electrocardiogram,
      52
    unipolar extremity leads,
      relation to, 14-15
  unipolar, 4, 6
  V. See Leads, precordial.
  VE, 13
  VF, 6, 9, 14
  VL, 6, 9, 14
  VR, 6, 9, 14
Left axis deviation, definition of, 36

-M-

Malignancy, metastatic to heart,
  274
Master's "two-step" test, 145
Membrane resting potential, 18
Mitral insufficiency, left ventricular hypertrophy, 98
  stenosis, cardiac hypertrophy,
    91
    electrocardiographic pat-
      terns, 275, 317, 338,
        343
    atrial flutter, 212
    ventricular hypertrophy,
      right, 110
  left atrial hypertrophy, 90
    electrocardiographic
      pattern, 92
    myocardial anoxia, 139
    right ventricular hypertrophy,
      108
  valvular disease, atrial fibrilla-
    tion, 215
    flutter, 211
MRP. See Membrane resting
  potential.
Muscular dystrophy, 273
Myocardial anoxia, 139-150
  vs. anxiety state, 88
  in atrial fibrillation, 217
    tachycardia, 207, 210
  bundle branch block, caused
    by, 195
  electrocardiographic patterns,
    143-144, 147
  exercise test, 349
  superimposed upon myo-
    cardial infarction, 196
  tobacco, due to, 282
  infarction, 151-196
    anterior, 159-171, 185
      bundle branch block, left,
        195
      right, 194
    electrocardiographic
      criteria, 171
      patterns, 323, 335, 344,
        347, 351, 360
    nodal rhythm, 233
    supraventricular tachy-
      cardia, 249
    vectorcardiogram, 322-
      323
  anteroapical, 167, 169
    electrocardiographic
      pattern, 343
  anterolateral, 167, 171
    electrocardiographic pat-
      tern, 339
    with peri-infarction block,
      293
  anteroseptal, 167-168
    electrocardiographic pat-
      tern, 334
  atrioventricular block,
    caused by, 220
  bundle branch block, 192
    with complete heart block,
      225
  diaphragmatic. See Myo-
    cardial infarction,
      inferior.
  endocardial, 154
  epicardial, 153

Myocardial infarction, Cont'd.
    focal intraventricular block,
        235-236
    inferior, 172-181, 186-188,
        189. See also Myocar-
        dial infarction,
                posterior.
        bundle branch block, left,
            195
            right, 194
        diaphragmatic peri-
            infarction block, 294
        electrocardiographic
            criteria, 181
            patterns, 325, 329, 340,
                352
        lateral, 180
            electrocardiographic
                pattern, 342
            vectorcardiogram, 324-
                325
            localization of, 158-196
    multiple, 185-188
        electrocardiographic pat-
            terns, 341, 348
        with peri-infarction block,
            295
    myocardial anoxia superim-
        posed, 196
    posterior; 172-181
        electrocardiographic pat-
            terns, 331, 333
        esophageal leads, 178
        "true," 178
    posterolateral, 325, 354
        vectorcardiogram, 326
    QS complex, 152
    simulated, 191
    ST segment, 156
    subendocardial electro-
        cardiographic patterns,
            337, 346
        infarction, 182-184
    transient left bundle branch
        block, 132
    transmural, 154-155
    T wave changes, 157
    ventricular aneurysm, 189
        fibrillation, 250
        premature beats, 237,
            244
        tachycardia, 245
    with Wolff-Parkinson-White
        syndrome, 263
        electrocardiographic
            pattern, 336
    irritability, effect of quinidine,
        198
Myocarditis, 169
    bundle branch block, left,
        transient, 132
    ventricular hypertrophy, 98
Myotonia atrophica, 273
Myxedema, 272
    coronary artery disease, 139

-N-

Negro, electrocardiographic
    patterns, 82, 86, 87
Neuromuscular diseases, 273
Nicotine. See Tobacco.
Nodal rhythm. See Atrioven-
    tricular rhythm.

Nodal, Cont'd.
    tachycardia, 234
Nonaugmented extremity leads.
    See Leads VF, VL, VR.

-O-

Orthogonal lead systems, 302

-P-

Pacemaker. See Cardiac pace-
    maker.
    in sinus arrest, 202
    wandering, 206
        with atrial tachycardia, 207
Pacing of the heart, electrical, 296
Pararrhythmias. See Arrhythmias.
Parasympathetic system, effect on
    cardiac rhythm, 198
Parasystole, 253-255
"Pardee T." See T wave, Pardee.
Paroxysmal tachycardia. See
    Arrhythmias.
Patent ductus arteriosus, ventricu-
    lar hypertrophy, left, 98
        right, 108
Pericardial effusion, 267
Pericarditis, 267-270
    electrocardiographic patterns,
        268-270, 345
Peri-infarction block, 293-295
    anterolateral, 293
    diaphragmatic, 294
    intraventricular block, left, 292
Physiological basis of electro-
    cardiography, 17-24
P-J interval, accelerated conduc-
    tion, 260, 262
P loop, vectorcardiogram, normal
    adult, 305-306
    mitrale, 92, 275, 349
Polycythemia, myocardial anoxia,
    139
Position of heart. See Heart
    positions.
Potassium, effect on electro-
    cardiogram, 283-288
Potential, electrical, normal
    muscle, 20-24
    in standard leads, 3
    intracellular, 17
    zero, 6
P-P interval, definition of, 27
Premature beats. See Arrhythmias.
    nodal, 228-231
    ventricular, 236-244
        indication of myocardial
            infarction, 244
P-R interval, accelerated con-
    duction, 260-266
    anxiety state, 88
    atrial premature beats, 203-204
    definition of, 27
    effect of emetine, 281
    first degree atrioventricular
        block, 220-222
    hypokalemia, 286
    myocarditis, 271
    myxedema, 272
    neuromuscular diseases, 273
    normal, 26, 27
    wandering pacemaker, 206
    Wenckebach phenomenon, 222,
        224

P-R interval, Cont'd.
    Wolff-Parkinson-White syn-
        drome, 260, 263
P'-R interval, atrial premature
        beats, 203-205
    tachycardia, 207
    wandering pacemaker, 206
Procainamide, cardiac rhythm,
        effect on, 198, 282
    electrocardiographic effects,
        282
P-R segment, definition of, 28
    normal, 54
Pt wave. See Ta wave.
Pulmonary hypertension, atrial
    hypertrophy, right, 90
        electrocardiographic
            pattern, 93
        cardiac hypertrophy, 91
        myocardial anoxia, 139
    infarction, bundle branch block,
        right, 116
    ventricular strain, right, 113
Pulmonic stenosis, ventricular
    hypertrophy, right, 108
Purkinje system, 40-41
P vector. See P loop.
    wave(s), atrial activation, 41
        depolarization, 25
        hypertrophy, left, 92
            right, 93, 115-116
        premature beats, 203-205
    complete atrioventricular
        dissociation, 256
    esophageal leads, 44, 178
    normal, 43-44, 45-62
        criteria, 91
        leads aVF, aVL, aVR, 54
        precordial leads, 54
        standard leads, 54
    parasystole, 254
    regular sinus rhythm, 200
    ventricular fibrillation, 250
        premature beats, 239
        tachycardia, 246
    wandering pacemaker, 206
P' wave(s), atrial flutter, 211-214
    premature beats, 203-205
    tachycardia, 207
    atrioventricular rhythm, 233
    interference dissociation, 257
    nodal premature beats, 228-231
        tachycardia, 234
    parasystole, 254
    reciprocal beats, 232
    ventricular premature beats,
        239
        tachycardia, 246
    wandering pacemaker, 206

-Q-

Qr complex, ventricular, cavity
        complex, right, 50
    epicardial complex, right, 45,
        47
QRS complex, atrial fibrillation,
        217
        flutter, 211
        premature beats, 203-205
        tachycardia, 207
    bundle branch block, 120
    complete heart block, 225-
        227

QRS complex, Cont'd.
  electrical alternans, 290
  hyperkalemia, 284
  left, bundle branch block,
      131-132
    intraventricular block, 291
    ventricular epicardial
        complex, 45-46
  myocardial infarction, 153-
      156
  myxedema, 272
  nodal premature beats, 228
  normal, leads aVF, aVL,
      aVR, 55-62
    precordial leads, 55-62
    standard leads, 55-62
  pericarditis, 267
  peri-infarction block, 293
  quinidine toxicity, 280
  reciprocal beats, 232
  ventricular activation, 42
    fibrillation, 250-252
    premature beats, 238-239,
        242
    tachycardia, 245-247
  Wolff-Parkinson-White syn-
      drome, 147, 260, 263
  interval, accelerated conduction,
      258-266
    bundle branch block, 120
    definition of, 28
    hyperkalemia, 284
    intraventricular block, left,
        291
      conduction defect, 235-236
    normal, 28, 54
    peri-infarction block, 293
    ventricular hypertrophy, 95-
        96
      left, 98
      right, 108
    premature beats, 238-239
    strain, left, 106
    Wolff-Parkinson-White syn-
        drome, 260, 263
  loop, vectorcardiogram, normal
      adult, 305, 307-309
  vector. See QRS loop.
    mean, 301
QS complex, myocardial infarction,
    152-156
  anterior, 159, 164, 171, 185-
      188
  anteroseptal, 168
  inferior, 181
  multiple infarcts, 185-188
  simulated by, 191
  ventricular cavity complex, left,
      49
    right, 50
    epicardial complex, right,
        45, 47
Q-T interval, definition of, 28
  digitalis effect, 275
  hypercalcemia, 289
  hypocalcemia, 289
  hypokalemia, 286
  hypothermia, 274
  myocarditis, 271
  normal, 28-29
  quinidine effect, 280
  refractory period, 198
Quinidine, 279-280
  atrial fibrillation, effect in, 218

Quinidine, atrial, Cont'd.
  flutter, caused by, 211
    effect on, 215
  atrioventricular block, caused
      by, 220
  bundle branch block, left,
      transient, caused by, 132
  cardiac rhythm, effect on, 198-
      199
  intraventricular conduction
      defect, caused by, 235
  nodal rhythm, caused by, 233
  sinus arrest, caused by, 202
  ventricular fibrillation, caused
      by, 250
    premature beats, caused by,
        236
    tachycardia, caused by, 245
Q-U interval, 28
  definition of, 28
  hypokalemia, 286
Q wave, abnormal, definition of,
    171, 181
  definition of, 25
  myocardial infarction, 152-156,
      157
    anterior, 159, 160-166, 171,
        185-188
    anteroapical, 169
    bundle branch block, left, 195
    inferior, 173-177, 181, 186-
        188
    multiple infarcts, 185-188
    posterior, 173, 178-179
    subendocardial infarction,
        182-184
  normal, 45-62

-R-

Radio amplifier, 2
Rate. See Heart rate.
Reciprocal beats, 232
Refractory period, 198
  blocked atrial premature beats,
      205
Refrigeration, electrocardiographic
    effect, 274
Renal hypertension. See Hyper-
    tensive cardiovascular
    disease.
Repolarization, 21-24
  atrial, 25
  muscle strip, 22-24
  ventricular, 55
    vectorcardiogram, T loop,
        305, 310
Respiration, electrocardiogram of
    left bundle branch block,
      effect on, 136
  normal electrocardiogram,
      effect on, 80
  and sinus arrhythmia, 201
Rheumatic fever, atrioventricular
    block, 220-221
      nodal rhythm, caused by,
          233
  myocarditis, electrocardio-
      graphic pattern, 271
Rhythm(s). See also Cardiac
    rhythm.
  bigeminal, 237, 243
  idioventricular, 225-227
  nodal. See Atrioventricular
    rhythm.

Rhythm(s), Cont'd.
  sinus, 200-202
    regular, 200
    simulated by atrial flutter,
        214
    tachycardia, 200
Right axis deviation, defined, 36
  bundle branch block. See
      Bundle branch block, right.
R-R interval, atrial premature
    beats, 203-205
  definition of, 27
rS complex, transitional zone
    ventricular epicardial
        complex, 48
  ventricular cavity complex,
      right, 50
    epicardial complex, right,
        45, 47
rSr' complex, ventricular cavity
    complex, right, 50
  epicardial complex, right, 45,
      47
RS-T junction, definition of, 28
  segment. See ST segment.
R wave(s), definition of, 25
  normal, 45-62
  ventricular hypertrophy, 95-96
    left, 95
    right, 108
    strain, left, 106
R' wave, definition of, 27

-S-

S-A node. See Sinoatrial node.
Sarcoidosis, pulmonary, ventricu-
    lar strain, right, 114-115
Schmitt system of vectorcardiog-
    raphy, 302
Septal defects, bundle branch block,
    left, 131
  right, 121
Serum sickness, pericarditis, 270
Sinoatrial node, 40-41
  blood supply, 158
  cardiac rhythm, 197
  sinus arrest, 202
Sinus arrest, 202
  arrhythmia, 201
  bradycardia. See Bradycardia.
  rhythms. See Rhythms, sinus.
  tachycardia. See Tachycardia.
Situs inversus, 84
  electrocardiographic pattern,
      334
Spatial vectorcardiogram. See
    Vectorcardiogram.
  vectorcardiograph, 301-327
Standardization of electrocardio-
    gram, 16
Stokes-Adams syndrome, 252
  complete heart block, due to,
      221
  ventricular fibrillation, 250
Strain, ventricular, electro-
    cardiographic criteria, 97
  left, 106
  right, 113-115
    electrocardiographic pattern,
        337
ST segment, accelerated conduction,
    258-266
  anxiety state, 88

ST segment, Cont'd.
  atrial fibrillation, 217
  bundle branch block, 120
    left, 131-132
  definition of, 28
  depression, ventricular hyper-
    trophy, 96
  digitalis effect, 275
  elevation, simulated, 94
  emetine, effect of, 281
  hyperthyroidism, 272
  hypocalcemia, 289
  hypokalemia, 286
  interval, 28
  myocardial anoxia, 139-144
    infarction, 156
      anterior, 159, 162-166,
        171
      anteroapical, 169
      inferior, 173-177, 181
        188
      left bundle branch block,
        195
      multiple infarcts, 187-188
      vs. pericarditis, 267
      posterior, 173, 178-179
      subendocardial infarction,
        182-184
  myocarditis, 271
  neuromuscular diseases, 273
  normal, 55-62
    variation in precordial leads,
      elevation, 86
  pericarditis, 267-268
  pseudodepression, 149-150
  quinidine effect, 279
  trauma to heart, 273
  ventricular aneurysm, 189
    hypertrophy, left, 98
      right, 108
    premature beats, 238
    strain, 97
      left, 106
      right, 113
    tachycardia, 245-247
  Wolff-Parkinson-White syndrome,
    260, 263
Supraventricular tachycardia, 234
S wave, definition of, 25
  normal, 45-62
  ventricular hypertrophy, left, 98
S' wave, definition of, 27
Sympathetic system, effect on
  cardiac rhythm, 198
Syphilis of the aorta. See Aortic
  insufficiency.
Syphilitic aortitis. See Aortitis.

-T-

Tachycardia. See also Arrhythmias.
  anxiety state, 88
  hyperthyroidism, 272
  nodal, 234
  sinus vs. atrial tachycardia, 210
    definition of, 200
  supraventricular, 234
Tartar emetic, effect on electrocardiogram, 281
Ta wave, atrial flutter, 211
  hypertrophy, 94
  repolarization, 25
  pseudodepression of ST segment,
    149-150

Tea, atrial premature beats,
  caused by, 205
Tetrahedron vector system, 302
Tetralogy of Fallot, electrocardiographic pattern, 354
  ventricular hypertrophy,
    112
Threshold potential, 19
Thrombi, atrial, in atrial fibrillation, 218
Thyrotoxicosis, 272
  atrial fibrillation, 215
  flutter, 211
  electrocardiographic voltage, 99
  myocardial anoxia, 139
T loop, vectorcardiogram, normal
  adult, 305, 310
Tobacco, atrial premature beats,
  caused by, 205
  electrocardiogram, effect on,
    282
Traumatic heart disease, 273
Tricuspid atresia, ventricular
  hypertrophy, left, 98
Tuberculosis, pulmonary, ventricular hypertrophy, right, 108
T vector. See T loop.
T wave(s), accelerated conduction,
  258-266
  anxiety state, 88
  atrial fibrillation, 217
    tachycardia, 207
  bundle branch block, 120
    left, 131-132
  "coronary," 157
  "cove-plane," 157
  digitalis effect, 275
  emetine, effect of, 281
  hyperkalemia, 283
  hyperthyroidism, 272
  hypocalcemia, 289
  myocardial anoxia, 141, 143-144
    infarction, 157
      anterior, 159, 162-166,
        171, 185-188
      anteroapical, 169
      anteroseptal, 168
      inferior, 173-177, 181,
        186-188
      multiple infarcts, 185-188
      posterior, 173
      subendocardial infarction,
        182-184
  myocarditis, 271
  myxedema, 272
  neuromuscular diseases, 273
  normal, 45-62
    adult Negro, inverted, 82
    children, inverted, 82
    leads aVF, aVL, aVR, 55-62
    precordial leads, 55-62
    standard leads, 55-56
  "Pardee," 157
  pericarditis, 267-270
  primary changes, ventricular
    gradient, 327
  quinidine effect, 279
  secondary changes, ventricular
    gradient, 327
  tartar emetic, effect of, 281
  trauma to heart, 273
  ventricular hypertrophy,
    inversion, 96
    left, 98

T wave(s), ventricular hypertrophy,
    inversion, Cont'd.
    right, 108
  premature beats, 238, 243
  repolarization, 27
  strain, 97
    left, 106
    right, 113
  tachycardia, 245-247
  Wolff-Parkinson-White syn-
    drome, 260, 263

-U-

Unipolar augmented extremity
  leads. See Leads aVF, aVL,
    aVR.
  leads. See Leads, unipolar.
  nonaugmented extremity leads.
    See Leads VF, VL, VR.
Uremia, electrocardiographic
  pattern of hyperkalemia, 284
U wave(s), definition of, 27
  in hypokalemia, 286

-V-

Vagal stimulation, in atrial arrhythmias, 211
  atrioventricular block, caused
    by, 220
Vagus nerve, effect on heart, 198
V. A. T. See Ventricular activation
  time and Intrinsic deflection.
Vector(s), cardiac, 31-38, 302
  frontal plane, 31-36
  horizontal plane, 37
  instantaneous, 31
  mean, 31
  sagittal plane, 38
Vectorcardiogram, 31, 301-327
  bundle branch block, left, 314-
    315
    right, 318-319
  myocardial infarction, anterior,
    322-323
    inferior, 324-325
    posterolateral, 325
  normal adult, 305-311
  ventricular hypertrophy, left,
    312-313
    right, 316-317
Vectorcardiography, 301-327
Ventricle. See Hypertrophy,
  ventricular.
  left, infarction, 151
  right, infarction, 151
Ventricular activation time, 22, 28
  bundle branch block, 120
    left, 131
  definition of, 28
  normal, in infants, 81
  ventricular epicardial com-
    plex, left, 45
    right, 45
  hypertrophy, 95-96
    left, 95
    right, 108
  strain, left, 106
aneurysm, 189
  electrocardiographic pattern,
    331
arrhythmias. See Arrhythmias,
  ventricular.

Ventricular, Cont'd.
    depolarization. See Depolar-
        ization, ventricular.
    fibrillation. See Arrhythmias.
    gradient, 327
    hypertrophy. See Hypertrophy,
        ventricular.
    premature beats, 236-244
    strain. See Strain.
    tachycardia, 245-249

Voltage, 29
    increased hyperthyroidism, 272
    low, myxedema, 272
        pericardial effusion, 267

-W-

Wandering pacemaker. See Pace-
    maker.
Wenckebach phenomenon, 222, 224

Wolff-Parkinson-White syndrome,
    234, 258, 260, 263, 336
    electrocardiographic pattern,
        332
    myocardial infarction, electro-
        cardiographic pattern,
        336
    vectorcardiogram, 321
    with ventricular tachycardia,
        245

NORMAL RANGES AND VARIATIONS IN THE ADULT
TWELVE-LEAD ELECTROCARDIOGRAM

A true understanding of the normal range and the normal variations of the electrocardiogram depends upon a basic understanding of both normal and abnormal cardiac electrophysiology. It must be remembered that many of the configurations tabulated below may represent cardiac abnormalities when interpreted in the context of the entire tracing and in the light of clinical history and physical examination. Therefore, the information contained in the following table is intended to be used only as a rough preliminary guide to the interpretation of ambiguous and borderline tracings.

Lead	P	Q	R	S	T	ST
I	Upright deflection.	Small. < 0.04 sec. and < 25% of R.	Dominant. Largest deflection of the QRS complex.	< R, or none.	Upright deflection.	Usually isoelectric; may vary from +1 to -0.5 mm. (see p. 86).
II	Upright deflection.	Small or none.	Dominant.	< R, or none.	Upright deflection.	,,
III	Upright, flat, diphasic, or inverted, depending on frontal plane axis (see p. 75).	Small or none, depending on frontal plane axis (see p. 75); or large (0.04-0.05 sec. or > 25% of R).	None to dominant, depending on frontal plane axis (see p. 75).	None to dominant, depending on frontal plane axis (see p. 75).	Upright, flat, diphasic, or inverted, depending on frontal plane axis (see p. 75).	,,
aVR	Inverted deflection.	Small, none, or large.	Small or none, depending on frontal plane axis (see p. 75).	Dominant (may be QS).	Inverted deflection.	,,
aVL	Upright, flat, diphasic, or inverted, depending on frontal plane axis (see p. 75).	Small, none, or large, depending on frontal plane axis (see p. 75).	Small, none, or dominant, depending on frontal plane axis (see p. 75).	None to dominant, depending on frontal plane axis (see p. 75).	Upright, flat, diphasic, or inverted, depending on frontal plane axis (see p. 75).	,,
aVF	Upright deflection.	Small or none.	Small, none, or dominant, depending on frontal plane axis (see p. 75).	None to dominant, depending on frontal plane axis (see p. 75).	Upright, flat, diphasic, or inverted, depending on frontal plane axis (p. 75).	,,
V_1	Inverted, flat, upright, or diphasic.	None (may be QS).	< S or none (QS); small r' may be present (see p. 47).	Dominant (may be QS).	Upright, flat, diphasic, or inverted.*	0 to +3 mm.
V_2	Upright; less commonly, diphasic or inverted.	None (may be QS).	< S or none (QS); small r' may be present (see p. 47).	Dominant (may be QS).	Upright; less commonly, flat, diphasic, or inverted.*	0 to +3 mm.
V_3	Upright.	Small or none.	R <, >, or = S	S >, <, or = R	Upright.*	0 to +3 mm.
V_4	Upright.	Small or none.	R > S	S < R	Upright.*	Usually isoelectric; may vary from +1 to -0.5 mm. (see p. 86).
V_5	Upright.	Small.	Dominant (< 26 mm.)	S < SV_4	Upright.	
V_6	Upright.	Small.	Dominant (< 26 mm.)	S < SV_5	Upright.	

*Inverted in infants, children, and occasionally in young adults (see pp. 82 and 87).

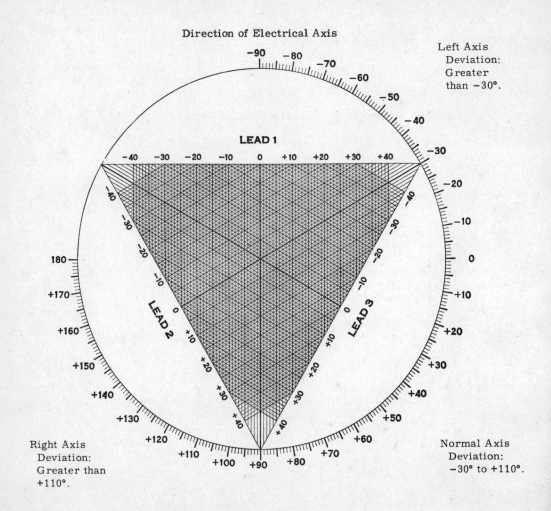

Direction of Electrical Axis

Determination of Frontal Plane Axis.

(1) Determine the algebraic sum of R and S in lead I. Plot this value on the lead I axis of the above diagram.

(2) Determine the algebraic sum of R and S in lead III. Plot this value on the lead III axis of the above diagram.

(3) Follow the perpendicular lines from the points plotted from (1) and (2) to the point of their intersection.

(4) Draw a line from the center of the diagram to intersection point (3) and continue this line to the circumference of the circle.

(5) Read the frontal plane electric axis as the point where line (4) crosses the circumference of the circle.